S0-BQM-383

CLINICAL PHARMACOLOGY OF ANTI-NEOPLASTIC DRUGS

Workshop on Methods in Cancer Research held in Lunteren, The Netherlands on April 24-25, 1978. Organized under the auspices of the Scientific Council of The Netherlands Cancer Society (Koningin Wilhelmina Fonds).

Editor

H. M. Pinedo

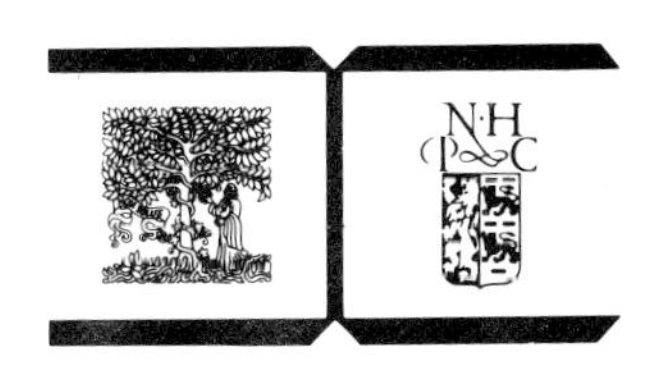

1978

ELSEVIER/NORTH-HOLLAND BIOMEDICAL PRESS
AMSTERDAM · NEW YORK · OXFORD

Published by:

Elsevier/North-Holland Biomedical Press B.V.
335 Jan van Galenstraat, P.O. Box 211
Amsterdam, The Netherlands

Sole distributors for the USA and Canada:

Elsevier North-Holland, Inc.
52 Vanderbilt Avenue
New York, N.Y. 10017

ISBN for the series: 0 444 80085 9
ISBN for the volume: 0 444 80086 7

Library of Congress Cataloging in Publication Data

Workshop on Methods in Cancer Research, 2d, Lunteren, 1978.
Clinical pharmacology of anti-neoplastic drugs.

(Applied methods in oncology ; v. 1)
Includes bibliographies and index.
1. Cancer--Chemotherapy--Congresses. 2. Anti-neoplastic agents--Congresses. 3. Methotrexate--Congresses. 4. Pharmacology--Congresses. I. Pinedo, H. M. II. Stichting Koningin Wilhelmina Fords. Scientific Council. III. Title. IV. Series.
[DNLM: 1. Antineoplastic agents--Pharmacodynamics--Congresses. W1 AP527 v. 1 /QV269 W926c 1978]
RC271.C5W68 1978 616.9'94'061 78-21509

ISBN 0-444-80086-7

PRINTED IN THE NETHERLANDS

CLINICAL PHARMACOLOGY OF ANTI-NEOPLASTIC DRUGS

APPLIED METHODS IN ONCOLOGY

Volume 1

Also published under the auspices of the Scientific Council of The Netherlands Cancer Society (Koningin Wilhelmina Fonds):

Cell Separation Methods

H. Bloemendal *(editor)*

CONTENTS

PART II FLUOROPYRIMIDINES, ADRIAMYCINS, BLEOMYCIN, CYCLOPHOSPHAMIDE, NITROSUREAS, VINCA ALKALOIDS AND CIS-PLATINUM

Introductory remarks

This volume is comprised of a collection of papers that were presented at the second international workshop held under the auspices of the Scientific Council of the Netherlands' Cancer Society (the "Koningin Wilhelmina Fonds", KWF). The meeting took place on April 24 and 25, 1978, in Lunteren, The Netherlands.
The Scientific Council is grateful for the enthousiastic willingness of Dr. H. Pinedo, Dr. O.Driessen and Dr. E. van der Kleijn to organize the program with the stimulating assistance of Dr. E. van Heemstra on behalf of the Council.

The workshop was the second in a series on applied methods in oncology. The purpose of the workshops is to get together leading scientists from the international scene with investigators in the field from our own country.
Concerning the clinical pharmacology of antineoplastic drugs, the Scientific Council was concerned in promoting research and application regarding the methodology of assaying drug levels in body fluids. A better understanding of the pharmacokinetics of anticancer agents will, as was mentioned in the lively discussions, minimize the administration of maximally tolerated doses to patients and letting them suffer from the accompanying toxicities.

The pharmacokinetics of methotrexate have been rigorously investigated and studies on selective reversal of toxicity have demonstrated promising results. Concluding the sessions on methotrexate was a critical discourse on the value of high dose methotrexate therapy. The very skillful chairmanship of Dr. J.Bertino during this part of the meeting should be acknowledged. Thanks also to the participation in the discussion of our guests from the U.S.A. and from Britain, disease states where a high dose regimen can be regarded good clinical practice were established.

On the second day, the pharmacology of other antineoplastic drugs including some newly developed agents was the subject of lectures and discussions. This, in particular, is the area from which the stimuli for development of cancer research in The Netherlands, and hopefully elsewhere, is being anticipated.

The meeting, however, looked further into the future. The relevance of drug serum levels to their antineoplastic activities at the cellular level was questioned. Another impressive point regards the tremendous variability between patients. The key-word might become pharmacogenetic, rather than pharmacokinetic, effects on anticancer drug development.

E. Boelsma
Applied Methods in Oncology,
editor

The financial support of the Netherlands' Cancer Society is gratefully acknowledged.

PART I: METHOTREXATE

Clinical Pharmacology of Anti-Neoplastic Drugs
H. M. Pinedo, editor

METHODS OF MEASURING METHOTREXATE IN BODY FLUIDS*

J.R. BERTINO** AND WILLIAM H. ISACOFF
Depts. of Medicine and Pharmacology, Yale University School of Medicine, New Haven, Ct. 06510 and Dept. of Medicine, University of California at Los Angelos - Harbor General Hospital, Torrance Ca. U.S.A.

*Supported by grants CA08010 and CA08341 from the National Cancer Institute and USPHS 5P01-CA-16042 and 1 R26 CA 21210 from the National Cancer Institute, National Institutes of Health
**American Cancer Society Professor of Medicine

ABSTRACT

Three satisfactory assay procedures for methotrexate in body fluids have been discussed in recent years:

1. an enzyme inhibition assay utilizing dihydrofolate reductase
2. a radioimmunoassay utilizing an antibody that binds MTX,
3. a competitive protein binding assay utilizing the enzyme dihydrofolate reductase as the macromolecular binder.

The latter two assays, employ either I^{125} labeled or tritiated MTX used as the radioactive ligand. They are rapid and have the capacity for the determination of a larger number of daily samples. The enzyme inhibition assay does not require radioactive counting equipment or radiolabeled MTX, but fewer samples can be processed per day by a technician. Not only is the assay of MTX in body fluids essential in regards to the high dose methotrexate regimens employed currently, but it is also clear that at least one major metabolite, 7-hydroxymethotrexate, results when larger doses are employed, and must be considered when the results of these assays are obtained.

INTRODUCTION

The recent use of methotrexate (MTX), a potent inhibitor of the enzyme dihydrofolate reductase (DHFR) in potentially lethal high doses, followed by leucovorin rescue (reviewed in (1)), have made quantitation of MTX in serum and in body fluids essential. By routinely monotoring plasma MTX levels during each course of therapy, the dose and duration of calcium leucovorin administration may be effectively adjusted in order to avoid clinical manifestations of drug induced toxicity. Accurate assessments of the calcium leucovorin can only be made when the rate of MTX plasma decay is known (2, 3).

Assays for this drug have been described since its introduction into the clinic, however, the microbiological assay described was tedious and cumbersome (4), and the fluormetric assay lacked sensitivity (5,6). Enzyme inhibition assays allowed measurements of MTX in body fluids to be made accurately and rapidly (7-10); however, the recently introduced "competitive binding assays" have added another dimension, i.e., the ease of larger numbers of sample determination per working day (11-13). This paper will review the more recent methods described namely the enzyme inhibition assay and the competitive protein binding assays, and will attempt to point out the principals of each type of assay and the advantages and disadvantages of each.

METHODS

The enzyme inhibition assay using dihydrofolate reductase.

Following the observation that MTX was an extremely potent inhibitor of the enzyme DHFR, Werkheiser pointed out that this inhibition, although reversible was "stoichiometric" when folic acid was used as a substrate, and could be utilized to quantitate MTX levels in unknown solutions (8). Bertino *et al.*, then described the pH dependency of this inhibition (15) and reported that this enzyme activity could be used to measure MTX levels in body fluids using the more convenient spectrophotometric assay using dihydrofolate as the substrate (7). This assay has been utilized in several laboratories since this time, and remains a sensitive, rapid method of quantitating MTX levels in serum and urine (1,15,16).

The assay is carried out either utilizing folic acid as a substrate, or with dihydrofolic acid as the substrate (Fig. 1).

$$(1)\ FH_2 + NADPH + H^+ \rightleftharpoons FH_4 + NADP^+$$
$$(2)\ F + NADPH + 2H^+ \rightleftharpoons FH_4 + 2NADP^+$$

Fig. 1. Reactions carried out by the enzyme dihydrofolate reductase. Abbreviations used are F, folic acid; FH_2, dihydrofolic acid; FH_4 tetrahydrofolic acid; NADP and NADPH, the oxidized and reduced forms of nicotinamide adenine diphosphate.

Use of dihydrofolate as the substrate has the advantage that less enzyme is requir-

ed, and a rapid continuous spectrophotometric assay may be employed (7,9,10). A standard curve is generated each day (Fig. 2), using a fixed amount of enzyme for each assay, and standard amounts of MTX. It should be emphasized that this assay should be run at pH 6.0 for maximum sensitivity, and that the concentration of dihydrofolate be as low as possible, also for maximum sensitivity. Since the inhibition of the enzyme is stoichiometric under these conditions, a straight line plot should be obtained until greater than 80% inhibition is produced (Fig. 2).
It follows also that when the unknown samples are analyzed the same amount of enzyme should be utilized, since the line will be displaced upward or downward on whether or not there is greater or less activity present, thus leading to inaccurate MTX estimations. Since pH and salt concentration, as well as the order of addition of reactants affect enzyme activity, careful attention should also be paid to these variables when unknown samples are assayed. The method we use employs a standard mix (buffer, KCI, enzyme, 2-mercaptethanol, NADPH) followed by addition of MTX (standard) or the unknown sample. After mixing and incubation at 37° for 2 minutes in the cuvette, the substrate, dihydrofolate, is pipetted into the cuvette and the reaction is started. The assay as performed routinely is capable of measuring as little as 10^{-6} μmol. MTX. We have recently described a new fluorometric assay that measures DHFR actively, accurately at one log less enzyme concentration, and should be capable of a correspondingly increased sensitivity for MTX assay (17). Of great convenience in the spectrophotometric assays is a continuous recording spectrophotometer such as the Gilford Model. A disadvantage of the assay is the relatively narrow range of sensitivity of the assay (20-80% inhibition). However, with the knowledge of the drug dose administered to the patient, and the interval at which the sample is obtained, estimates of the required dilutions can be made, thus reducing the time required for the assay. A detailed description of this assay has been published and is recommended for laboratories attempting to use this method (10). A major metabolite of MTX noted in patients receiving high dose MTX is the 7-hydroxy derivative, especially during the second 12 hours following high dose MTX (18). This compound is only about 1/100th as potent as an inhibitor of DHFR (19), and would not be expected to interfere appreciably with the enzyme assay, even during the time period when its excretion reaches 10-33% of the total MTX excreted in the urine.

Ligand - Binding Radioassays.

In recent years, two types of radioreceptor assays have been described for the routine measurement of MTX in biologic fluid. The radioimmunoassay is based on the competition between an isotopically labeled antigen and unlabeled antigen for

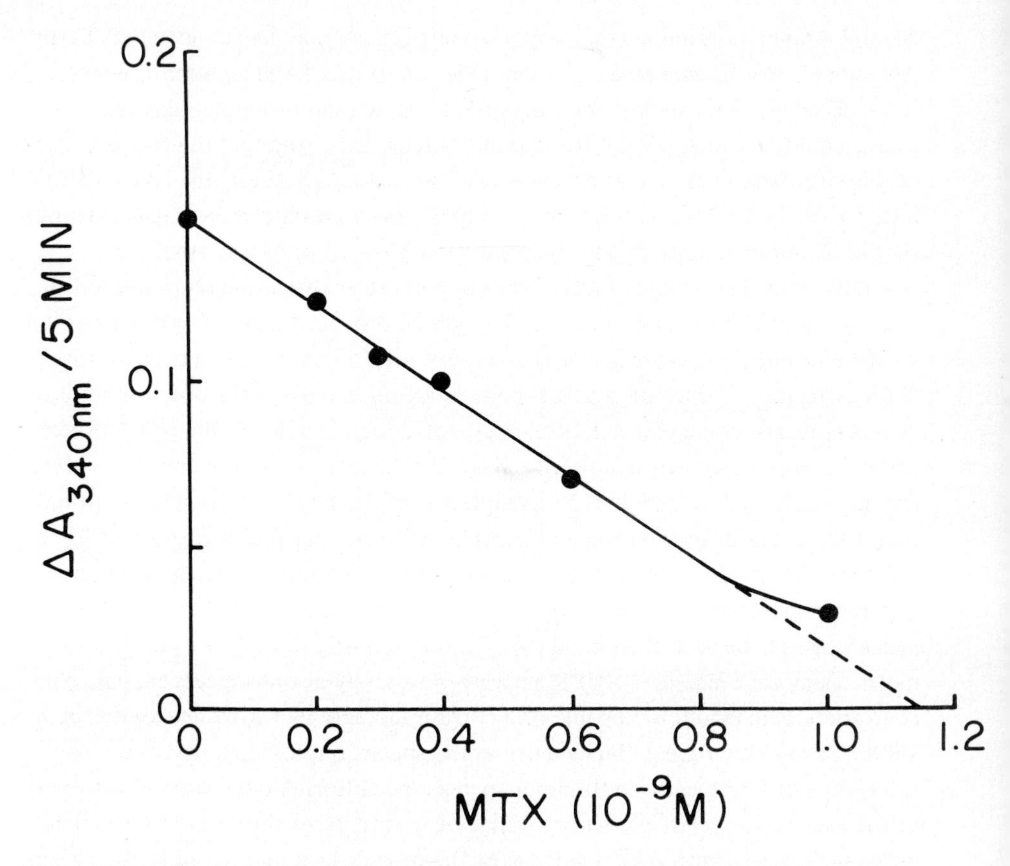

Fig. 2. Inhibition of dihydrofolate reductase activity by increasing amounts of methotrexate (standard curve). The reaction mix, in a 1.2 ml cuvette with a 10 mm light path, contained: tris-HCL buffer, 100 μmoles, pH 7.0; KCL, 150 μmoles; NADPH, 0.08 μmole, enzyme and water. After adding the MTX in the amounts indicated, the components were mixed, and incubated at 37° for 2 minutes. Dihydrofolate, 0.02 μmole containing 10 μmoles of 2-mercaptoethanol was then added, and the contents mixed. The final volume was 1 ml. A blank cuvette which did not contain dihydrofolate was also utilized and the change in absorbancy of the complete system was corrected by subtracting this value. The absorbancy chance at 340 mm was monitored with a Gilford 2000 equipped with and automatic cuvette changer.

binding sites on a specific antibody to the antigen. The ligand-binding radioassay is a general term which may be applied when there is competition for specific binding sites on a macromolecule by small labeled and unlabeled molecules called ligands. In radio-receptor assays which are termed "non-competitive", the binding sites of the macromolecule are first saturated by the radioactive ligand. Addition of unlabeled ligand will result in displacement of the radioactivity from the macromolecule-ligand complex. The degree of displacement of the radioligand will be proportional to the amount of non-radioactive ligand added. In a "competitive" radio-receptor assay the macromolecular protein binder is added to a mixture of radiolabeled ligand and unlabeled ligand.

The general principle of a ligand-binding radio-assay may be illustrated by the following equation:

$$\begin{array}{ccc} (L^*) + (B) & \rightleftharpoons & (L^* - B) \\ + & & \\ (L) & & \\ \upharpoonleft\downharpoonright & & \\ L\text{-}B & & \end{array}$$

where B is the macromolecular binder of the ligand,
L* is the radioactive labeled ligand, L is the unlabeled ligand and (L*- B) is the bound radioligand - macromolecular complex (20). If the concentration of (B) and (L*) are known and kept constant at relatively low concentrations, the quantity of (L*- B) that is formed will be inversely proportional to the amount of (L) present in the reaction mixture. As the concentration of (L) increases the amount of (L* - B) formed will decrease. If (L* - B) is the amount of bound radioactivity and (L*) the amount of free radioactivity then the ratio of "bound/free" will be a function of the molar concentration (L). By plotting "bound/free' radioactivity against known molar concentration of (L), the unknown concentration of (L) in a patient sample may be obtained by finding the ligand concentration that corresponds to the "bound/free" ratio observed in the unknown sample.

Two types of radioassays are described below: the first type uses an antibody to bind the ligand MTX; in this case the more specific term radioimmunoassay may be used to describe the radioassay. The second type that will be described uses another binding macromolecule, dihydrofolate reductase (DHFR), in this instance, the more general term competitive ligand or competitive protein binding assay is used to describe the assay.

The essential requirements for a radioreceptor assay procedure are:

1) a radioactive form of the ligand. Since the method requires the radio-labeled

ligand to be present in extremely low concentration, the higher the specific activity of the tracer, the greater the sensitivity of the assay.

2) a specific binding protein with high affinity for the ligand. The binding protein may be an antibody, naturally occurring plasma protein, or a target tissue binding site such as dihydrofolate reductase,
3) a method for extracting or purifying the sample,
4) finally, a rapid and precise method for separating the bound from the free or unbound radio-labeled ligand (21).

Radiolabeled ligand, MTX is available as either tritiated labeled of high specific activity ($3^1, 5^1, 9^3H)^1$ or as I^{125} labeled material in kit form for the assay. The I^{125} material has the advantage that it can be counted with a gamma counter and therefore does not require scintillation fluid and counting.

Radioimmunoassay for MTX.

This assay was first described in 1975 (11). Antibody to MTX covalently coupled to methylated bovine serum albumin was raised in rabbits, and the resultant antiserum is used for the binder. Radio-labeled MTX, the hapten or ligand, together with increasing amounts of unlabeled MTX , are used to construct a standard curve according to the principles outlined above, and MTX in the unknown sample is estimated, using the standard curve as a reference. The free and bound radio-labeled MTX are separated either using a nitrocellulose filter disc, or dextran or albumin coated charcoal or by precipitating the MTX-antibody complex, *e.g.*, using isopropanol (22), and counting the radioactivity in the precipitate. In the latter case a direct plot of counts precipitated vs. the amount of unlabeled MTX may be made, and serves as the standard curve (Fig. 3). This assay is relatively simple and convenient, if care is taken to remove the supernatant fluid completely after centrifugation. It has the advantage of not requiring a charcoal step, which can be a source of difficulty. The assays employing charcoal or nitrocellulose filters on the other hand have the advantage that a fraction of the supernatant not bound to charcoal or retarded by the nitrocellulose filter may be counted, and does not require quantitative precipitation of the hapten by the antibody. In this circumstance the percent radio-labeled MTX bound is plotted against the unlabeled MTX concentration added to give the standard reference curve. The percent bound is obtained by dividing the amount of radioactivity in the sample with an unlabeled MTX added divided by the radioactivity obtained without unlabeled MTX added.

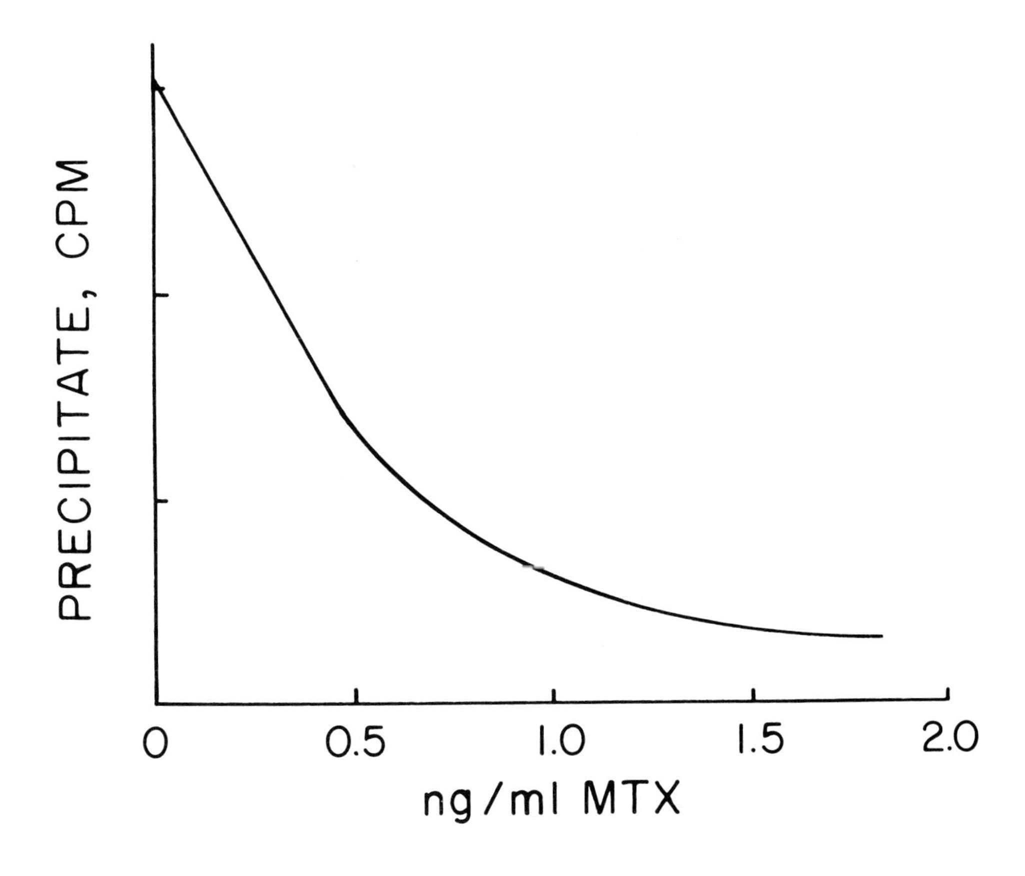

Fig. 3. Standard curve obtained with a radioimmunoassay utilizing precipitation of the I^{125} methotrexate antibody complex using isopropanol precipitation.

Ligand Binding Radioassay to Measure MTX Using DHFR as the Binder.

DHFR may be used as the macromolecular binder because of its high affinity for MTX (7,8). This enzyme may be obtained in relatively pure form for this purpose for *L. casei* or from various mammalian sources (7-10). A crude lysate from the L1210 tumor, rat liver, or guinea pig liver will also suffice for these assays. The advantage of this enzyme as the macromolecular binder is of course that it is easier to obtain than antiserum to MTX. When DHFR is used as the binder, it is necessary to include NADPH (2 mg/ml) in the final reaction mixture to enhance the binding between MTX and DHFR. At pH 6.0, binding of MTX to DHFR is optimum and approaches stoichiometric binding (14), and the assays should be run at or near this pH.

For the assay to be sensitive and easily reproducible the final reaction mixture should contain enough DHFR to bind approximately 50-60% of the radiolabeled MTX in a buffer at pH 6.0 which contains the appropriate concentration of NADPH. The nature of a competitive binding assay is such that DHFR, the binder, is added to a mixture of labeled and unlabeled ligand. Therefore, each reaction mixture will contain a known but fixed amount of radiolabeled MTX along with an unknown amount of unlabeled MTX to which DHFR is added. The excess unbound radiolabeled MTX is removed by adsorption to dextran-coated charcoal. The total amount of charcoal added to the reaction mixture should not exceed 4 mg/ml. Since Plasma MTX protein binders have been identified in patient's plasma receiving multiple course of MTX therapy, a simple boiling extraction procedure must be done before the assay can be accurately performed (23). These plasma proteins, if present, are capable of binding the radiolabeled MTX and thereby resulting in a false elevation of the "bound/free" ratio, which would lead to a significant underestimation of the actual amount of MTX in the patient sample. The extraction by boiling may be avoided if the plasma sample is diluted 10-100 fold. This would simply dilute the concentration of the plasma binding protein.

DISCUSSION

Advantages and Disadvantages of the Ligand Binding Assays Over the Enzyme Inhibition Method.

The ligand binding assays are relatively specific, and have the advantage that a large number of samples may be processed during a working day. As mentioned (*vide supra*) the enzyme inhibition assay is relatively insensitive to 7-hydroxy MTX, a metabolite noted in patients receiving high doses of MTX. This compound also competes minimally with MTX in the radioimmunoassay, and the competitive reductase binding assay, and produced 30% competition at 12-15 fold the concentration of MTX required for 50% inhibition (25). However, another metabolite of MTX, 2-4 diamino, N^{10} methyl pteroic acid (DAMPA) produced equal inhibition to MTX in the radioimmunoassay (10,24), but only minimal inhibition in the competitive reductase binding assay (24). Thus when MTX levels are assayed at time intervals when blood concentrations are low, these assays may give different results, because of the presence of metabolites such as DAMPA (24).

The enzyme inhibition assay has the advantage that it does not employ radio-isotopes, and therefore does not require radioactive counting equipment, and that it is rapid and accurate. However, it is less well suited to larger numbers of determination, since a technician can only run 10-12 samples per day.

REFERENCES

1. Bertino, J.R. (1977) Seminars in Onc. 4; 203-216.
2. Isacoff, W.H. et al. (1976) Medical and Pediatric Oncology 2; 319-325.
3. Isacoff, W.H. et al. (1977) Cancer Treatment Reports 61; 1665-1674.
4. Burchenal, J.H. (1953) Proc. Exp. Biol. Med. 83; 369-373.
5. Freeman, M.J. (1957) J. Pharmacol. 120; 1-8.
6. Kincade, J.M. et al. (1974) Method Biochem. Med. 10; 337-350.
7. Bertino, J.R. and Fisher, G.A. (1964) Methods Med. Res. 1; 297-307.
8. Workheiser, W.C. et al. (1962) J. Pharmacol. Exp. Ther. 137; 1620.
9. Overdijk, B. et al. (1975) Clin. Chim. Acta 59; 177.
10. Falk, L.C. et al. (1976) Clin. Chem. 22; 785-788.
11. Raso, V. and Schreiber, R. (1975) Cancer Res. 35; 1407-1410.
12. Myers, C.E. et al. (1975) Proc. Natl. Acad. Sci. U.S.A. 72; 3683-3686.
13. Arons, E. et al. (1975) Cancer Res. 35; 2033-
14. Bertino, J.R. et al. (1964) J. Biol. Chem. 239; 479-485.
15. Tatterssall, M.H.N. et al (1975) Cancer Chemother. Rep. 6 Part 3; 19-
16. Chabner, B.A. and Young, R.C. (1973) J. Clin. Invest. 52; 1804-
17. Lindquist, C.A. et al. (1977) Anal. Biochem. 83; 20-25.
18. Jacobs, S.A. et al. (1976) J. Clin. Invest. 57; 534-538.
19. Johns, D.G. and Loo, T.L. (1976) J. Pharm. Sci. 56; 356-359.
20. Berson, S.A. and Yalon, R.S.: Principles of Immunoassay of Peptide Hor-

mones in Plasma. In Clinical Endocrinology. (Astwood, E.B. and Cassidy, Eds.) New York, Grune and Stratton 1968, 699-721.

21. Rothenberg, S.P. et al. (1977) Cancer Treatment Rep. 61; 575-584.

22. Circular for Diagnostic Biochemistry Inc. I^{125} Methotrexate-RIA Kit.

23. Da Costa, M. et al. (1977) Blood 50 (Supp. 1) 190.

24. Donehower, R. et al. (1978) Proc. Am. Assoc. Cancer Res. 19; 172.

Clinical Pharmacology of Anti-Neoplastic Drugs
H. M. Pinedo, editor

ASSAY OF METHOTREXATE AND 7-HYDROXYMETHOTREXATE BY HIGH PRESSURE LIQUID CHROMATOGRAPHY AND ITS APPLICATION TO CLINICAL PHARMACOKINETICS

JAN LANKELMA, EPPO VAN DER KLEIJN AND EMIEL F.S. TERMOND
Department of Clinical Pharmacy, St. Radboud Hospital, University of Nijmegen, Geert Grooteplein Zuid 10, Nijmegen, The Netherlands.

ABSTRACT

Methotrexate concentrations can be determined rapidly in plasma, urine and cerebrospinal fluid by means of high pressure liquid chromatography combined with an on-column concentration procedure. The limits of the method are 2.10^{-8} M and 10^{-5} M respectively; in between a linear concentration dependency exists. The range is sufficiently wide to include therapeutic concentrations. The method has been proven to be useful for the measurement of 7-hydroxymethotrexate as well. Plasma concentration versus time curves have been determined during and after low, medium high and high dose infusions as well as after low dose oral administration and subsequent intrathecal injections. Changes in pharmacokinetics of both methotrexate and the metabolite in the course of therapy are reported and the clinical implications are discussed.

INTRODUCTION

The use of cytostatic drugs is often accompanied by serious side-effects. The main side-effects of methotrexate (MTX) are mucositis and bone marrow depression. Chabner et al. (1) found a 50% inhibition of DNA synthesis in mouse bone marrow cells and in intestinal epithelium at plasma concentrations of 10^{-8} M and 5.10^{-9} M respectively. In man Stoller et al. (2) showed that plasma methotrexate values during treatment with high doses of methotrexate predict the development of toxicity (see also Hande, this volume). A rapid clearance of the drug was not accompanied by toxicity. Pinedo et al. studied myeloid precursor cells (CFU-C) of mice by *in vitro* culture after continuous *in vivo* exposure to various plasma concentrations of methotrexate during different time intervals (5). They found that toxicity was not only related to the duration of exposure, but also to methotrexate plasma concentrations. Goldman reported similar findings in fibroblasts in culture (6).

Citrovorum factor (CF; synonyms leucovorin and 5-formyl tetrahydrofolate) is studied in relation to reversal of methotrexate toxicity (Pinedo, this volume). High methotrexate plasma concentrations can affect the passage of CF through the cell membrane (3,4). When methotrexate is given orally or intrathecally the passage from the compartment of administration into the blood can influence plasma methotrexate concentrations.

An optimal therapy requires monitoring of the plasma concentration and this may also provide an insight into the factors that are important for the design of new regimens.

Methotrexate is currently determined by either radioimmunoassays, using $[^{3}H]$-[7] or $[^{125}I]$-[8] labelled methotrexate, competitive protein binding assay (9), by fluorescence measurement (10) or through the inhibition of dihydrofolate reductase (11), as reviewed by Bertino (this volume).

The disadvantage of the radioimmunoassays is that the presence of metabolites can give misleading results. The enzyme inhibition assay needs a standard plot, because of variations in enzyme activity or a decrease in dihydrofolate concentration with time. The standard plot has to be prepared daily. A minor disadvantage is that the assay covers a limited range (1 log) of concentrations. The low detection limit (3.10^{-9} M) is however, an advantage for pharmacokinetic studies.

The use of high pressure liquid chromatography following an oxidation reaction has been reported by Nelson et al. (12). After deproteinization oxidation is carried out by means of potassium permanganate. No suitable organic extraction solvent for methotrexate has yet been reported. The reaction product is eluted over a reversed phase column and detected by means of a fluorescence method. For the analysis 250 μl of deproteinized plasma is injected on to the column.

It is not certain whether the column can be used for a great number of determinations. Wahlund (13) reported a maximum of 400 μl of deproteinized serum on a similar column after which the column deteriorated.

In the method reported here we chose to concentrate the methotrexate on a reversed phase column, whereby elution was aimed at high retention of methotrexate. By switching over to an eluent that flows reversely through the same column, methotrexate is transported directly on to an analytical column on which methotrexate can be separated from other concentrated compounds by an anion exchange resin. The system is presented schematically in Fig. 1.

With adequate conditions to achieve respectively high retention on the reversed phase column and a moderate retention on the analytical column higher concentration and better purification of the sample can be achieved than when a single column is used. During concentration the sample is purified, as non-retained components

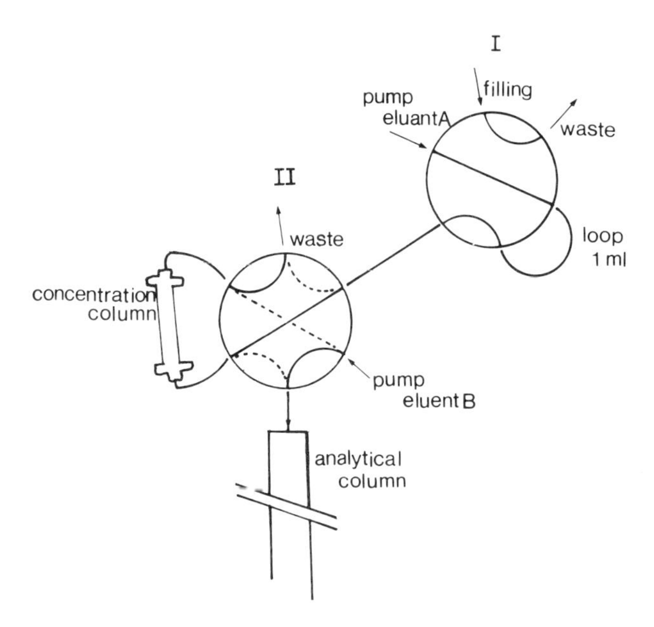

Fig. 1. Principle of the chromatographic determination of methotrexate. The sample is brought into the loop of the high pressure valve I and is transported by eluent A to the concentration column. After switching valve II into the injection position (dotted line) eluent B flows in the reverse direction through the concentration column and brings the concentrated methotrexate onto the analytical column.

are washed out. In this way the analytical column can be kept free of the many potential plasma contaminants. With this system it appeared to be possible to use one analytical column for the analysis of over a 1000 samples. The concentration column is replaced easily and no high quality is needed since the only condition is that it should have a high retention. Considerations about the choice of the optimal conditions for this system have been reported in the literature (14) The lower detection limit of our method is 2.10^{-8} M and the measurable concentrations range up to 10^{-5} M, so the method covers a large area of the concentrations presently achieved during clinical use of methotrexate. The relative standard deviation is 3.5%. After blood sampling a methotrexate concentration can be known within half an hour.

MATERIALS AND METHODS

Plasma and cerebrospinal fluid (CSF) from patients under treatment with methotrexate were obtained from several clinical departments.

The standard methotrexate (purity 97.5%) was kindly provided by Lederle (American Cyanamid, P.O. Box 500, Kenilworth, N.J.07033, U.S.A.). All chemicals used were of analytical grade.

Procedure

Plasma and CSF samples are deproteinized by adding a solution of trichloroacetic acid in 0.1 N hydrochloric acid. The denaturated proteins are removed by centrifugation and the clear supernatant is injected directly onto the concentration column. The eluent of the concentration column is tap water, the eluent of the analytical column is a mixture of sodium phosphate buffer (0.05M, pH 4.95) and methanol (v/v 4:1). The concentration column (length 4.6 cm, ID 3 mm) and the analytical column (length 25 cm, ID 4.6 mm) are packed with RP 8 (Merck, Darmstadt, G.F.R., particle size 10 μm) respectively. More details on the chromatography have been reported elsewhere (14).

For measuring concentrations below 2.10^{-8} M we used the enzyme inhibition method (11). Using 10 times more of the sample (200 μl) than prescribed in the literature a detection limit can be reached of 3.10^{-9} M. The method shows a standard deviation of 3% at 8.10^{-9} M and of 20% at 3.10^{-9} M.

RESULTS AND DISCUSSION

From the plasma concentration versus time curves a pharmacokinetic model can be derived (15). In such a pharmacokinetic study the body is divided into compartments. The drug passes from one compartment into another. Two, three and more compartment models have been described for methotrexate (16-19). For clinical applications a one or two compartment model is often useful. Plasma concentrations during and after 24 h infusions in patients treated for head and neck cancers (20) were found to fit a two compartment model. This is illustrated in Fig. 2.
The curve has been drawn through the data according to the stripping method as described by Wagner (15). The peripheral compartment is an equivalent of the drug outside the central compartment. From the plasma curve an estimate can be made of the amount that is present in the peripheral compartment.

In this case the steep slope (α) of the first part of the curve is mainly determined by renal excretion of the drug. The second slope (β) is determined by passage of the drug from the peripheral compartment into the blood. If we presume equal concentrations in both compartments in the equilibrium state, the volume of the peripheral

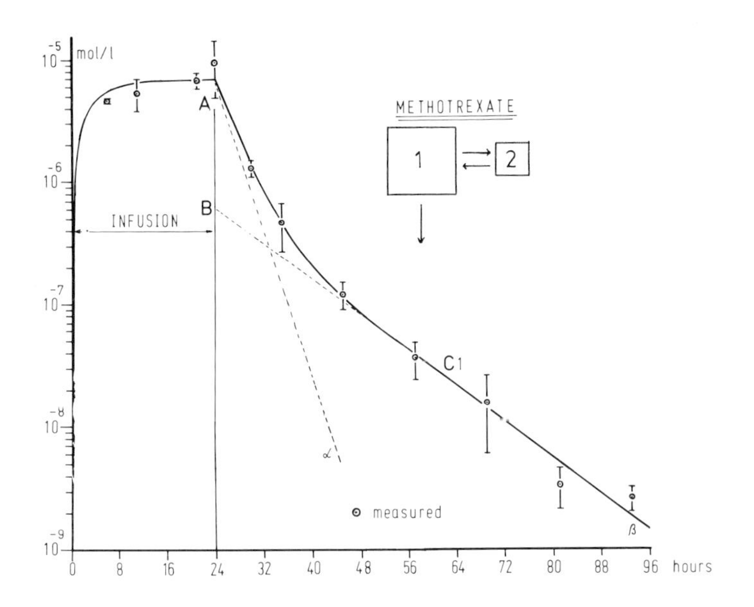

Fig. 2. MTX plasma concentration versus time curve in a patient receiving an infusion of 460 mg MTX in 24 h.
∘ mean values of three subsequent infusions;
the drawn line fits a two compartment model, corresponding to the following pharmacokinetic parameters:
$\alpha = 0.30\ h^{-1}$
$\beta = 0.08\ h^{-1}$
volume of distribution of compartment 1:21.4 l, of compartment 2:3.5 l.
The tangents α and β (dotted lines) of the corresponding phases α and β intercept the termination of the infusion line at A and B respectively, where plasma concentrations are 7.1×10^{-6} M/l and 6.1×10^{-1} M/l respectively.

compartment appears to be smaller than that of compartment 1. This indicates that only small amounts of the drug are distributed over the peripheral tissues. A deviation of the linearity between tissue and plasma concentrations below a plasma concentration of 2.10^{-7} M is reported in mouse studies (21). If this would also be the case in man, even after the time this concentration has been reached, a rough estimate with possible clinical use could be made. As the therapeutic cytostatic activity takes place in the peripheral compartment an estimation of the pharmacokinetic parameters may give valuable information to predicting the amount and the rate of disappearance from the peripheral compartment. When the drug is administered orally it is absorbed from another compartment, namely from compartment zero: in pharmacokinetic studies this compartment is not considered as part of the body. Plasma concentrations achieved after oral administration of low doses of methotrexate in patients with psoriasis (22) are shown in Fig. 3.

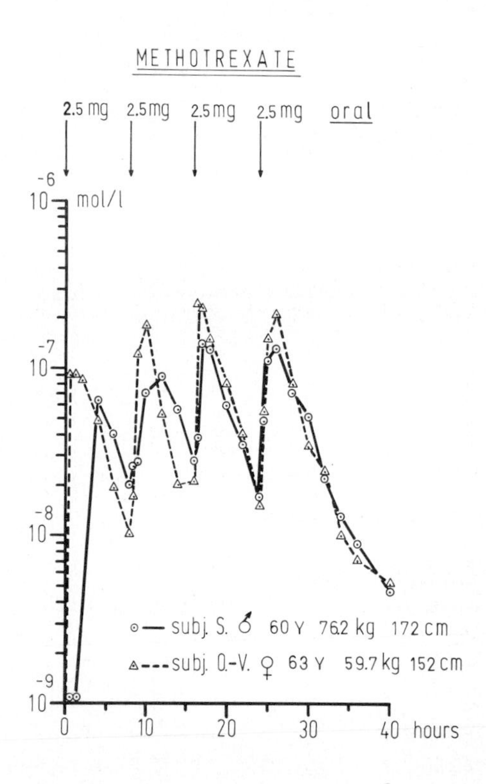

Fig. 3. Methotrexate plasma concentrations after oral administration in two patients who were treated for psoriasis.

A gradual rise in the first part of the curve can be explained by a slow absorption from the compartment of administration. This slope can vary from patient to patient as exemplified by the determinations after the first oral dosage of 2.5 mg methotrexate. (Fig. 3). When the greater part of the dose has left the compartment of administration, the rest of the curve is determined by the distribution over the other compartments. The second slope does not show here, because the concentrations were too low to be determined. Differences in absorption and their clinical implications are reported elsewhere (23).

An analogous model is shown after subsequent intrathecal injections during the profylactic treatment of meningeal leukemia (24). The appearance of methotrexate in plasma after intrathecal administration of the drug is a phenomenon comparable to that as occurring after oral administration. The plasma concentration is a function of time and can be determined with the following equation:

$$C(t) = A_0.e^{-k_{01}.t} + A_1.e^{-\alpha t} + A_2.e^{-\beta t}$$

in which : $C(t)$ = plasma concentration;

A_0 = initial concentration in compartment of administration,

k_{01} = rate constant determining the rate of drug transport from compartment 0 into 1,

α and β represent the slopes of the disappearance curves,

α and β are related to the reaction transfer rate constants by the following equations (15)

$\alpha.\beta = k_{21}.k_{13}$ (2) and

$\alpha + \beta = k_{12} + k_{21} + k_{13}$, (3)

in which : k_{21} = rate constant, determining the rate of drug transport from compartment 2 into 1,

k_{13} = rate constant determining the rate of drug transport from compartment 1 into 3, etc.

The plasma concentration versus time curves of five subsequent intrathecal injections have been determined in ten children and eight adults. In five of the children the curves of the first two injections revealed a lower rate of transport from the CSF into the plasma than the last two curves did. This is illustrated in Figs 4a and 4b for one of the children. In the adults only a limited number of plasma concentration curves have been determined. The conclusion can be reached that the rate of absorption increases in the adults when the values obtained of the first two injections are compared with those after the last two injections. When α and β are taken from Fig. 4b and when k_{01} is varied, the plasma curves will vary as presented in Fig. 5.

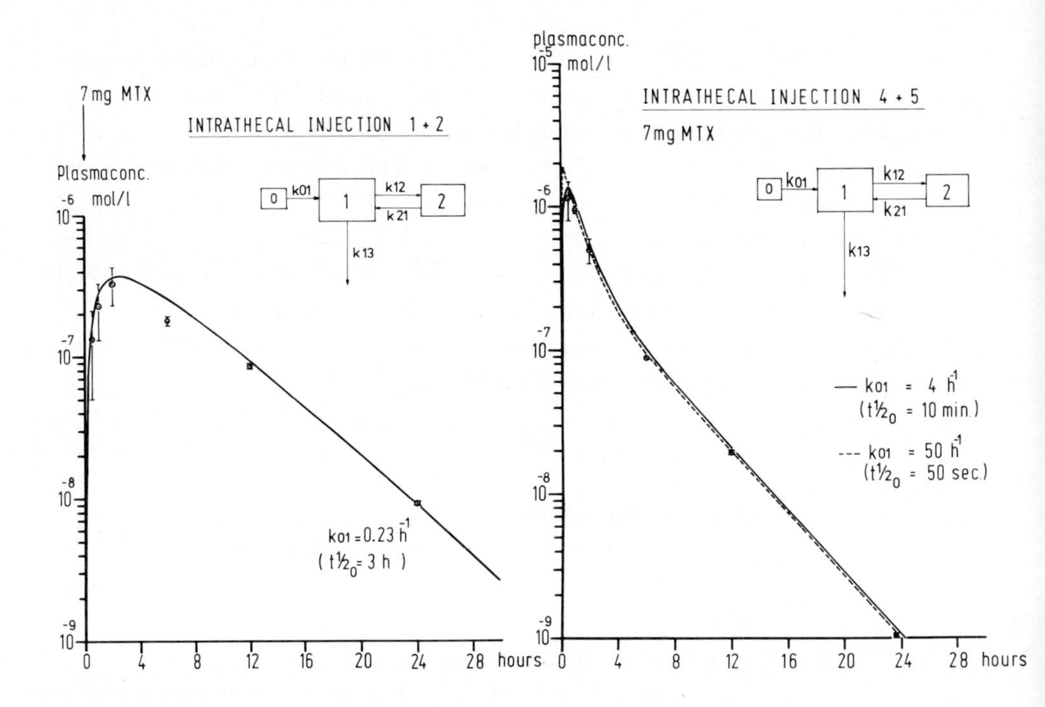

Fig. 4a Fig. 4b

Methotrexate plasma concentrations in a 3-year old child who received 5 intrathecal injections. Curves have made fit a two compartment model with an extra compartment of administration. The averaged values of the first two injections (Fig. 4a) show a slower absorption than those of the last two injections. (Fig. 4b).

As is to be seen from Fig. 5 the shape of the plasma concentration curve of the first two injections (Fig. 4a) can be explained pharmacokinetically by a lower value of the k_{01} of the first two injections as compared to the last two injections. At the third injection the value of k_{01} is in between the values of the injections 1 and 2 and of 4 and 5.

The amount of drug in the CSF compartment as a function of time is described by the following equation

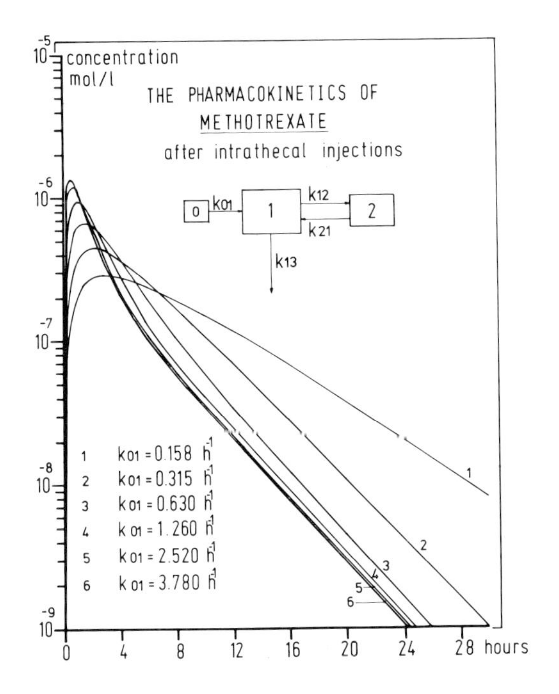

Fig. 5. Predicted methotrexate plasma concentrations for same patient as Fig. 4, with varying k_{01} values.

$$Q = Q_0 \cdot e^{-k_{01} \cdot t} \qquad (4)$$

wherin:

Q = amount of drug,

Q_0 = amount of drug at time 0.

When applying this equation and the values obtained from the fitted curves of Figs. 4a and b we calculated that 2 hours after the last two injections only less than 0.1% of the amount left of the first two injections remained in the CSF.

In the model the assumption is made that the resorption of drug to the CSF is negligible, which is justified when taking in mind that the CSF concentrations are much higher than the blood concentrations (25).

The changes in absorption rates and their possible clinical implications have been reported for children as well as for adults (26).

METABOLISM

Under the chromatographic conditions as described for the determination of methotrexate, a metabolite of methotrexate can be determined in the same sample. By means of UV spectroscopy, field desorption mass spectrometry and NMR spectroscopy this compound could be identified as 7-hydroxymethotrexate (27). Jacobs (28) reported the occurrence of this metabolite in the urine of man a high dose of methotrexate (>50 mg/kg). The analysis was carried out with a DEAE cellulose column and UV detection at 300 nm.

In this presentation is shown that a significant concentration of 7-hydroxymethotrexate appears in the plasma during low dose methotrexate infusions (29) as well. (Fig. 6)

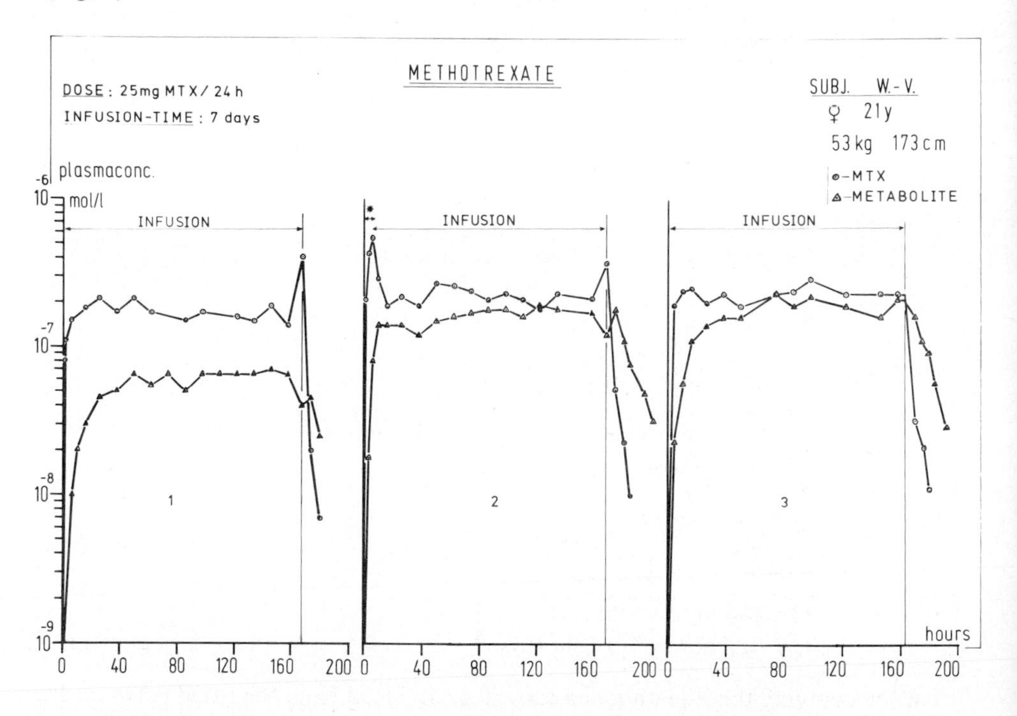

Fig. 6. Plasma concentrations of methotrexate and 7-hydroxymethotrexate in the treatment of chorioncarcinoma. The metabolite concentration reaches a higher plateau after the second infusion, which is maintained after subsequent infusions.
$\overset{*}{\leftrightarrow}$ = higher infusion rate.

Both compounds were detected at a wavelength of 306 nm (30).
After termination of the infusion the metabolite plasma curve shows a slope which

is less steep than that of the methotrexate curve. A similar slope of 7-OH methotrexate has been observed after medium high dose (Fig. 7) and high dose infusions (Fig. 8).

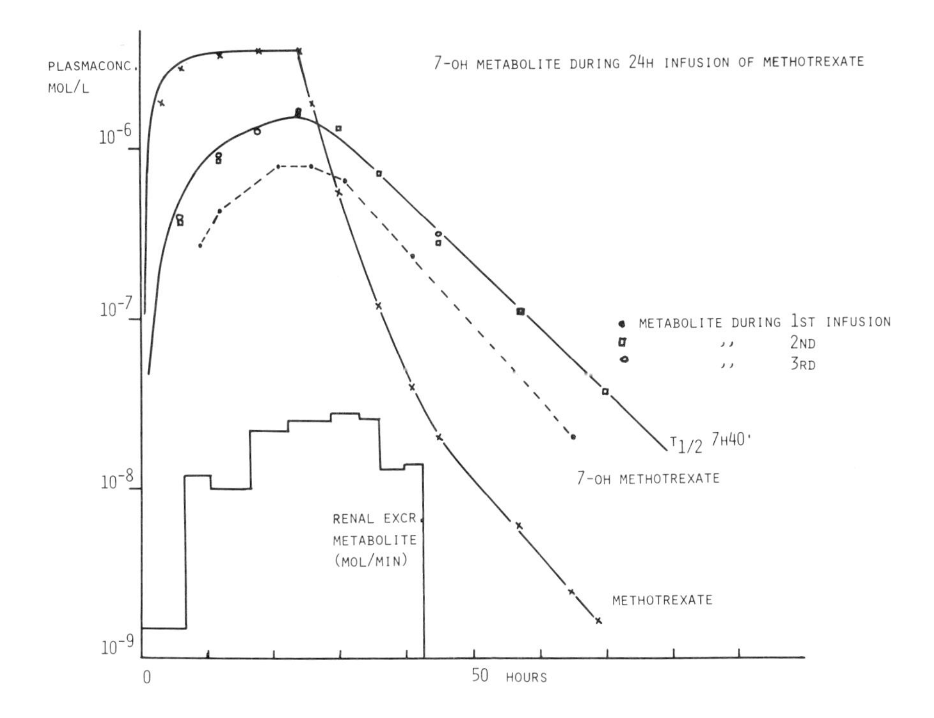

Fig. 7. Methotrexate plasma concentrations and 7-OH methotrexate concentrations in a patient receiving 378 mg methotrexate in 24 h.
Methotrexate concentrations have been averaged from three subsequent infusions (x).
The dotted line represents the 7-OH methotrexate curve obtained from the 1st infusion (.).
Concentrations of 7-OH methotrexate from the 2nd and 3rd infusion have been averaged (□ and o).
See Fig. 6. The renal excretion of 7-OH methotrexate from the 3rd infusion is plotted.

The activity of the 7-OH metabolite as an inhibitor of mammalian dihydrofolate reductase is 200 times less as compared to the activity of methotrexate (28).

However, plasma concentrations of the metabolite can be higher than that of

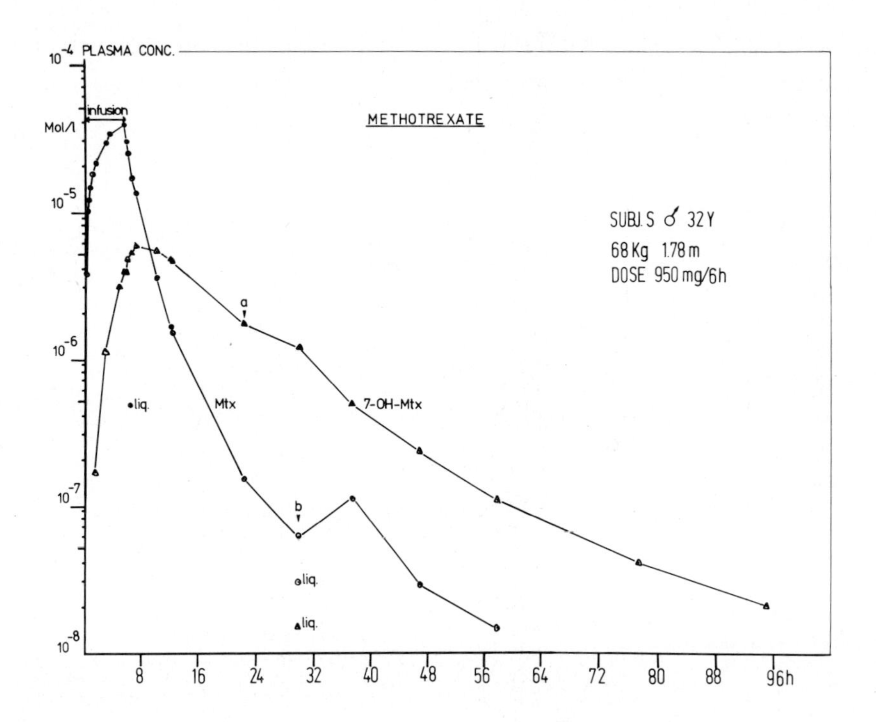

Fig. 8a. Plasma concentration curves of methotrexate and 7-OH methotrexate during and after a high dose infusion (950 mg in 6 h). Concentrations in two CSF samples are presented. 30 h after starting the infusion a dose of 5 mg methotrexate was administered intrathecally.

methotrexate (Figs 7 and 8). Therefore, the cytostatic activity of 7-hydroxymethotrexate should not be neglected in all cases.

Such a high concentration of the folate analogue 7-OH methotrexate might compete with methotrexate at the cell membrane level with regard to entrance into the cell. This is well known for 5-formyl tetrahydrofolate and for 5-methyl tetrahydrofolate (3,4). If this would also be the case for 7-hydroxymethotrexate determination might be helpful in the development of rational "rescue" regimens.

Another remarkable phenomenon is the increased concentration of 7-OH methotrexate during the second and next infusion as compared to the first one. This can be explained by induction of the liver enzyme responsible for the conversion of methotrexate into the metabolite after the first methotrexate infusion.

Analysis of the medium high dose infusion data (Fig. 7) shows that 91% of the administered dose was excreted unchanged as methotrexate, while 5% was found as the hydroxymetabolite.

As shown in Fig. 8 the metabolite was detected in the CSF as well.

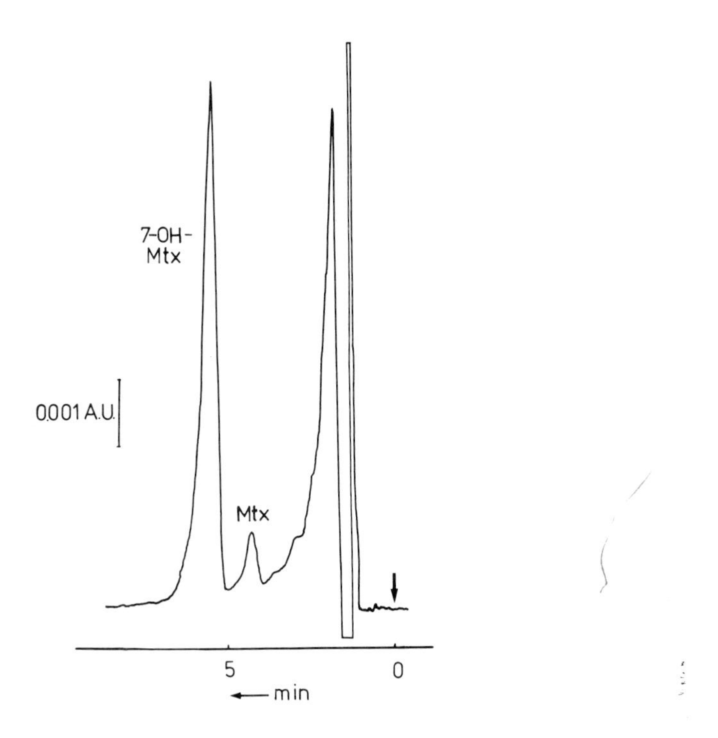

Fig. 8b. Chromatogram of a sample taken 24 h from the start. Note the higher concentration of 7-OH methotrexate as compared to that of methotrexate.

CONCLUSIONS

On-column concentration on reversed phase material, combined with analysis on an anion exchange resin under high pressure liquid chromatography provides a rapid determination technique for methotrexate as well as for its 7-OH metabolite.

A rapid determination of methotrexate is useful in high as well as in low dose therapy with methotrexate.

A systemic change in the pharmacokinetics during five subsequent intrathecal injections in the prophylactic treatment of leukemia has been observed. It is mainly attributable to an increase absorption by the plasma. Pharmacokinetic calculations have shown that two hours after the last two injections considerable less methotrexate is present in the CSF than after the first two injections. Assuming a dose dependent cytostatic effect, the prophylactic potency of the highest concentrations may be lower from the last two injections than from the first two.

The method reveals the occurrence of higher concentrations of 7-OH methotrexate than of the parent drug in the plasma after termination of the infusion. The inhibitory effect of the metabolite and its influence on the transport of methotrexate across the cell membrane will be studied by *in vitro* exposure to human bone marrow cells.

ACKNOWLEDGMENTS

Samples from patients were provided by Dr. A. Drenthe-Schonk, Dr. R.J.J. Lippens, Dr. J.H. Pasmooy and Dr. J.G. Stolk from the St. Radboud Hospital and by Dr. F. Smit from the Pieter Pauw Hospital (Wageningen, The Netherlands).

This investigation has been made possible by a grant of the Netherlands' Cancer Society (the Koningin Wilhelmina Fonds, KWF).

REFERENCES

1. Chabner, B.A. and Young, R.C. (1973) J. of Clin. Inv., 52, 1804-1811.

2. Stoller, R.G., Hande, K.R., Jacobs, S.A., Rosenberg, S.A. and Chabner, B.A. (1977) New Eng. J. Med., 297, 630-634.

3. Sirotnak, F.M., Donsbach, R.C., Dorick, D.M. and Moccio, D.M. (1977) Canc. Treatm. Rep., 61, 565-574.

4. Goldman, I.D. (1975) Canc. Chemother. Rep., part 3, 6, 62-72.

5. Pinedo, H.M., Zaharko, D.S., Bull, J. and Chabner, B.A. (1977) Canc. Res. 37, 445-450.

6. Goldman, I.D. (1974) Mol. Pharm. 10, 257-274.

7. Levine, L. and Powers, E. (1974) Res. Commun. Chem. Pathol. Pharm. 9, 543-554.

8. Description of RIA kit, Diagnostic Biochemistry, Inc. 10457 Roselle Street, San Diego, California 92121, U.S.A.

9. Myers, C.E., Lippman, M.E., Eliot, H.M. and Chabner, B.A. (1975) Proc. Nat. Acad. Sci. U.S., 72, 3683-3686.

10. Kinkade, J.M., Vogler, W.R. and Dayton, P.G. (1974) Biochem. Med. 10, 337-350.

11. Falk, R.C., Clark, D.R., Kahlman, S.M. and Long, T.F. (1976) Clin. Chem., 22, 785-788.

12. Nelson, J.A., Harris, B.A., Decker, W.J. and Farquhar, D. (1977) Cancer Res., 37, 3970-3973.

13. Wahlund, K. and Lund, U. (1976) J. Chromatogr. 122, 269-276.

14. Lankelma, J. and Poppe, H. (1978) J. Chromatogr. 149, 255.

15. Wagner, J.G. (1975) Fundamentals of Clinical Pharmacokinetics, Drug Intell. Publ. Inc., Hamilton, Ill. 62341.

16. Stoller, R.G., Jacobs, S.A., Drake, J.C., Lutz, R.J. and Chabner, B.A. (1975) Canc. Chemother. Rep., 6, 19-24.

17. Huffman, D.H., Wan, S.H., Azarnoff, D.L. and Hoogstraten, B. (1973) Clin. Pharm. & Therap., 14, 572-579.

18. Bischoff, K.B., Dedrick, R.L., Zaharko, D.S. and Longstreth, J.A. (1971) J. Pharm. Sci., 60, 1128-1133.

19. Reich, S.D., Bachur, N.R., Goebel, R.H. and Berman, M. (1977) J. Pharm. & Biopharm., 5, 423-433.

20. Capizzi, R.L., DeConti, R.C., Marsh, J.C. and Bertino, J.R. (1970) Canc. Res., 30, 1782-1788.

21. Oliverio, V.T. and Zaharko, D.S. (1971) Ann. N.Y. Acad. Sci. 186, 387-399.

22. Halprin, K.M., Fukui, K. and Ohkawara, A. (1971) Arch. Dermatol., 103, 243-249.

23. Smit, F., Lankelma, J. and Van der Kleijn, E., in preparation.

24. Geiser, C.F., Bishop, Y., Jaffe, N., Furman, L., Traggis, D. and Frei, III. E. (1975) Blood, 45, 189.

25. Bleyer, W.A. and Dedrick, R.L. (1977) Canc. Treatm. Rep., 61, 703-708.

26. Lippens, R.J.J., Drenthe-Schonk, A., Lankelma, J., Van der Kleijn, E. and Termond, E.F.S., submitted for publication.

27. Lankelma, J. and Van der Kleijn, E., submitted for publication.

28. Jacobs, S.A., Stoller, R.G., Chabner, B.A. and Johns, D.G. (1977) Canc. Treatm. Rep., 61, 651-656.

29. Bagshawe, K.D. (1969) Choriocarcinoma, Edward Arnold Ltd, (London).

30. Johns, D.G. and Valerino, D.M. (1971) Ann. N.Y. Acad. Sci., 186, 378-386.

Clinical Pharmacology of Anti-Neoplastic Drugs
H. M. Pinedo, editor

CLINICAL AND KINETIC PARAMETERS THAT INFLUENCE THE RESPONSE AND TOXICITY TO METHOTREXATE.

P.M. WILKINSON[1], E.R. MORICE[1] AND S.B. LUCAS[2].
[1]Christie Hospital and Holt Radium Institute, Manchester M20 9BX.
[2]Faculty of Medicine, Computational Group, Manchester University, M13 9PL., U.K.

INTRODUCTION

Methotrexate (MTX) was first used for the treatment of acute lymphatic leukaemia in 1948 following the observation that folates aggravated the disease process (1). While superseded by other drugs in this disease, it is still used extensively in a variety of solid tumours, particularly choriocarcinoma (2) and head and neck carcinoma (3,4,5). A variety of dose schedules have been proposed with not unexpectedly a variation in response rates. Following the observations in animals that lethal doses followed by rescue with Citrovorum factor was superior to methotrexate used alone (6), high dose MTX with rescue was introduced into clinical practice. However, despite the initial encouraging results, the overall response rate in, for example, head and neck carcinoma, although less toxic, is not significantly better than MTX used alone (7,8,9,10). It is perhaps relevant therefore that the clinical pharmacology of MTX when used alone should be reviewed to try and clarify those factors that determine response and toxicity.

MECHANISM OF ACTION AND RESISTANCE

MTX is an "S" phase specific drug that acts by preventing the conversion of folic acid to tetrahydrofolate by stoichiometric inhibition of the enzyme dihydrofolate reductase (DHFR) (11). The binding to DHFR is both reversible and competitive (12) but complete inhibition of DNA synthesis requires the presence of free intra-cellular drug as well as the proportion bound to DHFR (13). A concentration of $> 10^{-6}$ M produces more than 95% inhibition of DNA synthesis both *in vivo* and *in vitro* (14) but removal of free drug results in a rapid reversal of inhibition despite the persistence of that fraction that remains bound to protein (13). The concentration necessary to produce inhibition is specific for each tissue and is related to the plasma concentration. A critical minimal extra-cellular concentration threshold exists for each target organ that must be exceeded before organ toxicity will occur (15). The degree of toxicity is a function of both concentration and duration of exposure during the initial period of rapid cell kill (16).

As with bacteria, it is quite probable that exposure to "suboptimal concentrations" are likely to encourage the growth of resistant cells which then replace those originally sensitive to the drug. Spontaneous mutations may also occur and whilst an initial response will be seen, the tumour will rapidly become resistant. Both MTX and folic acid share the same active transport process (17) and thus one mechanism of resistance is decreased transport (18,19). Resistance may also develop by increased synthesis of DHFR within the cell (20) and there is evidence that subspecies of DHFR may be synthesised that show a markedly decreased affinity for MTX (21). Part of the rationale for high dose MTX was that the increased serum concentrations achieved would overcome transport resistance and increase enzyme synthesis and whilst "resistant" osteogenic sarcoma will respond to higher doses (22) the case remains umproven for other tumours.

CLINICAL PHARMACOLOGY IN MAN

In view of the above experimental observations, it is not surprising that the various doses of MTX used in clinical practice have produced variable response rates. Usually fixed repeated doses are prescribed and the response rate evaluated. Such treatments are satisfactory if the between patient variation in drug handling is minimal but this may be considerable with MTX. Hansen and co-workers (1971) observed that the dose required to produce toxicity without rescue varied by a factor of eighteen in a heterogeneous group of patients (23). Thus if the dose required to produce tumour regression is similar to that required to produce toxicity, a considerable dose range would be necessary for optimal response. The explanation for this variation must, in part, be due to those factors that influence absorption, distribution, metabolism and excretion.

Absorption

Absorption from the gastro-intestinal tract is complete only with small doses. Both MTX and folic acid are absorbed by an active transport process which is saturated with oral doses of > 30 mg/m^2 (24,25), and doses in excess of this must be administered intravenously. An oral dose of 30 mg/m^2 will produce a serum concentration of approximately 10^{-6} M that decays with a half time of twenty-five hours (26). This is greater than the threshold concentration that is toxic to both the bone marrow and gastro-intestinal epithelium (15) and explains why frequent oral doses produce cumulative toxicity to both these organs. It is not clear though whether this particular concentration is lethal to tumour cells which may account for the variable response seen following oral administration. Whilst satisfactory in leukaemia (27), the majority of schedules for solid tumours recommended the administration of MTX i.v. which is also the author's preference. In addition to achieving higher serum concentrations initially, this avoids difficulties with patient compliance and overcomes between patient variation in absorption.

Kinetics and Distribution

Following the i.v. administration of [^{3}H]-MTX the serum concentration/time curve decays as a triphasic function and the half time of the third phase is twenty-seven hours (26). However, this latter value may be an over-estimate because spontaneous degradation of radio-labelled compound occurs *in vivo* (28). More reliable methods of assay are now available and MTX concentrations can be determined fluorometrically (29), enzymatically (30), by radioimmunoassay (31,32,33) or by a competitive binding procedure suitable for large numbers of samples (34). (see also Bertino, this volume).

Serum concentrations determined by radioimmunoassay and enzymatic assay at this institute has confirmed the triphasic decay of MTX following i.v. administration. The concentration/time curve following the single administration of 100 mg/m^2 is shown in Fig. 1. Here the time scale is plotted logarithmically and the serum concentrations arithmetically because of the wide between patient variation in the latter. The concentration half times ranged from 2-8 minutes for the first phase, 0.9 - 2 hours for the second phase and 5.3 - 11.0 hours for the third phase. These times are similar to those reported with high dose MTX (35). A concentration of more than 10^{-6} M was maintained for twelve hours and a concentration of 10^{-7} M $>$ 36 hours. The initial decay phase is explained by redistribution of drug into the tissues, the second phase is by both metabolism and excretion and the gradual release of drug from within the cell results in the third phase.

The initial volume of distribution or central compartment volume was 3.5 litres which is less than the extra-cellular volume. Approximately 50% of drug within the central compartment is bound to plasma albumen (25) and the remainder distributes within the tissues. As MTX is a weakly acidic drug that part bound to albumen will be displaced by drugs of a similar nature leading to an increased concentration of free drug (36). The apparent volume of distribution was 95 litres which is similar to that observed by other workers (26).

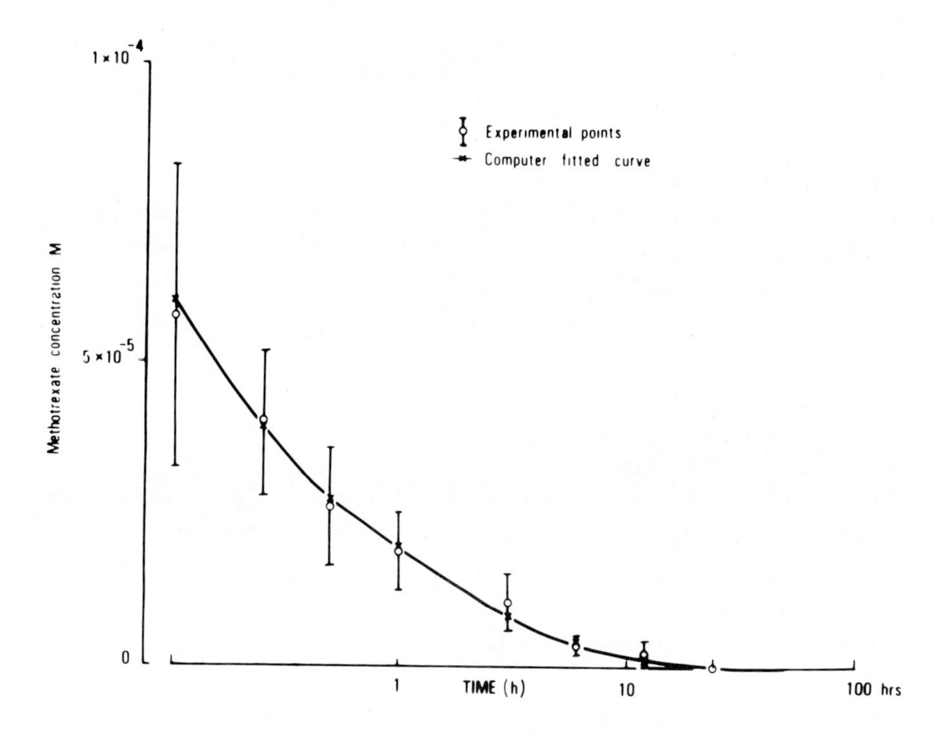

Fig. 1. Decay of methotrexate (M) (mean ± S.E.M.) during the first 48 hours after the administration of 100 mg/m^2 to eight patients with malignant disease.

The distribution of drug within the tissues is probably not uniform. Although there is some diffusion into the CSF, conventional doses achieve sub-optimal concentrations (37). This can be overcome by intrathecal injection or by using high dose MTX (37,38). The CSF concentrations are prolonged in those patients with CNS disease which results in increased toxicity (38). The presence of ascitic or pleural fluid increases the distribution volume and acts as a drug reservoir. Drug is gradually released back into the serum, prolongs the third phase and results in increased toxicity (24,26).

Metabolism and Excretion

A small proportion of MTX is metabolised following conventional i.v. administration (26). However, if the drug is given by mouth then several metabolites are produced due to bacterial degradation within the intestinal tract (39,40,41). Administration of high dose MTX results in more biotransformation and up to 30% of the administered dose may be excreted in the urine as 7-hydroxymethotrexate (42). To date, none of these metabolites have been shown to possess activity, although they may account for up to one third of the total plasma concentrations during the third phase (26). It is unknown whether between patient variation in metabolism is important both in terms of response and toxicity.

Excretion

MTX is eliminated predominantly be renal excretion by both glomerular filtration and renal tubular secretion. The proportion excreted varies from 37-100% (26), and this is probably accounted for by variation in urine pH. Being a weak acid, the proportion of MTX excreted increases with increasing pH and urinary pH is rarely, if ever, measured during treatment. Whilst renal toxicity is rare with doses of < 1 g (43), the importance of urinary alkalisation and diuresis were recognised in early trials of high dose MTX to overcome this problem (44).

MTX is actively secreted into the bile and the small proportion (0.4-6%) secreted varies inversely with the dose (46,47). The proportion of drug excreted into the gastro-intestinal tract undergoes entero-hepatic circulation and biotransformation by bacteria.

Toxicity

The dose required to produce toxicity varies considerably (9,23). Attempts to correlate toxic reactions with the kinetics of MTX indicate that a minimal extracellular concentration must be exceeded before organ toxicity will occur (15). The most sensitive tissues are bone marrow and the gastro-intestinal epithelium but the kidney, liver, skin and lungs may also be affected. There is little published data on comparative toxicities on the same dose of MTX given either as an i.v. infusion or as an i.v. push, and the factors that determine between patient variations in sensitivity are as yet unknown. Various factors have, however, been advocated. These include the level of DHFR within the cell (48), variations in membrane permeability (49) and folate status prior to treatment.

KINETIC APPLICATIONS

Several models are described to account for the distribution of MTX (50,51) but for the general clinician these are probably too complicated for routine use. Most centres have assay facilities and therefore various selected kinetic parameters can readily be determined from the concentration/time curve and related to response and toxicity. In a study of this type at this institute it was observed that the smaller the area under the third phase of the decay curve, the greater the probability of response suggesting that some patients retained proportionately more drug within the cell. No kinetic parameter would successfully predict for toxicity but a significant inverse correlation was observed between the proportion of dose eliminated in the urine and the observed degree of toxicity (Fig. 2).

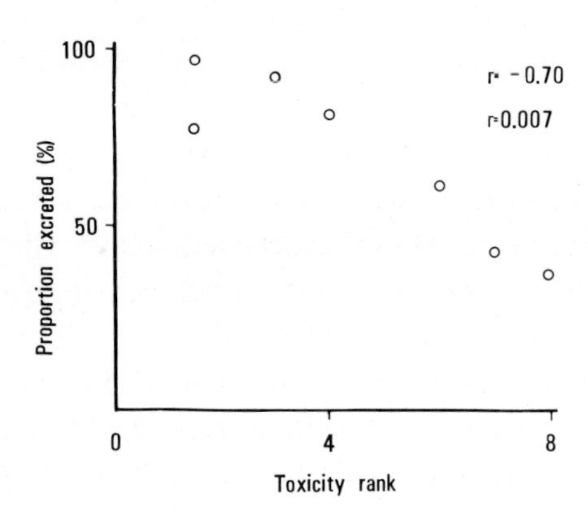

Fig. 2. Correlation between urinary excretion of methotrexate and toxicity in eight patients who received 100 mg/m^2. Patients were ranked from 1 to 8, where 1 represents the least and 8 the most severe degree of observed toxicity.

Those patients who excreted less than 50% of the dose within fortyeight hours experienced toxicity but there was no significant correlation between creatinine clearance or clearance of MTX.

In summary, it is difficult to suggest an optimal dose of MTX. In the study quoted here the overall response rate in 20 patients with head and neck cancer who received 100 mg/m^2 at intervals of two weeks was 66% which is comparable to high dose schemes. It remains to be seen whether dose manipulations using information obtained from concentration/time curves will increase the responsc rate but reduce toxicity; kinetic studies have been of value with high dose schemes in predicting toxicity but not response (35,52). Although such studies are time consuming, because of the between patient variability, they may be necessary in order to achieve the optimum response to MTX when used alone.

REFERENCES

1. Farber, S., Cutler, E.C., Hawkins, J.W., Harrison, J.H., Pierce, E.C. and Lenz, G.G. (1947) Science. 106; 619-621.

2. Hertz, R., Lewis, J.Jr., and Lipsett, M.B. (1961) Am.J.Obstet. Gynaecol. 82; 631-640.

3. Papac, R.J., Jacobs, E.M., Foye, L.V. and Donohue, D.M. (1963) Cancer Chemother. Rep. 32; 47-54.

4. Lane, M., Moore, J. and Levin, H. (1968) JAMA 204; 561-563.

5. Leone, L., Abala, M. and Rege, V. (1968) Cancer 21; 828-832.

6. Goldin, A., Mantel, N., Greenhouse, S.W., Venditti, J.M. and Humphreys, S.R. (1953) Cancer Res. 13; 843-850.

7. Djerassi, I., Rominger, C.J., Kim, J.S., Turchi, J., Suvansri, U. & Hughes, D. (1972) Cancer 30; 22-30.

8. Capizzi, R.L., DeConti, R.C., Marsh, J.C. and Bertino, J.R. (1970) Cancer Res. 30; 1782-1788.

9. Levitt, M., Mosher, M.B., DeConti, R.C., Farber, L.R., Skeel, R.T., Marsh, J.C., Mitchell, M.S., Papac, R.J., Thomas, E.D. and Bertino, J.R. (1973) Cancer Res. 33; 1729-1734.

10. Khandekar, J.D. and Wolff, A. (1977) Proc. Am. Assoc. Cancer Res. 18; 281.

11. Werheiser, W.C. (1961) J. Biol. Chem. 236; 888-893.

12. Bertino, J.R. (1974) In "Antineoplastic and immunosuppressive agents" (Handbook of experimental pharmacology) Vol. 38, Part 2. Ed. Sartorelli, A.C. and Johns, D.S. New York. Springer-Verlag 468-483.

13. Goldman, I.D. (1974) Mol. Pharmacol. 10; 257-274.

14. Hryniuk, W.M. and Bertino, J.R. (1969) J. Clin. Invest. 48; 2140-2155.

15. Chabner, B.A. and Young, R.C. (1973) J. Clin. Invest. 52; 1804-1811.

16. Pinedo, H.M., Zaharko, D.S., Bull, J. and Chabner, B.A. (1977) Cancer Res. 37; 445-450.

17. Goldman, I.D., Lichtenstein, N.S. and Oliverio, V.T. (1968) J. Biol. Chem. 243; 5007-5017.

18. Kessel, D., Hall, T.C. and Roberts, D. (1968) Cancer Res. 28; 564-570.

19. Bender, R.A., Bleyer, W.A., Frisby, S.A. and Oliverio, V.T. (1975) Cancer Res. 35; 1305-1308.

20. Bertino, J.R., Donohue, D.R., Gabrio, B.W., Silber, R., Alenty, A., Meyer, M. and Huennekens, F.M. (1962) Nature 193; 140-142.

21. Albrecht, A.M., Biedler, J.L. and Hutchinson, D.J. (1972) Cancer Res. 32; 1539-1546.

22. Jaffe, N. (1972) Cancer 30; 1627-1631.

23. Hansen, H.H., Selawry, O.S., Holland, J.F. and McCall, C.B. (1971) Br. J. Cancer 25; 298-305.

24. Wan, S.H., Huffman, D.H., Azarnoff, D.L., Stephens, R. and Hoogstraten, B. (1974) Cancer Res. 34; 3487-3491.

25. Henderson, E.S., Adamson, R.H. and Oliverio, V.T. (1965) Cancer Res. 25; 1018-1024.

26. Huffman, D.H., Wan, S.H., Azarnoff, D.L. and Hoogstraten, B. (1973) Clin. Pharm. Ther. 14; 572-579.

27. Acute Leukaemia Group B. (1969) JAMA 207; 923-928.

28. Calvert, A.H., Bondy, P.K. and Harrap, K.H. (1973) Cancer Treat. Rep. 9; 1647-1656.

29. Freeman, M.J. (1957) J. Pharmacol. 120; 1-8.

30. Bertino, J.R. and Fischer, F.A. (1964) Meth. Med. Res. 10; 297-307.

31. Raso, V. and Schreiber, R. (1975) Cancer Res. 35; 1407-1416.

32. Loeffler, L.J., Blum, M.R. and Nelsen, M.A. (1976) Cancer Res. 36; 3306-3311.

33. Aherne, G.W., Piall, E.M. and Marks, V. (1977) Br. J. Cancer 36; 608-617.

34. Myers, C.E., Lippman, M.E., Eliot, H.M. and Chabner, B.A. (1975) Proc. Nat. Acad. Sci. 72; 3683-3686.

35. Stoller, R.G., Hande, K.R., Jacobs, S.A., Rosenberg, S.A. and Chabner, B.A. (1977) N. Engl. J. Med. 297; 630-634.

36. Liegler, D.G., Henderson, E.S., Hahn, M.A. and Oliverio, V.T. (1969) Clin. Pharm. Ther. 10; 849-857.

37. Shapiro, W.R., Young, D.F. and Mehta, B.M. (1975) N. Engl. J. Med. 293; 161-166.

38. Pitman, S.W. and Frei, E. III (1977) Cancer Treat. Rep. 61; 695-701.

39. Zaharko, D.S., Bruckner, H. and Oliverio, V.T. (1969) Science 166; 887-888.

40. Levy, C.C. and Goldman, P. (1967) J. Biol. Chem. 242; 2933-2938.

41. Pratt, R.G., Crawford, E.J. and Friedkin, J.J. (1963) J. Biol. Chem. 243; 6367-6372.

42. Jacobs, S.A., Stoller, R.G. and Chabner, B.A. (1976) J. Clin. Invest. 57; 534-538.

43. Condit, P.T., Chanes, R.E. and Joel, W. (1969) Cancer 23; 126-131.

44. Pitman, S.W., Parker, L. and Tattershall, M.N.H. (1975) Cancer Chemother. Rep. 6; 43-49.

45. Kates, R.E. and Tozer, T.N. (1976) J. Pharm. Sci. 65; 1348-1352.

46. Creaven, P.J., Hansen, H.H., Alford, D.A. and Allen, L.M. (1973) Br. J. Cancer 28; 589-591.

47. Bleyer, W.A. (1977) Cancer Treat. Revs. 4; 87-101.

48. Bertino, J.R., Cashmore, A.R. and Hillcoat, B.L. (1970) Cancer Res. 30; 2372-2378.

49. Jarabak, J. and Bachur, N.R. (1971) Biochem. Med. 5; 430.

50. Zaharko, D.S., Dedrick, R.L., Bischoff, K.B., Longstreth, J.A. and Oliverio, V.T. (1971) J. Nat. Cancer Inst. 46; 775-784.

51. Bischoff, K.B., Dedrick, R.L., Zaharko, D.S. and Longstreth, J.A. (1971) J. Pharm. Sci. 60; 1128-1133.

52. Nirenberg, A., Mosende, C., Mehta, B.M., Gisolfi, A.L. and Rosen, G. (1977) Cancer Treat. Rep. 61; 779-783.

Clinical Pharmacology of Anti-Neoplastic Drugs
H. M. Pinedo, editor

REVERSAL OF METHOTREXATE TOXICITY TO MOUSE BONE MARROW AND L1210 LEUKEMIA CELLS GROWN *IN VITRO*

ALBERT LEYVA, LIESBETH VAN DE GRINT AND HERBERT M. PINEDO
University Hospital, Catharijnesingel 101, 3511 GV Utrecht, The Netherlands.

ABSTRACT

The use of nucleotide derivatives for the reversal of methotrexate (MTX) toxicity may provide selective rescue of normal versus tumor tissues. We performed a comparative study of mouse bone marrow cells and L1210 leukemia cells grown in culture. The proliferation of the marrow granulocyte precursor cells (CFU-C*) and L1210 cells was examined according to colony formation 7 to 9 days after continuous exposure to MTX, leucovorin or nucleic acid precursors in a semisolid medium. At 10^{-8} M, MTX produced a partial reduction in colony formation while higher concentrations were markedly cytotoxic. Inhibition of CFU-C colony formation at 10^{-8} and 10^{-7} M was completely blocked by equimolar concentrations of leucovorin. However, at higher MTX concentrations full reversal of drug cytotoxicity required that the concentration of leucovorin exceed that of MTX approximately 100-fold. The same competitive reversal of MTX cytotoxicity by leucovorin was observed with L1210 cells. Combinations of thymidine plus a purine, but neither individually, reversed noncompetitively the MTX-mediated inhibition of colony formation. Adenine and hypoxanthine, but not guanine, derivatives were effective with thymidine. Equimolar concentrations of thymidine and a purine at 10^{-5} and 10^{-4} M protected bone marrow cells from MTX toxicity independent of drug concentration. Conversely, L1210 cells exposed to 10^{-8} M MTX were spared only with 10^{-5} M thymidine and inosine. At higher MTX concentrations, nucleosides had a minimal protective effect as L1210 colony formation did not exceed 20% of control. In addition to these cell culture experiments, normal mouse plasma was examined by high performance liquid chromatography to determine the levels of purine and pyrimidine bases and nucleosides. Thymidine was found at 1.3 to 3.5 x 10^{-6} M concentrations, while the only purine consistently detected was hypoxanthine at levels still below 1.0 x 10^{-6} M. These data indicate that at least *in vitro*, reversal of MTX cytotoxicity with thymidine plus a purine has advantages over the use of leucovorin, providing

1) more efficient protection of bone marrow cells at high MTX concentrations,

*CFU-C, colony forming unit (in) culture.

2) more selective protection of bone marrow cells compared to leukemia cells. Data of plasma levels of nucleobases and nucleosides suggest that normally the availability of both thymidine and purines limits the reversal of MTX cytotoxicity.

INTRODUCTION

MTX, a folate antimetabolite, inhibits dihydrofolate reductase leading to a depletion of reduced folates in the cell which are necessary for 1-carbon transfer in *de novo* thymidylate synthesis and *de novo* purine nucleotide synthesis (1). The potent inhibitory effect of MTX on nucleic acid synthesis and cell growth accounts for this drug's antineoplastic properties and extensive clinical use. However, MTX toxicity to normal proliferating tissues such as bone marrow and intestinal mucosa is often encountered limiting the antitumor effectiveness of the drug. The toxic side effects have been largely prevented or alleviated by the use of a "rescue" agent, leucovorin. Leucovorin, a folate derivative, is capable of replenishing intracellular pools of reduced folates affected by the MTX-mediated inhibition of dihydrofolate reductase. Recently in experimental chemotherapy, an attempt has been made to replace leucovorin with thymidine with the prospect of exploiting potential differences between normal and neoplastic cells regarding the antipurine effect of MTX (2). Although an enhanced antitumor effect has been demonstrated by the administration of MTX plus thymidine, the ability of thymidine alone to protect normal tissues from drug toxicity has not been clearly shown (2-4). Studies of various mammalian cells in culture have been reported showing the reversal of MTX cytotoxicity by thymidine plus a purine and a partial effect by thymidine alone (5-10). The depletion of nucleotides resulting from the inhibitory effects of MTX on *de novo* thymidylate synthesis and *de novo* purine synthesis can in principle be circumvented by the re-utilization of preformed pyrimidines and purines via salvage pathway enzymes. The effectiveness of this by-pass process would be dependent on various factors, including the availability of nucleobases and nucleosides plus other required substrates. Although evidence has been reported indicating that the liver via the blood supplies purines and pyrimidines to non-hepatic tissues (11-12), there is little information to date on the concentrations of these metabolites in blood.

We present here a comparative study on the cytotoxicity of MTX to mouse bone marrow (13) and L1210 leukemia cells grown in culture and the potential of leucovorin and nucleosides to reverse drug toxicity. Also presented are data on the chromatographic analysis of mouse plasma for the presence of nucleobases and nucleosides in order to determine what influence these endogenous metabolites might have on MTX toxicity *in vivo*. The results are discussed in light of relevant studies reported by others and regarding the implications to MTX therapy in the treatment of experimental tumors and human cancer using leucovorin versus nucleoside rescue.

MATERIALS AND METHODS

Cell culture.

The short-term culture of bone marrow cells in semisolid medium has been described (13,14). Bone marrow was obtained from the femurs of healthy, untreated C57BL mice and pooled. Nucleated marrow cells (10^5 per culture dish) were added to culture medium containing 2.1% methyl cellulose, 10% dialyzed fetal calf serum, bovine serum albumin and dialyzed L-cell supernatant (colony stimulating factor) in McCoy's medium. Any drugs or rescue factors were added to the medium before the addition of cells. After a 7-day incubation period at 37° C, colonies consisting of 50 cells or more were counted using light microscopy. The mean number of colonies per plate was determined for groups of 4 plates each and expressed relative to the number of colonies in control cultures without MTX or rescue agents.

L1210 leukemia cells were maintained in suspension culture in RPMI 1640 medium with 10% fetal calf serum. However, exposure to MTX and rescue factors was carried out in semisolid medium culture in the same manner as for bone marrow cells, except for the absence of any colony stimulating factor. Also, 500 cells obtained from log phase cultures were plated per culture dish and colonies were counted after a 9-day incubation period. Compared to CFU-C, L1210 cloning efficiency was higher (30-40%) and colonies were larger and more compact. The more distinct appearance of these colonies made it possible to assess L1210 colony formation by the use of a computerized, electronic image analyzer capable of counting colonies at different minimal diameter sizes ranging from 0.05 to 0.70 mm. Colony number expressed as percent of colony number recorded at the highest sensitivity (0.05 mm) was plotted against the different sensitivity settings giving a size distribution curve. L1210 colony formation was also evaluated as described for bone marrow cells, i.e. the mean number of colonies counted at a chosen sensitivity was determined for groups of 4 plates each and expressed relative to the number of colonies in control cultures, counted at the same sensitivity.

High performance liquid chromatography (HPLC)

The concentrations of purine and pyrimidine bases and nucleosides in mouse plasma were measured by HPLC using a Pye Unicam LC-20 chromatograph. Stainless-steel columns, 10 cm x 4.6 mm ID, were packed with Aminex A28 (Bio-Rad), a strong anionic exchange resin with a particle diameter size of 7-11 microns. These columns were equipped with water jackets for temperature control. Detection was performed with a Perkin Elmer L15 UV detector at a fixed wavelength of 254 nm or with a Pye Unicam LC-3 variable wavelength detector. Isocratic elution was carried out according to Eksteen et al. (15) with modifications designed to improve separation, especially for plasma samples. Two chromatographic systems were used both with an eluant composed basically of 0.01 M sodium phosphate and 0.005 M sodium citrate. In chromatographic system 1 the pH of the eluant was adjusted to 7.7 and ethanol was added to 30%. Elution was performed at 60° C and at a flow rate of 0.3 ml/min. In system 2 the pH of the eluant was adjusted to 9.6 and ethanol was added to 20%. Elution in this case was performed at 70° C and at a flow rate of 0.5 ml/min.

Prior to chromatography, plasma samples were deproteinized by either ultrafiltration through Amicon CF-25 cones or by precipitation with 0.4 M perchloric acid followed by neutralization with potassium bicarbonate. Volumes of 20 to 25 μl of the prepared samples were injected. Peaks were identified by retention times and also absorbance ratio at different wavelengths, comparison being made with standard solutions. Quantitation of bases and nucleosides was made by comparison of peak height with those determined for standard solutions at various concentrations. The lower limit of detection for early eluting peaks was about 1×10^{-11} M and for later peaks about 5×10^{-11} M.

RESULTS

Inhibition of CFU-C proliferation by MTX

The exposure of cells to MTX in culture medium containing biologically derived components of undefined composition can lead to altered drug toxicity. The potential presence of thymidine and purine metabolites can interfere with the inhibitory effects of MTX on thymine nucleotide and purine nucleotide synthesis. The growth of cells in culture generally requires the presence of serum, and for bone marrow cells a colony stimulating factor (L-cell supernatant) as well. If fetal calf serum and L-cell supernatant were used undialyzed inhibition of colony formation with MTX was observed only above 10^{-6} M, 50% inhibition occurring at 10^{-4} M (data not shown). When these medium components were dialyzed before use, a high sensitivity to MTX resulted, 50% less colonies appearing at 10^{-8} M MTX. This finding agrees with previous data indicating that DNA synthesis in bone marrow is inhibited *in vivo* at or above plasma MTX concentrations of 10^{-8} M (16). Analysis of the fetal calf serum and the colony stimulating factor by HPLC after dialysis has shown a marked reduction in UV-absorbing peaks corresponding with thymidine and purine bases and nucleosides (13). In dialyzed samples these pyrimidines and purines were undetectable, levels being less than 5 x 10^{-7} M. Further dilution of any residual amounts of these compounds after addition to the medium would reduce their levels to less than 10^{-8}M In order to eliminate the influence of fetal calf serum and L-cell supernatant on MTX cytotoxicity, these medium components were always used dialyzed.

Under the conditions described, in which 10^5 nucleated bone marrow cells were plated, the mean number of colonies in control cultures was 90. Most of the colonies consisted of more than 100 cells. The use of dialyzed versus undialyzed fetal calf serum and colony stimulating factor yielded a higher number of colonies in control cultures, most likely explained by the removal of inhibitory substances by dialysis. At MTX concentrations of 10^{-8} to 10^{-6} M a notable decrease in the number of colonies consisting of at least 50 cells was observed, although clusters of less than 50 cells were also present. Higher MTX concentrations caused complete inhibition of cell proliferation indicated by the absence of any colonies or clusters. At 10^{-9} M MTX slight stimulation of cell proliferation, i.e. increased colony number compared to control cultures, was consistently observed. This latter finding is potentially significant and has been designated for further examination in future planned studies.

Effects on leucovorin on bone marrow cells

The ability of leucovorin to protect cultured bone marrow cells from the inhibitory effects of MTX at various concentrations was studied (Fig. 1).The partial inhibition of colony formation by 10^{-8} M MTX and the complete inhibition by 10^{-7} M MTX could be reversed by the presence of 10^{-7} M leucovorin. However, at higher MTX concentrations leucovorin was less effective. Prevention of toxicity to CFU-C exposed to 10^{-6} and 10^{-5} M MTX was observed with 10^{-4} and 10^{-3} M leucovorin, respectively. At 10^{-4} M MTX, the highest concentration studied, no sign of toxicity reversal was apparent by leucovorin even at 10^{-3} M.

Effects of nucleosides on bone marrow cells

As shown in Table 1, neither thymidine nor adenosine alone at concentrations of 10^{-9} to 10^{-4} M was capable of reversing the 50% inhibition of colony formation produced by 10^{-8} M MTX. Other purine metabolites, inosine, guanosine and hypoxanthine, gave results similar to those described for adenosine. Although adenosine itself showed no toxicity at concentrations up to 10^{-4} M, thymidine at 10^{-4} M caused a decrease in colony number and at 10^{-3} M thymidine no colonies appeared. The combination of thymidine with the purine derivatives was found to give complete protection in CFU-C cultures containing 10^{-8} to 10^{-4} M MTX. Fig. 2 illustrates these results for thymidine and inosine when added in equimolar concentrations.

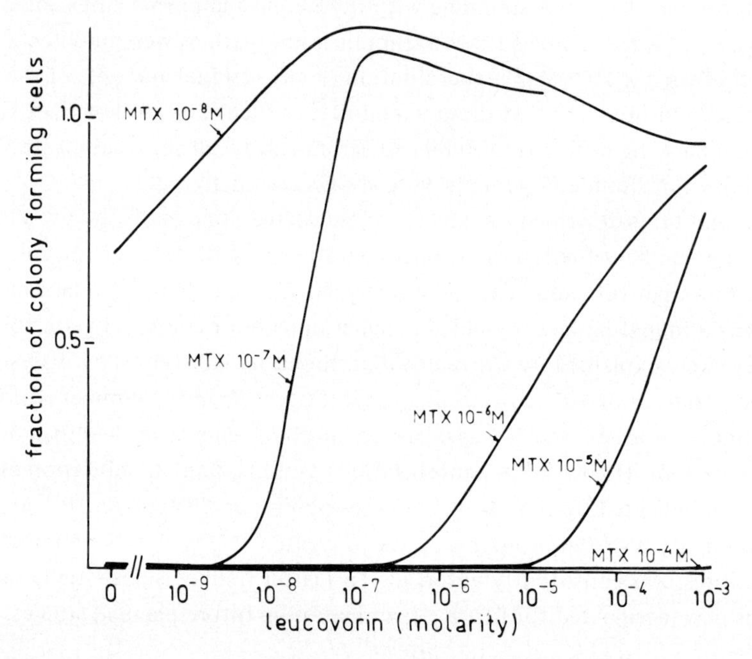

Fig. 1. Effect of leucovorin on MTX cytotoxicity in CFU-C cultures at different MTX concentrations.(Data from reference 13, Pinedo et al.)

TABLE 1
EFFECTS OF THYMIDINE AND ADENOSINE ON CFU-C PROLIFERATION IN THE PRESENCE AND ABSENCE OF MTX.

Final molar concentrations in medium			Colonies
MTX	Thymidine	Adenosine	(% control)
10^{-8}	- [a]	-	50
10^{-8}	10^{-9} - 10^{-5}	-	50
10^{-8}	10^{-4}	-	30
10^{-8}	10^{-3}	-	0
10^{-8}	-	10^{-9} - 10^{-4}	50
-	10^{-9} - 10^{-5}	-	100
-	10^{-4}	-	30
-	10^{-3}	-	0
-	-	10^{-9} - 10^{-4}	100

[a] , MTX or nucleoside omitted (Data from reference 13, Pinedo et al.).

Complete reversal of the inhibitory effects of MTX, regardless of MTX concentration, appeared to be at 10^{-5} M. A lesser degree of reversal was obtained with 10^{-4} M thymidine and inosine, whereas with less than 10^{-5} M or greater than 10^{-4} M nucleosides no appreciable reversal was observed. Similar results were noted with equimolar combinations of thymidine and adenosine or hypoxanthine, however, MTX toxicity persisted with thymidine plus guanosine present. Although the purine bases and nucleosides alone were not toxic at concentrations as high as 10^{-4} M, thymidine alone was toxic at 10^{-4} M resulting in colony formation 30% that of control (Table 1).

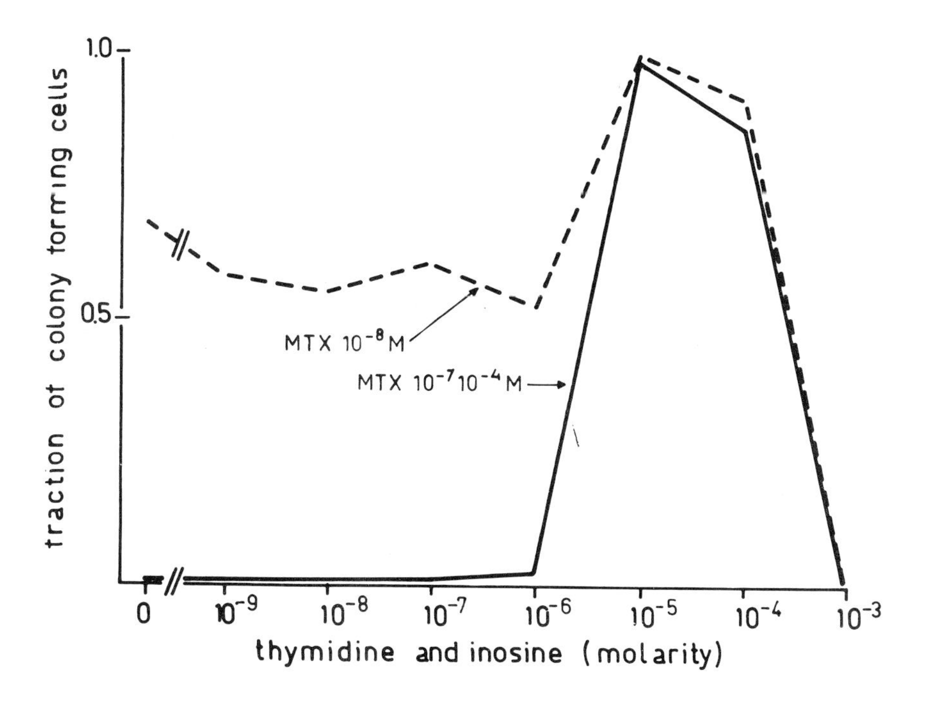

Fig. 2. Effect of equimolar concentrations of thymidine and inosine on MTX cytotoxicity in CFU-C cultures. Broken line represents experiments performed at 10^{-8} M MTX, whereas solid line represents experiments at 10^{-7} to 10^{-4} M MTX. (Data from reference 13,Pinedo et al.).

It is likely that thymidine toxicity was responsible for the decrease in the reversal potential of thymidine and purine combinations above 10^{-5} M.

Inhibition of L1210 cell proliferation by MTX

When L1210 cells were plated in a semisolid medium with MTX added, inhibition of colony formation differed from that observed in bone marrow cultures. Even at MTX concentrations as high as 10^{-6} M the number of colonies formed was only slightly decreased compared to control cultures, although colony size and density were clearly reduced. The aid of an electronic image analyzer facilitated the quantitative evaluation of the inhibitory effects of MTX on L1210 cell growth in the semisolid culture system. Fig. 3 (control curve) illustrates the size distribution of the colonies formed in the absence of MTX. The exposure of L1210 cells to 10^{-6} M MTX resulted in a marked shift of the colony size distribution curve to the left and a more than 80% decrease in the number of colonies detected at the highest sensitivity or 0.05 mm minimal diameter (Fig. 3).

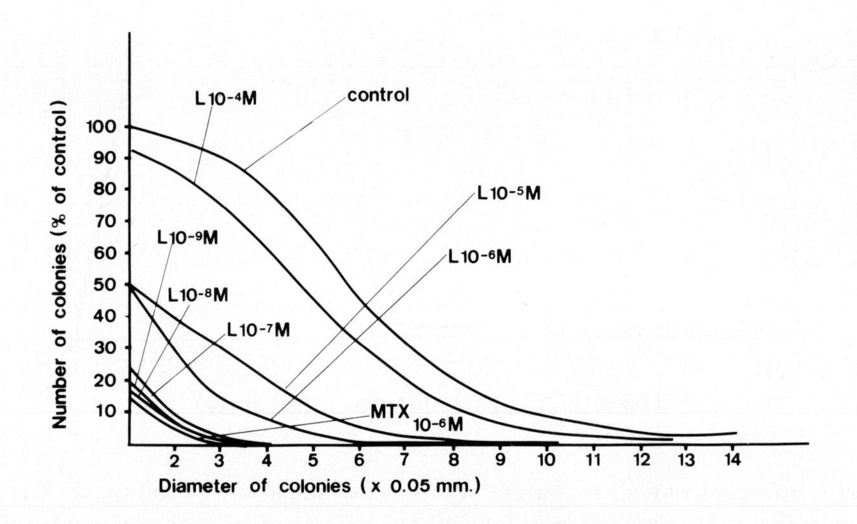

Fig. 3. Effect of leucovorin on L1210 colony formation in the presence of 10^{-6} M MTX. Except for line marked control, all lines represent experiments performed in the presence of 10^{-6} M MTX. Leucovorin (L) was tested at 10^{-9} to 10^{-4} M.

The distribution curve representing colony formation in the presence of 10^{-8} M

MTX (data not shown) indicated that there was little effect on the number of colonies detected at the highest sensitivity. However, a reduction in colony size was demonstrated by a shift of the size distribution curve to the left.

Effects of leucovorin on L1210 cells

Fig. 3 demonstrates the reversal of the MTX-induced inhibition of L1210 colony formation by the presence of leucovorin. A shift in colony size distribution approaching that of control was observed in cultures exposed to MTX and increasing concentrations of leucovorin. The ability of leucovorin to protect L1210 cells exposed to MTX was found to be dependent on the concentration of MTX present. This is illustrated in Fig. 4 in which assessment of colony formation was made by recording the number of colonies with a diameter size of 0.15 mm or larger. In the absence of MTX or leucovorin 90% of the total number of colonies detected were in this size range.

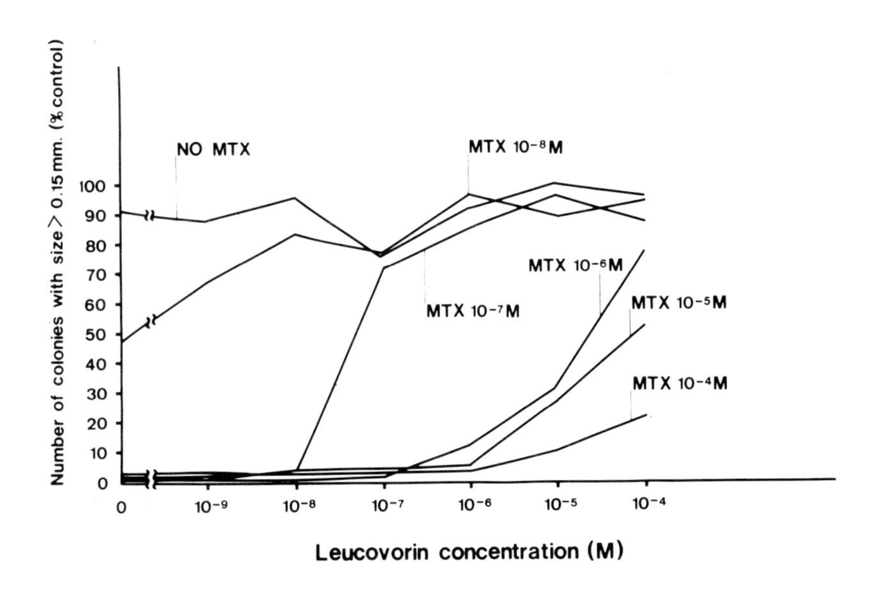

Fig. 4. Leucovorin-mediated reversal of MTX toxicity to L1210 cells at different MTX concentrations.

Leucovorin alone had no appreciable effect on colony number. A 48% reduction in colony number was observed with 10^{-8} M MTX, while no colonies were detected at 10^{-7} M or higher concentrations of MTX. The concomitant addition of leucovorin and MTX resulted in the complete protection of L1210 cells from the inhibitory effects of 10^{-8} and 10^{-7} M MTX, while leucovorin at higher MTX concentrations was only partially effective.

Effects of nucleosides on L1210 cells

The inhibitory effect of MTX on L1210 colony formation was not prevented by the presence of thymidine alone or a purine nucleoside alone as observed with CFU-C cultures (data not shown). Also, thymidine at 10^{-4} M caused a further reduction in colony number. Thymidine at lower concentrations than 10^{-4} M plus purine nucleosides at 10^{-9} to 10^{-4} M concentrations resulted in no apparent toxicity. Comparable to experiments with CFU-C cultures, equimolar combinations of thymidine and purine nucleoside were added to L1210 cell cultures exposed to MTX in attempt to revers MTX cytotoxicity (Fig. 5). A decrease in colony formation with 10^{-8} M MTX was nearly completely reversed by the addition of 10^{-5} M thymidine and inosine. whereas lower nucleoside concentrations were less effective and at 10^{-4} M additional toxicity was observed. At higher concentrations of MTX at which no colonies with a minimal diameter of 0.15 mm were formed, only 10^{-5} M thymidine and inosine produced reversal; however, in this case the number of colonies increased to no more than 15% of control values. A marked reduction in colony formation resulted consistently at 10^{-4} M thymidine and inosine whether MTX was present or not.

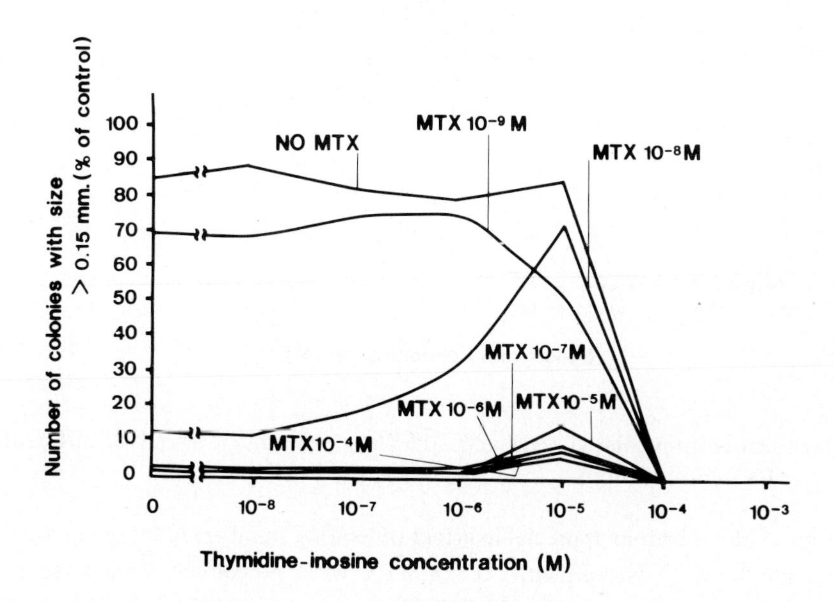

Fig. 5. Nucleoside-mediated reversal of MTX toxicity to L1210 cells at different MTX concentrations.

Analysis of purines and pyrimidines in mouse plasma

In order to determine the potential of tissues *in vivo* to overcome MTX cytotoxicity by the use of endogenous thymidine and purine bases and nucleosides, the presence of these metabolites was examined in mouse plasma. Figs 6 and 7 illustrate the HPLC separations of normal mouse plasma using two different elution systems.

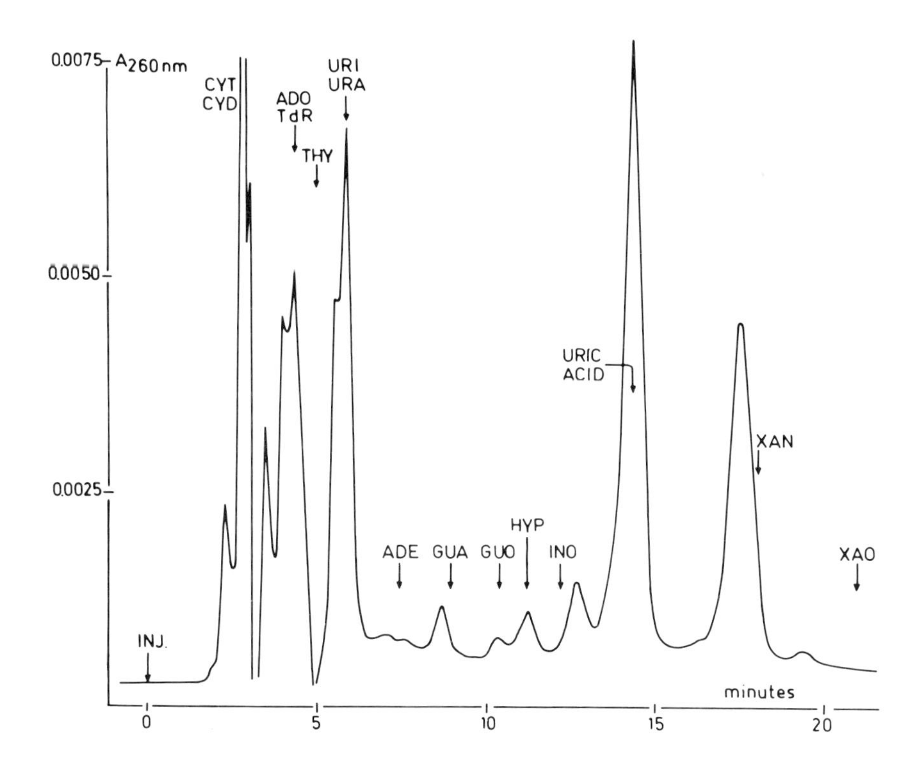

Fig. 6. HPLC analysis of nucleobases and nucleosides in normal mouse plasma — chromatographic system 1 (see MATERIALS AND METHODS). Elutions times of standard compounds are indicated. Abbreviations: CYT, cytosine; CYD, cytidine; THY, thymine; TdR, thymidine; URA, uracil, URI, uridine; ADE, adenine; ADO, adenosine; GUA, guanine; GUO, guanosine; HYP, hypoxanthine; INO, inosine; XAN, xanthine; XAO, xanthosine.

The elution profile shown in Fig. 6 depicts the presence of several UV-absorbing peaks most of which are near the limit of detection. A major peak of uric acid was always present and a minor peak identifiable with hypoxanthine was found in several plasma samples examined. No peaks identifiable with thymine, adenine, guanine, guanosine, inosine, xanthine or xanthosine were clearly detected. Using a second chromatographic system (Fig. 7), which provided better resolution of thymidine and adenosine, a peak corresponding to thymidine was observed. The presence of adenosine is indicated in Fig. 7, however, this was not a common occurrence. Other peaks detected by both chromatographic systems included uracil and uridine, while cytosine derivatives were not easily resolved due to poor retention. The analysis of plasma of 6 mice indicated the presence of thymidine at concentrations of 1.3 to 3.5 x 10^{-6} M, while thymidine was not detected (< 0.5 x 10^{-6} M).

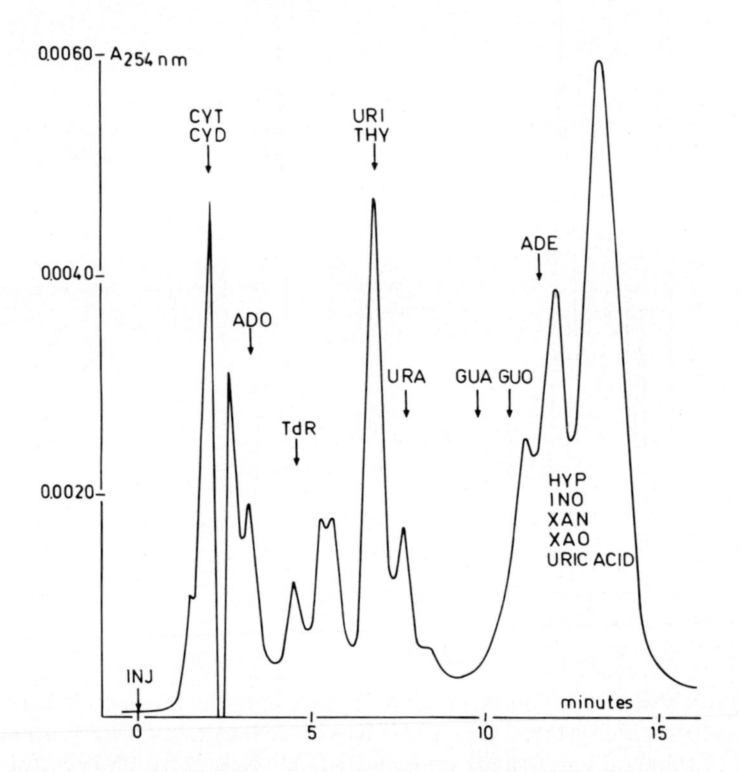

Fig. 7. HPLC analysis of nucleobases and nucleosides in normal mouse plasma — chromatographic system 2 (refer to legend of Fig. 6)

Hypoxanthine levels were < 0.5 to 0.9 x 10^{-6} M. Other purine metabolites were found to be consistently below minimal detection levels: adenosine and inosine, < 1.0 x 10^{-6} M; adenine, guanine and guanosine, each < 0.5 x 10^{-6} M; xanthine and xanthosine, < 2.0 x 10^{-6} M.

DISCUSSION

A comparison of the *in vitro* protection of bone marrow cells and L1210 leukemia cells from MTX cytotoxicity is presented in this paper. Leucovorin reversal of the inhibition of cell proliferation by MTX in the two cell types was shown to be quantitatively similar and appeared to occur by a competitive mechanism. Conversely, reversal of drug toxicity with thymidine plus a purine occurred non-competitively in the two cell types, and was less effective in L1210 cells.

An important feature of the studies reported here is the long exposure of cells to MTX and rescue agents for 7 to 9 days, in contrast to hours in studies reported by others. In the latter cases MTX was furthermore usually washed out after a short-term exposure before testing for cytotoxic effects. Long-term exposure to drugs as described in our experiments could be considered more relevant to *in vivo* chemotherapy. The critical role of free intracellular MTX, unbound to high-affinity sites (dihydrofolate reductase), in effecting maximal suppression of DNA synthesis has been proposed (17). The maintenance of free intracellular MTX levels *in vivo* may serve to achieve a more efficient tumor cell kill. Also, in high dose MTX therapy (> 50 mg/kg) the aim has been to attain more elevated concentrations of MTX to overcome potentially developed tumor resistance which may be related to high levels of dihydrofolate reductase or poor transport of MTX across the cell membrane. MTX therapy involving long-term exposure to MTX at toxic levels (> 10^{-8} M), resulting from either continuous drug infusion or the administration of high doses of MTX, must include some form of protection of normal tissues from severe toxicity. Leucovorin has been conventionally used in the clinic to achieve rescue. Our studies *in vitro* involved the examination of the ability of leucovorin and nucleosides to prevent MTX cytotoxicity during such prolonged periods of drug exposure.

It should be noted that in high dose MTX therapy, leucovorin is administered during a 4- to 6-hour MTX infusion, generally after a 2- to 4-hour delay. During the first 18 hours of this treatment, plasma MTX levels range between 10^{-5} and 10^{-3} M (18). The results of the *in vitro* bone marrow experiments reported here indicate that toxicity to myeloid precursor cells at MTX concentrations below 10^{-6} M is readily reversed by equimolar concentrations of leucovorin, but that reversal of toxicity at higher concentrations requires much more than equimolar levels of leucovorin. At 10^{-4} M MTX, which may *in vivo* exist in plasma for 8 to 12 hours after the start of high dose infusion, leucovorin was ineffective *in vitro*. If these findings reflect the *in vivo* situation, it is illogical to start leucovorin rescue immediately or shortly after terminating MTX high dose infusion. Sirotnak et al. (19) have reported in mice successful prevention of toxicity with retention of antitumor effectiveness using high, lethal doses of MTX (400 mg/kg) followed by leucovorin rescue 16 to 20 hours later. Such understanding of the quantitative aspects of leucovorin rescue may be important in the handling of high dose treated patients with abnormally high levels of MTX, in regard to providing appropriate doses of leucovorin for efficient rescue. The monitoring of plasma MTX concentration during high dose MTX therapy is valuable in screening for patients with delayed drug clearance and also gives an indication of the leucovorin dose required (20).

Rescue with thymidine and a purine base or nucleoside, as an alternative to leucovorin, is suggested by these experiments to be superior for two reasons. First, the re versal of MTX cytotoxicity with thymidine and purines, at least for bone marrow cells *in vitro*, appears to occur noncompetitively. Relatively low concentrations of nucleosides (10^{-5} M) were found to be sufficient for the complete protection of CFU-C in the presence of MTX as high as 10^{-4} M. Secondly, potential differences in the utilization of thymidine and purines by salvage pathways may exist in normal and tumor tissues. Our finding that L1210 could not be efficiently protected by thymidine plus inosine at MTX concentrations above 10^{-8} M supports this possibility.

The reversal of the lethal effects of MTX by nucleosides (and bases) in cell culture has been described by various investigators indicating a requirement for both thymidine and a purine (5-10). The potential for differential protection or rescue of cells from MTX cytotoxicity by pyrimidines and purines is realized by the reported variability in results for different cell lines depending on concentrations of thymidine and purines used and the choice of purine. While experiments on L-cells by Borsa and Whitmore (6) and those described here on mouse bone marrow have indicated that combinations of thymidine and guanine derivatives are ineffective, partial reversal by such pyrimidine and purine combinations has been demonstrated for sarcoma 180 cells (5) and L5178Y cells (8). The greater degree of toxicity of thymidine to L1210 cells compared to bone marrow described in the present report indicates the potential of thymidine plus a purine in providing selective rescue to bone marrow from MTX toxicity. A partial reversal of the MTX-mediated inhibition of cell growth with thymidine alone has been observed by Tattersall et al. (10) and found to be variable in five mammalian cell lines. This may suggest that the antipurine effect of MTX differs from one cell type to another. However, this latter study involved the use of medium containing undialyzed fetal calf serum and should be viewed with some reservation. Caution against the use of medium components of undefined composition, especially in regard to purine and pyrimidine content is warranted based on experiments reported here. It should be noted that although Tattersall and coworkers described a partial reversal in L1210 cells with thymidine alone, under our experimental conditions using the same cell type this was not observed.

Animal studies have suggested the importance of purines and pyrimidines in determining MTX cytotoxicity. Grindey and Moran (21) showed that the concurrent administration of allopurinol and MTX to L1210 leukemia-bearing mice reduced the therepeutic effectiveness of MTX. Based on the known inhibitory effect of allopurinol on purine catabolism and its purported ability to increase the availability of preformed purines for re-utilization, it was suggested that in the mouse the antitumor activity of MTX is a result of a depletion of purine nucleotides and is less dependent on the induction of a thymineless state. Tattersall et al. (2) reported a striking finding that the use of thymidine in MTX treatment of L1210 leukemia-bearing mice enhanced the therapeutic effectiveness of MTX. This improvement in antitumor effect could not be demonstrated with a combination of MTX, thymidine and allopurinol. It is conceivable that normal tissues in the mouse exposed to MTX undergo a depletion of thymidine nucleotides rather than purine nucleotides which can be alleviated by an exogenous supply of thymidine in addition to that already available in plasma. Conversely, L1210 does not appear to be protected from MTX toxicity by thymidine alone requiring in addition a source of purines. Although in this same study an indication was noted that thymidine treatment could protect normal mice against MTX toxicity, Straw and coworkers (3) demonstrated that thymidine prevented MTX toxicity to bone marrow and gut in tumor-bearing but not normal mice. Similarly, despite the loss of antitumor activity of MTX induced by allopurinol, no effect by allopurinol on MTX toxicity was observed in normal mice. This suggests that L1210 leukemia cells may be more efficient than normal tissues in re-utilizing circulating purines and pyrimidines, or that in the absence of actively growing tumor tissue both a thymineless and purineless state may be induced by MTX. It is possible that there is an increased presence of purines and pyrimidines in the plasma of tumor-bearing animals as a result of active tumor purine metabolic turnover or initial tumor cell death due to MTX treatment. In order to fully understand the involvement of endogenous thymidine and purines in MTX cytotoxicity, further studies will be required, including the determination of these metabolites in the circulation of tumor-bearing animals.

It appears that *in vivo*, nucleotide synthesis via salvage pathways plays an important role in nucleic acid metabolism despite evidence that many tissues have the capacity to synthesize purines and pyrimidines *de novo*. The liver is highly active in the production of nucleotides by *de novo* pathways and there have been several studies reported indicating that a key function of the liver is supplying other tissues with nucleic acid precursors in the form of nucleosides and bases transported by the circulation (11,12). Our analysis of normal mouse plasma demonstrates the presence of thymidine at levels of 1.3 to 3.5 x 10^{-6} M and even lower concentrations of purines, only hypoxanthine being detectable although below 1 x 10^{-6} M. These data indicate that in the mouse the availability of purines and pyrimidines from the plasma is rather limited. However, it cannot be excluded that red blood cells may be more directly involved in the transport of nucleobases and nucleosides to peripheral tissues.

A current study in our laboratory of the concentrations of nucleobases and nucleosides in human plasma reveals that in several normal individuals and patients with neoplastic disease the plasma levels of these metabolites are generally found to be approximately 1 x 10^{-6} M or less. Among the purine metabolites hypoxanthine and inosine were found in the highest concentrations although only in the range of 1 to 4 x 10^{-6} M. Recently, Howell et al. (22) have reported finding in cancer patients even lower plasma concentrations of less than 0.5 x 10^{-6} M for hypoxanthine, inosine and adenosine. Interestingly, despite the presence of low concentrations of purines in plasma, initial clinical trials of thymidine rescue from MTX cytotoxicity have proved successful without the administration of purines (22,23) and unpublished results. Moreover, thymidine rescue has been achieved with plasma thymidine levels of less than 2 x 10^{-6} M.

CONCLUSIONS

We conclude on the basis of the results of this study that in the *murine* system:

1) protection against MTX cytotoxicity can be better achieved by the noncompetitive reversal of drug toxicity with thymidine plus a purine, compared to the use of leucovorin,
2) the use of thymidine plus a purine for the reversal of MTX cytotoxicity is more effective in bone marrow cells than in leukemia cells, while leucovorin does not offer such selectivity,
3) the concentrations of thymidine and purines in mouse plasma are below optimal for the reversal of MTX cytotoxicity thus allowing the control of drug toxicity through the administration of these nucleic acid precursors.

ACKNOWLEDGMENTS

This study was supported in part by the Netherlands' Cancer Society (Koningin Wilhelmina Fonds, KWF; project number UUKC Int. 77-3) and the Maurits and Anna de Kock Foundation. We wish to thank Dr. H. Nederbragt and Ms. A. Baan-Gout for their assistance with cell culture studies. We are grateful for Dr. J.M.M. Roelofs' help with the examination of L1210 colonies using the electronic image analyzer. HPLC analyses were performed with assistance from Ms. E. Italiaander-

Kwakkel. We are also thankful for the secretarial assistance provided by Ms. M.M.A. Spliet and Ms. H. Wesselo.

REFERENCES

1. Bertino, J. and Johns, D.G. (1967) Ann. Rev. Med., 18, 27-34.

2. Tattersall, M.H.N., Brown, B. and Frei, E. III (1975) Nature, 253, 198-200.

3. Straw, J.A., Talbot, D.C., Taylor, G.A. and Harrap, K.R. (1977) J. Nat. Cancer Inst., 58, 91-97.

4. Zaharko, D.S., Fung, W.P. and Yung, K.H. (1977) Cancer Res., 37, 1602-1607.

5. Hakala, M.T. and Taylor, E. (1959) J. Biol. Chem., 234, 126-128.

6. Borsa, J. and Whitmore, G.F. (1969) Cancer Res., 29, 737-744.

7. Hryniuk, W.M. (1972) Cancer Res., 32, 1506-1511.

8. Hryniuk, W.M. (1975) Cancer Res., 35, 1085-1092.

9. Hryniuk, W.M., Brox, L.W., Henderson, J.F. and Tamaoki, T. (1975) Cancer Res., 35, 1427-1432.

10. Tattersall, M.H.N., Jackson, R.C., Jackson, S.T.M. and Harrap, K.R. (1974) Eur. J. Cancer, 10, 819-826.

11. Murray, A.W. (1971) Ann. Rev. Biochemistry, 40, 811-826.

12. Levine, R.L., Hoogenraad, N.J. and Kretchmer, N. (1974) Pediat. Rev., 8, 724-734.

13. Pinedo, H.M., Zaharko, D.S., Bull, J.M. and Chabner, B.A. (1976) Cancer Res., 36, 4418-4424.

14. Brown, C. and Carone, P.P. (1971) Cancer Res., 31, 185-190.

15. Eksteen, R., Kraak, J.C. and Linssen, P. (1978) J. Chromatog. 148, 413-427.

16. Chabner, B.A. and Young, R.C. (1973) J. Clin. Invest., 52, 1804-1811.

17. Goldman, D. (1975) Cancer Chemother. Rep., Part 3, 6, 51-61.

18. Stoller, R.G., Jacobs, S.A., Drake, J.C., Lutz, R.J. and Chabner, B.A. (1975) Cancer Chemother. Rep., Part 3, 6, 19-24.

19. Sirotnak, F.M., Moccio, D.M. and Dorick, P.M. (1978) Cancer Res. 38, 345-353.

20. Pinedo, H.M., Zaharko, D.S., Bull, J.M. and Chabner, B.A. (1977) Cancer Res., 38, 445-450.

21. Grindey, G.B. and Moran, R.G. (1975) Cancer Res., 35, 1702-1705.

22. Howell, S.B., Ensminger, W.D., Krishan, A. and Frei, E. III (1978) Cancer Res., 38, 325-330.

23. Ensminger, W.D. and Frei, E. III (1977) Cancer Res., 37, 1857-1863.

Clinical Pharmacology of Anti-Neoplastic Drugs
H. M. Pinedo, editor

THE SELECTIVE REVERSAL OF METHOTREXATE TOXICITY IN TUMOUR-BEARING ANIMALS

K.R. HARRAP and J. RENSHAW
Department of Biochemical Pharmacology, Institute of Cancer Research, Sutton, Surrey, U.K.

ABSTRACT

Techniques for the reversal of methotrexate toxicity in tumour-bearing animals are reviewed in relation to the known mechanisms of action of antifolates. The low antitumour selectivity of these compounds is contrasted with their successful role as antibacterial and antiprotozoan agents. The review is concerned primarily with those techniques which rely on a direct metabolic reversal of the intracellular molecular defects induced by methotrexate, and discusses the use of:

(i) Reduced folates
(ii) Preformed purine and/or pyrimidines
(iii) Carboxypeptidase G_1

The discussion focusses on the biochemical properties which may determine the enhanced therapeutic efficacy of methotrexate when used in conjunction with these procedures.

INTRODUCTION

Many drug development programmes have focussed on pathways of folate metabolism, and in particular on the enzyme dihydrofolate reductase [EC 1.5.1.3]. The diaminopyrimidines, notably trimethoprim and pyrimethamine have found clinical application in the treatment of protozoan and bacterial infections respectively. The selective properties of these agents are determined primarily by their greater affinity for the dihydrofolate reductase of the parasite/bacterium than for that of host tissues (1). Also of importance is the failure of preformed reduced tetrahydrofolates to penetrate the cell walls of pathogenic microorganisms, while remaining fully permeable to cells comprising the tissues of the host. Thus the metabolic block imposed by the diaminopyrimidines on folate reduction can be by-passed in host cells, but not in bacteria. It is possible to enhance further the selective antibacterial properties of the diaminopyrimidines by using them in binary combination with a sulphonamide: the latter inhibits the *de novo* biosynthesis of folate, essential to the survival of microorganisms. Host tissues on the other hand are not dependent on this pathway and rely upon preformed folates in order to mediate one-carbon transfer reactions essential to *de novo* purine and pyrimidine nucleotide biosynthesis (2). As a result, the sequential blockade of folate synthesis and reduction in the bacterium leads to potentiative bacterial cell kill without inducing potentiative host toxicity.

Such qualitative differences in folate metabolism are not apparent in tumour cells. The tumour arises from the host's own tissues, and it is perhaps not surprising that only quantitative phenotypic differences exist between host and tumour cells (3). Accordingly, the widely used antifolate drug methotrexate (MTX) is far less selective in its antitumour properties than are the diaminopyrimidines in their antibacterial and antiprotozoan activities. Methotrexate kills proliferating cells in both host and tumour tissues. Its therapeutic effectiveness is probably determined by differences between tumour and host tissues in: cytokinetics; enzyme kinetic parameters; transport properties; and "salvage" pathways. In attempting to enhance the therapeutic effectiveness of methotrexate, we and others have concentrated on the development of techniques for selectively protecting normal proliferating host tissues from the toxic consequences of exposure to this drug. The availability of such methods should permit its more intensive utilisation, hopefully with accompanying therapeutic benefit.

In this presentation we will discuss briefly the molecular mode of action of MTX as a basis for a review of the various methods available for reversing the whole body toxicity of the drug.

Mechanism of action of methotrexate

The closely-related antifolates aminopterin and methotrexate were synthesized by Seeger et al. (4,5). The first clinical use of aminopterin was by Farber et al. in 1948 for the successful treatment of acute lymphocytic leukaemia (6). Subsequently, methotrexate was made available ine purer form and became the drug of choice for clinical studies. These developments heralded the modern era of cancer chemotherapy and many laboratories throughout the world have contributed to the present status of knowledge concerning the mode of action of MTX.

Molecular aspects. MTX is a tight-binding inhibitor of dihydrofolate reductase, the nature of this affinity having been described as "Stoichiometric" by Werkheiser (7). For drug-sensitive L1210 cells the Ki for the MTX-dihydrofolate reductase inhibition is 5.3×10^{-12} M (8). Relevant biochemical pathways are outlined in

Fig. 1.

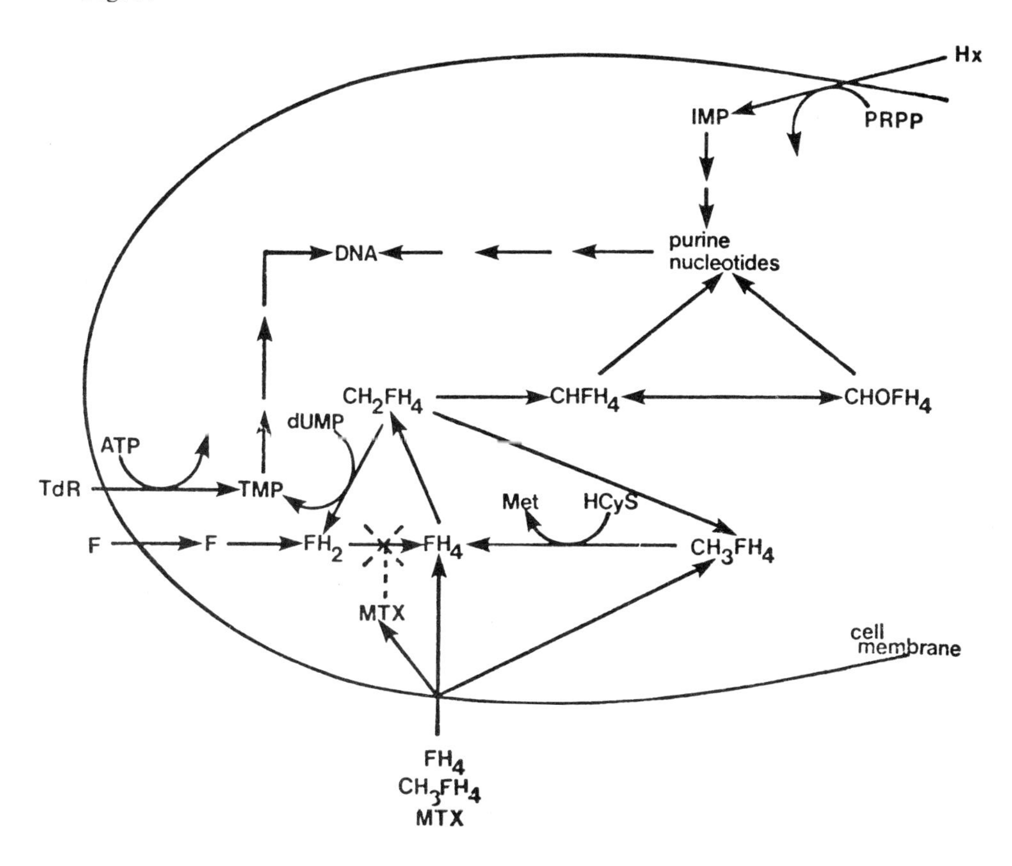

Fig. 1. Pathways of cellular folate metabolism and of purine and pyrimidine "salvage".

Abbreviations: FH_4, tetrahydrofolate; FH_2, dihydrofolate; F, folic acid; CH_3FH_4, 5-methyl tetrahydrofolate; CH_2FH_4, 5, 10-methylene tetrahydrofolate; $CHFH_4$, 5, 10-methenyl tetrahydrofolate; $CHOFH_4$, 10-formyl tetrahydrofolate; dUMP, deoxyuridylate; TMP, thymidylate; TdR, thymidine; Hx, hypoxanthine; ATP, adenosine triphosphate; PRPP, 1-phosphoribosyl-5 pyrophosphate; IMP, inosinic acid; HCys, homocysteine; Met, methionine.

It must be emphasized that dihydrofolate reductase is not the rate limiting enzyme in folate pathways leading to thymidylate biosynthesis. This role is fulfilled by thymidylate synthetase [EC 2.1.1.b], which in L1210 cells is present at approximately 1/20th the quantity of dihydrofolate reductase (9). Thus in cells exposed to MTX, no reduction in the rate of TMP biosynthesis will be seen until dihydrofolate reductase has become rate limiting: this will occur when enzyme activity has been reduced by approximately 95%. Hence only 5% dihydrofolate reductase activity is required to maintain adequate pools of tetrahydrofolates. Even though the affinity of MTX for dihydrofolate reductase is very high, the kinetics of the inhibition are reversible, and when 95% inhibition of enzyme activity has been achieved, some "free" (unbound) MTX appears in the cell (9,10). The relationship between free intracellular MTX and cytotoxicity has received extensive attention (11,12). Once dihydrofolate reductase has been made rate-limiting, the cell loses its ability to regenerate tetrahydrofolate from dihydrofolate, the latter being a product of the thymidylate synthetase reaction. Dihydrofolate builds up behind the MTX-imposed block, and the pools of one-carboncarrying tetrahydrofolates, essential substrates for the *de novo* synthesis of methionine, serine, thymidylate and purines, become exhausted. In terms of substrate pools available for DNA synthesis, the cell may become deficient in purine, or pyrimidine, or both. The exact nature of the deficiency state *in vivo* will depend on the ability of methotrexate-inhibited cells to utilize preformed purines and pyrimidines present in the extracellular environment. Failure of *de novo* methionine and serine biosynthesis is unlikely to be of great consequence in animals, where these amino acids are adequately supplied in the diet.

Several low affinity binding sites have been implicated in MTX cytotoxicity. These include thymidylate synthetase, serine hydroxymethyl transferase [EC 2.1. 2.1]and the membrane transport of reduced folates (13,14,15). Of these, the intracellular low affinity site of major significance is thymidylate synthetase, though this is relevant only when considerable MTX resistance has been generated through increased dihydrofolate reductase activity (16).

This discussion has implied that the monoglutamyl folates are the proximal substrates for the *de novo* biosynthesis of purine and pyrimidine nucleotides, and of serine and methionine. However, evidence is accumulating that the polyglutamyl forms of these cofactors are the preponderant species present in tissue culture cells and in tissues (17,18,19,20). Further, deletion of the folate polyglutamate synthesizing system in Chinese Hamster cells is a lethal mutation (21). Such considerations have led Ensminger et al. recently to propose that the polyglutamyl forms of tetrahydrofolates are probably the authentic cofactors for the reactions discussed above (22).

MTX transport. MTX enters cells by a concentrative carrier-mediated process which is temperature-dependent and energy requiring. Reduced folates, such as 5-methyl tetrahydrofolate and 5-formyl tetrahydrofolate (folinic acid) share the same transport mechanism, and in the presence of MTX will compete for uptake. However, folic acid enters the cell via an independent route (23,24,25,26).

Resistance to MTX. The development of resistance to MTX can be associated with impaired transport of the drug, with elevated levels of the target enzyme dihydrofolate reductase, or with the enhanced utilization of preformed purine and pyrimidine precursors of DNA synthesis ("salvage").

Transport-determined resistance has been observed by a number of workers. In L5178Y cells, MTX resistance was attributed to reduced drug uptake, the level of dihydrofolate reductase and its affinity for MTX remaining unchanged (27,28). Similar properties were observed in MTX-resistant Walker 256 carcinosarcoma cells (29). In a MTX-resistant subline of L1210 cells, Sirotnak et al. showed that resistance was due to impaired drug uptake by virtue of an increased Km for carrier binding (30). These membrane changes are confined to the mechanism concerned with reduced folate uptake: folate transport is unchanged in MTX-transport resistant L1210 mutants (31).

Acquired resistance to MTX can also be associated with elevation in dihydrofolate reductase activity (32). The enzyme occurs in two forms: as free enzyme (Type I) and in a form containing an equimolar amount of noncovalently bound NADPH (Type II) (33). Both accelerated synthesis and delayed turnover could account for the accumulation of enzyme. The accelerated synthesis of dihydrofolate reductase in MTX-resistant mutants has been attributed to the presence of elevated quantities of mRNA for the enzyme (34). Delayed enzyme turnover has been attributed either to the stabilisation of Type II enzyme by bound NADPH or to the stabilisation of both modifications by bound MTX (35).

In some cases both impaired transport and elevated dihydrofolate reductase activity can occur simultaneously in association with acquired MTX-resistance (13).

It is appropriate also to note that the kinetic properties of dihydrofolate reductase can be modified, notably by a reduction in affinity of MTX for the enzyme, during the development of acquired resistance (16). Further, *intrinsic* resistance to MTX, has been associated with reduced affinity of MTX for cellular dihydrofolate reductase (8).

Some cells exhibit the potential to circumvent the metabolic block applied by

MTX: elevation in thymidine kinase activity and an enhanced utilization of the pyrimidine nucleoside "salvage" pathways for DNA biosynthesis have been demonstrated in tumour cells exposed to MTX (36,37).

Toxicity and antitumour activity of MTX in rodents

The toxicity of MTX in the mouse is related to the time for which free drug, i.e. that in excess of the dihydrofolate reductase concentration, persists in tissues "at risk". The tissue most sensitive to MTX in the mouse is the gastro-intestinal mucosa: non-dividing tissues such as liver and kidney are relatively resistant to the effects of the drug (29). Thus the persistance of free MTX in the gastro-intestinal epithelium for periods in excess of 24 hr leads to irreversible inhibition of DNA synthesis and death of the animal (38,39,40,41).

As with its toxicity to intestinal epithelial cells, so the antitumour effectiveness of MTX correlates with the time for which free drug persists in the tumour. A major component of the drug's therapeutic selectivity is its rate of egress from tumour compared with that from the gastro-intestinal mucosa: in the case of L1210 tumour-bearing animals, the rates of MTX uptake into tumour and gastro-intestinal mucosa are comparable. However, due to a lower rate of efflux from the tumour, higher levels of free drug are maintained in this tissue than in gastro-intestinal mucosa. Hence, for the L1210 tumour, MTX is selectively cytotoxic (42,43). This should be regarded as a special case: in general, unacceptable host toxicity is encountered with doses of MTX which are sufficient to induce high tumour cell kill. This underlines the continuing efforts made to reduce selectively the systemic toxicity of MTX.

Modulation of methotrexate cytotoxicity

From the above discussion it will be apparent that the molecular events arising from the exposure of cells to MTX may be reversed (or prevented) either by replenishing the depleted tetrahydrofolate pools with an appropriate reduced folate, or by by-passing the metabolic block with preformed purine and/or pyrimidine. Co-administration of MTX and the reversing agent(s) is referred to as "protection", while delayed use of the latter has been termed "MTX rescue". Another reversal method is to restrict the time for which the animal is exposed to MTX by administering carboxypeptidase, which results in the rapid degradation of circulating MTX. These three techniques will receive separate discussion below.

It is also possible to modulate the toxicity of MTX with asparaginase. Gastro-intestinal toxicity is avoided and additive tumour toxicity is maintained in L5178Y tumour-bearing mice. The mechanism underlying these effects is not well understood: it may depend on the induction of a non-proliferative G0 state in gastro-intestinal cells due to asparaginase deprivation (44). Since this procedure does not involve a strict metabolic reversal of MTX toxicity, it will not be considered further in this presentation.

Reversal of MTX toxicity with tetrahydrofolates

(i) Folinic acid. Some confusion has arisen over the synonymous use of the terms "Leucovorin", "citrovorum factor" and "folinic acid": a brief note on the origin of these terms may not be inappropriate. A naturally occurring factor, necessary for the growth of *Leuconostic citrovorum ATCC 8081* was first described by Sauberlich and Bauman in 1948 (45) and referred to as "citrovorum factor". Reduction products of 5-formyl folic acid also supported the growth of *L. citrovorum* and reversed aminopterin toxicity in the mouse (46,47). "Folinic acid" was isolated from liver and shown to promote the growth of several folate-dependent microorganisms (48). "Folinic acid" was subsequently synthesized and shown to be 5-formyl 5, 6, 7, 8, tetrahydro pteroyl glutamic acid (49,50). Broquist et al. had named citrovorum factor "Leucovorin", which subsequently was identified as 5-formyl 5, 6, 7, 8, tetrahydro pteroyl glutamic acid (51, 52, 53). Hence "Leucovorin", citrovorum factor and folinic acid refer to the same compound, namely 5-formyl 5, 6, 7, 8, tetrahydro pteroyl glutamic acid. This exists in two enantiomeric forms (54): the commercially available material is supplied as the calcium salt of dl-L-5 formyl tetrahydrofolate, which possesses half the biological activity, on a molar basis, of the naturally occurring compound (1-L-5 formyl FH_4).

The ability of 5-formyl tetrahydrofolate both to protect against the systemic toxicity of aminopterin and to potentiate its antitumour activity was established by Goldin et al. These authors also showed that the administration of 5-formyl tetrahydrofolate, simultaneously with, or prior to, administration of the antifolate also reversed its antitumour effect. Delayed folinic acid rescue produced a considerably enhanced therapeutic index, while multiple antifolate treatments, in association with delayed rescue, were accompanied by further improvements in drug efficacy. Moreover, the protection afforded by delayed folinic acid permitted the use of higher doses of MTX, with further therapeutic advantage (55,56,57,58,59,60). This work and its historical background has been reviewed recently by Goldin (61).

Metabolism of folinic acid. Folinic acid is the most stable chemical form of all the naturally occurring reduced folates (53,62) and is therefore best suited for clinical use. Nixon and Bertino have followed in man the plasma disappearance, metabolism and urinary excretion of folinic acid following both intravenous and oral administration (63). Under fasting conditions 90% of an orally administered dose was absorbed and converted rapidly to 5-methyl tetrahydrofolate, the major circulating reduced folate in man and rats (64,65). Metabolism of oral 5-formyl tetrahydrofolate to serum 5-methyl tetrahydrofolate was presumed to occur during transfer from the gastro-intestinal tract to the systemic circulation, since conversion was more rapid after oral than after intravenous dosage.

Conversion of intravenously administered folinic acid to 5-methyl tetrahydrofolate occurred more slowly, though 5-methyl tetrahydrofolate remained the major metabolite. Hence after oral administration of folinic acid the proximal rescue agent would appear to be 5-methyl tetrahydrofolate. However, after parenteral administration, both folinic acid and 5-methyl tetrahydrofolate persist in the circulation. Enzymatic conversion of 5-formyl tetrahydrofolate to 10-formyl tetrahydrofolate has been reported (66,67) and this may contribute, in addition to 5-methyl tetrahydrofolate, to an expansion of intracellular reduced folate pools depleted by exposure to MTX.

(ii) 5-Methyl FH_4. As indicated in Fig. 1, 5-methyl tetrahydrofolate does not equilibrate with the pools of other one-carbon carrying reduced folates, since the equilibrium for the reduction of 5, 10-methylene tetrahydrofolate to 5-methyl tetrahydrofolate, catalyzed by the enzyme 5, 10-methylene tetrahydrofolate reductase [EC 1.1.1.68], lies predominantly in the forward direction (68). Thus for 5-methyl tetrahydrofolate to reverse in the intracellular effects of MTX, it is necessary that tetrahydrofolate be released from the rescue agent. The only metabolic pathway by which this can be achieved is via the *de novo* synthesis of methionine from homocysteine, for which 5-methyl tetrahydrofolate acts as the methyl donor. The enzyme catalysing this reaction is 5-methyl tetrahydrofolate: homocysteine methyl transferase [EC 2.1.1.13], or methionine synthetase.

Mead et al. (69) found that 5-methyl tetrahydrofolate was as effective as folinic acid in reversing MTX toxicity in mice. However, the therapeutic effectiveness of MTX/5-methyl tetrahydrofolate in L1210 tumour-bearing animals was no greater than that of MTX/folinic acid. Blair and Searl (70) and Kisliuk et al. (71) have confirmed these findings. In addition, the former authors proposed that the effects of folinic acid derive from its metabolic conversion to 5-methyl tetrahydrofolate.

Further interest in the use of 5-methyl tetrahydrofolate as an alternative to folinic acid was stimulated by Halpern et al. (72). These authors were unable to reverse MTX cytotoxicity with 5-methyl tetrahydrofolate in several cultured malignant cell lines, though reversal was possible in cultures of normal fibroblasts. Folinic acid rescued both normal and malignant cell lines from MTX cytotoxicity with comparable efficacy. It was proposed that these effects were determined by the presence in tumour cell lysates of lower methionine synthetase activity than could be detected in normal cell extracts (73). It was also of interest that in a medium, supplemented with vitamin B_{12} and folic acid, in which homocysteine had replaced methionine, normal fibroblast lines grew well, but tumour cells failed to survive (72). Chello and Bertino (74) reported that media containing 5-methyl tetrahydrofolate would support the growth of L5178Y cells only when supplemented with large amounts of vitamin B_{12} and transcobalamin II. Presumably increased amounts of methionine synthetase holoenzyme were formed, leading to an enhanced utilization of 5-methyl tetrahydrofolate.

Now apo-methionine synthetase requires vitamin B_{12} in the form of methyl cobalamin for assembly of the holoenzyme (75). Kerwar et al. (76) reported that although HeLa cells synthesized apo-methionine synthetase, they contained insufficient vitamin B_{12} to satisfy the enzyme's cofactor requirements, unless the cells were grown in the presence of the vitamin. These results would indicate that methionine synthetase holoenzyme levels might be limiting in some tumour cells. However, Hoffman and Erbe (77) conclude that tumour cells do not differ markedly from normal cells in the absolute levels of either apo or holo methionine synthetase, though the proportion of holo enzyme present in normal cells is greater than that in tumour cells.

There is clearly a continuing controversy on the functional activity of methionine synthetase in some tumour cell lines, particularly in relation to methionine requirements. Some tumour cell lines, in contrast to normal cells, grow inadequately in vitamin B_{12} - and folate-supplemented media, where homocysteine has been substituted for methionine (74,77). They clearly possess a limiting requirement for preformed methionine, which is not the case with normal cell lines. It is possible that these observations may relate to effects of methionine on reduced folate transport. Methionine appears to potentiate the transport of reduced folates in vitamin B_{12} deficiency (78): further, the low tetrahydrofolate levels found in the liver of vitamin B_{12}-deficient sheep can be elevated following the administration of methionine (79,80). It is also noteworthy that bone marrow cultures from vitamin B_{12} deficient patients cannot be rescued from MTX toxicity with 5-methyl tetrahydrofolate, though folinic acid is an effective rescue agent (81).

Recent studies in this department indicate that MTX, followed by 5-methyl tetrahydrofolate rescue of L1210 tumour-bearing animals leads to an enhanced median survival time and a higher proportion of long term survivors than MTX/folinic acid (82).

Reversal of MTX toxicity with preformed purines and pyrimidines

Molecular aspects. Nucleic acid synthesis is rapidly halted when cells are exposed to MTX, as indicated by inhibition [^{14}C] formate, [^{3}H] uridine and [^{3}H] thymidine incorporation into these macromolecules (12,26,37,83). These effects are accompanied by a fall in the intracellular levels of ATP and GTP (83). These antipurine effects of MTX are also reflected in lowered deoxynucleoside triphosphate pools: thus dATP and dGTP levels are reduced (together with those of dTTP). In many cells, dGTP is limiting, and the reduction in levels of this deoxynucleoside triphosphate, following exposure to MTX, probably accounts for the observed inhibition of DNA synthesis (37,26,84,86). It is apparent from these measurements, therefore, that MTX, through an erosion of tetrahydrofolate cofactors, can lead to inhibition of both purine and pyrimidine nucleotide biosynthesis *de novo*, with consequent reduction in the levels of substrates available for DNA synthesis.

However, cells differ both qualitatively and quantitatively in the nature of the DNA precursor deficiency established by MTX. Work in this area has involved the addition of thymidine or a purine (or both) to cells cultured in presence of MTX in order to identify the precursor deficiency. Working with a parent line of S-180 cells, and two sublines, selected for resistance to MTX, Hakala et al. showed that a combination of thymidine and hypoxanthine invariably protected all cell lines against MTX cytotoxicity. Partial protection could be obtained in the parent line with hypoxanthine alone, as was also the case in one resistant line; in the third line, partial protection was afforded with thymidine alone (87,88,89). Comparable results were obtained by Tattersall et al. in five tumour cell lines (Yoshida, L5178Y, L cells, W1-L2, L1210): combinations of thymidine and hypoxanthine protected all cell lines from MTX toxicity, while good protection was afforded by thymidine alone in the case of Yoshida and W1-L2 cells (86). Borsa and Whitmore, working with L60TM cells, and Roberts and Warmath with CCRF-CEM cells also showed that MTX cytotoxicity could be partially reversed with thymidine (90,91). Hryniuk has studied the identity and time-course of DNA precursor deficiency induced by MTX in cultured L5178Y cells (92). Initially MTX induced a purineless condition, which could be reversed with hypoxanthine, though subsequently a thymineless state developed.

Thus it is apparent that thymidine alone can afford partial protection against MTX cytotoxicity in some cell types. It is possible that different rates of catabolism and anabolism of the rescue agents may account for the observed rescue properties in different cells: Jackson and Weber (93), studying a range of cultured hepatoma cell lines, have demonstrated that more differentiated tumours retain the capacity of normal liver to catabolise thymidine, and hence require higher concentrations of the pyrimidine for reversal of MTX toxicity.

Reversal of MTX toxicity in rodents

The observation that some tumour cell lines were protected ineffectively from MTX toxicity by preformed thymidine or purines prompted the speculation that such techniques might enhance the selectivity of the drug in tumour-bearing animals. Such speculation, of course, depended on the ability to devise an appropriate rescue combination which effectively protected host tissues from MTX toxicity. It was first necessary to identify the nature of the metabolic defect induced by MTX in normal proliferating tissues. Work from this laboratory (94), showed that single non-toxic doses of MTX induce a rapid (within 1 h) combined deficiency of pyrimidine and purine in gastro-intestinal mucosa, which was maintained for 24 h. Although a pyrimidineless condition was established with equal rapidity in bone marrow, purine deficiency in this tissue was only observed at 24 h. Both defects could be reversed by administration of thymidine/hypoxanthine combinations, with full maintenance of DNA synthesis at control values in the two named tissues. It was apparent, therefore that the efficient protection of the gastro-intestinal mucosa from MTX-induced damage required a rescue combination containing both thymidine and a purine. In practice this was shown to be the case: animals receiving a single lethal dose of MTX (400 mg/K) were protected against the toxic effects of the drug with a rescue protocol containing 500 mg/kg thymidine + 50 mg/kg hypoxanthine + 10 mg/kg allopurinol. Rescue was started either 12 h or 24 h after MTX administration and was continued daily for 4 days. Thymidine alone was ineffective as a rescue agent (94,95). These results contradict those of Tattersall et al., who were able to protect mice from MTX toxicity with thymidine alone (96). However, these authors did encounter sporadic toxicity with their MTX/thymidine protocols, which in the present authors' experience was never the case so long as the rescue schedule contained a purine (hypoxanthine or inosine) in addition to thymidine. In L1210 tumour-bearing animals the therapeutic efficacy of MTX followed by thymidine/hypoxanthine (or inosine) rescue was much greater than that of MTX/folinic acid (97).

Grindey and co-workers have used intravenous infusions of thymidine to modulate the antitumour effectiveness of MTX given by the same route. They have shown that co-infusion of MTX (16 mg/kg/day for 48 h) and thymidine (5 g/kg/day for 96 h) resulted in 125% increase in life span without incurring host toxicity. Higher concentrations of either MTX or thymidine resulted in loss of antitumour activity (98,99).

Thymidine has been shown both to protect and to rescue patients from MTX toxicity. Ensminger and Frei found that co-infusion of MTX (at maximum doses of 6 g/m^2 for 72 h) and thymidine (at 8 g/m^2/day for 120 h) produced no untoward toxic side-effects (100). When used as a "rescue" agent it was found that thymidine (8 g/m^2/day), infused for 3 days following the termination of high dose infusions of MTX, satisfactorily reversed MTX toxicity (101).

Carboxypeptidase G_1

McCullough et al. isolated carboxypeptidase G_1 from a strain of *Pseudomonas stutzeri.* This enzyme catalyses the hydrolysis of the carboxyl-terminal glutamate from both reduced and non-reduced folate derivatives including MTX, aminopterin, folic acid, folinic acid and 5-methyl tetrahydrofolate: Km values fall in the range 1.1 - 18.1 x 10^{-6} M[102]. With MTX as substrate, the product is 4-amino-4 deoxy N-10-methyl pteroic acid (APA) which is a moderately effective inhibitor of dihydrofolate reductase (apparent Ki = 1.3 x 10^{-9} M). APA was found to be considerably less toxic than MTX in mice, though where purified enzyme is used *in vivo* to degrade high circulating concentrations of MTX, APA toxicity might be expected. The caecal contents of mice can cleave MTX to APA *in vitro*, and this cleavage reaction is largely prevented by antibiotic pretreatment of the animals. APA is also found in the faeces of MTX-treated mice, derived probably from metabolism of the drug by the intestinal flora (103).

This enzyme has been shown to possess antitumour activity against some murine leukaemias as a result of its ability to lower serum folate levels (104). When carboxypeptidase G_1 was administered to mice 24 h after a lethal dose of MTX (1,000 mg/kg), the serum level of MTX was rapidly lowered and 50% of the animals survived. However, MTX reappeared in the plasma between 12-24 h after enzyme administration, and a second enzyme treatment at 48 h increased the survival to 94%. The antitumour effectiveness of MTX, followed 24 h later with carboxypeptidase G_1 rescue was equivalent, in L1210 tumour-bearing mice, to that achieved with MTX followed by delayed folinic acid rescue (105). Presumably the efficiency of this technique relies upon the rapid enzymic hydrolysis of extracellular MTX, permitting the efflux of free MTX from cells and some dissociation of the inhibitor from its binding to dihydrofolate reductase. As a result sufficient dihydrofolate reductase becomes available for the regeneration of tetrahydrofolates and subsequent DNA synthesis.

Carboxypeptidase G_1 has been administered to acute leukaemia patients, when serum folate levels could be suppressed by 50-90% for periods up to 12 h. Only transient effects were observed on the proliferation of leukaemic cells. Carboxypeptidase G_1, administered 24 h after high dose MTX treatment, successfully protected against drug toxicity. However a complication was the appearance of anaphylaxis (106).

ACKNOWLEDGEMENTS

The authors are most grateful to Dr. G.B. Grindey (Roswell Park Memorial Institute, Buffalo) for much valued informal discussion and also for making available preprints of publications currently in press.

This work was supported by grants from the Cancer Research Campaign.

REFERENCES

1. Burchal, J.J. and Hitchings G.H. (1965) Mol. Pharmacol. 1, 126-136.

2. Hitchings, G.H. (1969) Cancer Res. 29, 1895-1903.

3. Harrap, K.R. (1976) in Biology of Cancer, Ambrose E.J. and Roe, F.J.K. eds., Ellis Horwood, Chichester, pp. 96-125.

4. Seeger, D.R., Smith, J.M.Jr. and Hultquist M.E. (1947) J. Amer. Chem. Soc. 69, 2567-2567.

5. Seeger, D.R., Smith, J.M.Jr. and Hultquist M.E. (1949) J. Amer. Chem. Soc. 71, 1753-1759.

6. Farber, S., Diamond, L.K., Mercer, R.D., Sylvester, R.F. and Wolff, J.A. (1948) New Eng. J. Med. 238, 787-793.

7. Werkheiser, W.C. (1961) J. Biol. Chem. 236, 888-893.

8. Jackson, R.C., Hart, L.I. and Harrap, K.R. (1976) Cancer Res. 36, 1991-1997.

9. Jackson, R.C. and Harrap, K.R. (1973) Arch. Biochem. Biophys. 158, 827-841.

10. Jackson, R.C., Niethammer, D. and Hart, L.I. (1977) Arch. Biochem. Biophys. 182, 646-656.

11. Goldman, I.D. (1974) Mol. Pharmacol. 10, 257-274.

12. White, J.C., Loftfield, S. and Goldman, I.D. (1975) Mol. Pharmacol. 11, 287-297.

13. Niethammer, D. and Jackson, R.C. (1975) Eur. J. Cancer 11, 845-854.

14. Niethammer, D. and Jackson, R.C. (1975) in Chemistry and Biology of Pteridines, Pfleidener W. ed., de Gruyter, Berlin, pp. 197-207.

15. Niethammer, D. and Jackson, R.C. (1976) in Molecular Base of Malignancy. New Clinical and Therapeutic Evidence, Deutsch E., Moser, K., Rainer, A. and Stacher, A., eds., Thienne, Stuttgart, pp. 90-99.

16. Jackson, R.C. and Niethammer, D. (1977) Eur. J. Cancer 13, 567-575.

17. Moran, R.G., Werkheiser, W.C. and Zakrzewski, S.F. (1976) J. Biol Chem. 251, 3569-3575.

18. Swendseid, M.E., Bethell, F. and Bird, O.D. (1951) Cancer Res. 11, 864-867.

19. Scott, J.M. (1976) Biochem. Soc. Trans. 4, 845-850.

20. Scott, J.M. (1977) Proc. of Workshop on Human Folate Requirements Nat. Acad. Sci. 43-55.

21. McBurney, M.W. and Whitmore, G.F. (1974) Cell 2, 173-182.

22. Ensminger, W.D., Grindey, G.B. and Hoglind, J.H. (1978) Adv. in Cancer Chemother. 1, in press.

23. Goldman, I.D. (1971) Ann. N.Y. Acad. Sci. 186, 400-422.

24. Nahas, A., Nixon, P.F. and Bertino, J.R. (1972) Cancer Res. 32, 1416-1412.

25. Goldman, I.D. (1975) Cancer Chemother. Rep. 6, 63-72.

26. Goldman, I.D. (1977) Cancer Treat. Rep. 61, 549-558.

27. Fischer, G.A. (1962) Biochem. Pharmacol. 11, 1233-1234.

28. Harrap, K.R., Hill, B.T., Furness, M.E. and Hart, L.I. (1971) Ann. N.Y. Acad. Sci. 186, 312-324.

29. Werkheiser, W.C. (1963) Cancer Res. 23, 1277-1285.

30. Sirotnak, F.M., Kurita, S. and Hutchinson, D.J. (1968) Cancer Res. 28, 75-80.

31. Jackson, R.C., Niethammer, D., Huennekens, F.M. (1975) Cancer Biochem. Biophys. 1, 151-155.

32. Johns, D.G. and Bertino, J.R. (1973) in Cancer Medicine, Frei, E. and Holland, J.F., eds., Lea and Febiger, Philadelphia, pp. 739-754.

33. Huennekens, F.M., Dunlap, R.B., Freisheim, J.H., Gundersen, L.E., Harding, N.G.L., Levison, S.A. and Mell, G.P. (1971) Ann. N.Y. Acad. Sci. 186, 85-99.

34. Chang, S.E. and Littlefield, J.W. (1976) Cell 7, 391-396.

35. Jackson, R.C. and Huennekens, F.M. (1973) Arch. Biochim. Biophys. 154, 192-198.

36. Wilmanns, W. (1971) Ann. N.Y. Acad. Sci. 186, 365-371.

37. Tattersall, M.H.N. and Harrap, K.R. (1973) Cancer Res. 33, 3086-3090.

38. Margolis, S., Philips, F.S. and Sternberg, S.S.V. (1971) Cancer Res. 31, 2037-2046.

39. Sirotnak, F.M., Donsbach, R.C., Dorick, D.M. and Moccio, D.M.(1976) Cancer Res. 36, 4672-4678.

40. Sirotnak, F.M., Donsbach, R.C., Dorick, D.M. and Moccio, D.M. (1977) Cancer Treat. Rep. 61, 565-574.

41. Zaharko, D.S., Dedrick, R.L. (1973) Proc. 5th Int. Congr. Pharmacol. 3, 316-324.

42. Sirotnak, F.M. and Donsbach, R.C. (1973) Cancer Res. 33, 1290-1294.

43. Sirotnak, F.M. and Donsbach, R.C. (1975) Cancer Res. 35, 1737-1744.

44. Capizzi, R.L. (1975) Cancer Chemother. Rep. 6, 37-41.

45. Sauberlich, H.E. and Baumann, C.A. (1948) J. Biol. Chem. 176, 165-173.

46. Shive, W., Bardos, T.J., Bond, T.J. and Rogers, L.L.(1950) J. Amer. Chem. Soc. 72, 2817-2818.

47. Brockman, J.A.Jr., Roth, B., Broquist H.P., Hulquist, M.E., Smith, J.M.Jr., Fahrenbach, M.J., Cosulich, D.B., Parker, R.P., Stockstad, E.L.R. and

Jukes, T.H. (1950) J. Amer. Chem. Soc. 72, 4325-4326.

48. Bond, T.J., Bardos, T.J., Sibley, M. and Shive, W. (1949) J. Amer. Chem. Soc. 71, 3852-3853.

49. Flynn, E.H., Bond, T.J., Bardos, T.J. and Shive, W. (1951) J. Amer. Chem. Soc. 73, 1979-1982.

50. Pohland, A., Flynn, E.H., Jones, R.G. and Shive, W. (1951) J. Amer. Chem. Soc. 73, 3247-3252.

51. Broquist, H.P., Stokstad, E.L.R. and Jukes, T.H. (1951) Fed. Proc. 10, 167.

52. Roth, B., Hultquist, M.E., Fahrenbach, M.J., Cosulich, B., Broquist, H.P., Brockman, J.A.Jr., Smith, J.M.Jr., Parker, R.D., Stokstad, E.L.R. and Jukes, T.H. (1952) J. Amer. Chem. Soc. 74, 3247-3252.

53. Cosulich, D.B., Roth, B., Smith, J.M.Jr., Martin, E., Hultquist, M.E. and Parker, R.P. (1952) J. Amer. Chem. Soc. 74, 3252-3263.

54. Cosulich, D.B., Smith, J.M.Jr. and Broquist, H.P. (1952) J. Amer. Chem. Soc. 74, 4215-4216.

55. Goldin, A., Greenspan, E.M., Venditti, J.M., Shoenbach, E.B. (1952) J. Nat. Cancer Inst. 12, 987-1002.

56. Goldin, A., Mantel, N., Greenhouse, S.W., Venditti, J.M. and Humphreys, S.R. (1953) Cancer Res. 13, 843-850.

57. Goldin, A., Mantel, N., Greenhouse, S.W., Venditti, J.M. and Humphreys, S.R. (1954) Cancer Res. 14, 43-48.

58. Goldin, A., Venditti, J.M., Humphreys, S.R., Dennis., D., Mantel, N. and Greenhouse, S.W. (1955) Cancer Res. 15, 57-61.

59. Goldin, A., Venditti, J.M., Humphreys, S.R., Dennis, D. and Mantel, N. (1955) Cancer Res. 15, 742-747.

60. Goldin, A., Venditti, J.M., Kline I. and Mantel, N. (1966) Nature 212, 1548-1550.

61. Goldin, A. (1978) Cancer Treat. Rep. 62, 307-312.

62. May, M., Bardos, T.J., Barger, F.L., Lansford, M., Ravel, J.M., Sutherland, G.L. and Shive, W. (1951) J. Amer. Chem. Soc. 73, 3067-3075.

63. Nixon, P.F. and Bertino, J.R. (1972) New England J. Med. 286, 175-179.

64. Herbert, V., Larrabee, A.R. and Buchanan, J.M. (1962) J. Clin. Invest. 41, 1134-1138.

65. Bird, O.D., McGlohon, V.M. and Vaitkins, J.W. (1965) Anal. Biochem. 12, 18-35.

66. Kay, L.D., Osborn, M.J., Hatefi, Y. and Huennekens, F.M. (1960) J. Biol. Chem. 235, 195-201.

67. Greenberg, D.M., Wynston, L.K. and Nogabhushanam, A.(1965) Biochemistry 4, 1872-1877.

68. Blakley, R.L. (1969) in The Biochemistry of Folic Acid and Related Pteridines, Neuberger, A. and Tatum, E.L., eds., North Holland Publishing Co., Amsterdam, London, pp. 197-201.

69. Mead, A.R., Venditti, J.M., Schrecker, A.W., Goldin, A. and Keresztesy, J.C. (1963) Biochem. Pharmacol. 12, 371-383.

70. Blair, J.A. and Searle, C.E. (1970) Br. J. Cancer 24, 603-609.

71. Kisliuk, R.L., Tattersall, M.H.N., Gaumont, Y., Pastore, E.J. and Brown, B. (1977) Cancer Treat. Rep. 61, 647-650.

72. Halpern, R.M., Halpern, B.C., Clark, B.R., Ashe, H., Hardy, D.N., Jenkinson, P.Y., Chou, S.C. and Smith, R.A. (1975) Proc. Nat. Acad. Sci. 72, 4018-4022.

73. Ashe, H., Clark, B.R., Chu, F., Hardy, D.N., Halpern, B.G., Halpern, R.M. and Smith, R.A. (1974) Biochem. Biophys. Res. Commun. 57, 417-425.

74. Chello, P.L. and Bertino, J.R. (1973) Cancer Res. 33, 1898-1904.

75. Blakley, R.L. (1969) Frontiers Biol. 13, 332-362.

76. Kerwar, S.S., Spears, C., McAuslam, B. and Weissbach, H. (1971) Arch. Biochim. Biophys. 142, 231-237.

77. Hoffman, R.M. and Erbe, R.N. (1976) Proc. Nat. Acad. Sci. USA 73, 1523-1527.

78. Gawthorne, J.M. and Smith, R.M. (1974) Biochem. J. 142, 119-126.

79. Smith, R.M. and Osborne-White, W.S. (1973) Biochem. J. 136, 279-293.

80. Smith, R.M., Osborne-White, W.S. and Gawthorne, J.M. (1974) Biochem. J. 142, 105-117.

81. Sauer, H. and Wilmanns, W. (1977) Brit. J. Haematol. 36, 189-198.

82. Calvert, A.H., Taylor, G.A., Dady, P.J. and Harrap, K.R. (1978) Unpublished results.

83. Hryniuk, W.M., Brox, L.W., Henderson, J.F. and Tamaoki, T. (1975) Cancer Res. 35, 1427-1432.

84. Skoog, L., Nordenskjöld, B., Hurula, S. and Hagerstrom, T. (1976) Eur. J. Cancer 12, 839-845.

85. Fridland, A. (1974) Cancer Res. 34, 1883-1888.

86. Tattersall, M.H.N., Jackson, R.C., Jackson, S.T.M. and Harrap, K.R. (1974) Eur. J. Cancer 10, 819-826.

87. Hakal, M.T. (1957) Science 126, 255.

88. Hakala, M.T. and Taylor, E. (1959) J. Biol. Chem. 234, 126-128.

89. Hakala, M.T., Zakrzewski, S.F. and Nichol, C.A. (1961) J. Biol. Chem. 236, 952-958.

90. Borsa, J. and Whitmore, G.F. (1969) Mol. Pharmacol. 5, 303-317.

91. Roberts, D. and Warmath, E.V. (1975) Eur. J. Cancer 11, 771-782.

92. Hryniuk, W.M. (1975) Cancer Res. 35, 1085-1092.

93. Jackson, R.C. and Weber, G. (1976) Biochem. Pharmacol. 25, 2613-2618.

94. Straw, J.A., Talbot, D.C., Taylor, G.A. and Harrap, K.R. (1977) J. Natl. Cancer Inst. 58, 91-97.

95. Harrap, K.R., Taylor, G.A., Talbot, D.C., Calvert, A.H., Stock, J.A., Stringer, M., Browman, G.P., Dady, P.J. and Cobley, T. (1978) in Advances in Tumour Prevention, Detection and Characterization, Davies, W. and Harrap, K.R., eds., Excerpta Medica Int. Congr. Series No. 420, Amsterdam, Oxford, Volume 4, pp. 93-105.

96. Tattersall, M.H.N., Brown, B.L. and Frei, E. III (1975) Nature 253, 198-200.

97. Harrap, K.R., Taylor, G.A. and Browman, G.P. (1977) Chem. -Biol. Interactions 18, 119-128.

98. Semon, J.H. and Grindey, G.B. (1976) Proc. AACR/ASCO 17, 82.

99. Grindey, G.B., Semon, J.H. and Pavelic, Z.P. (1978) in Antibiotics and Chemotherapy, Schabel, F.M., ed., Karger, S, Basel, Volume 23, pp. 295-304.

100. Ensminger, D.E. and Frei, E. III (1977) Cancer Res. 37, 1857-1863.

101. Howell, S.B., Ensminger, W.D., Krishan, A. and Frei, E. III (1978) Cancer Res. 38, 325-330.

102. McCullough, J.L., Chabner, B.A. and Bertino, J.R. (1971) J. Biol. Chem. 23, 7207-7213.

103. Valerino, D.M., Johns, D.G., Zaharko, D.S. and Oliverio, V.T. (1972) Biochem. Pharmacol. 21, 821-831.

104. Chabner, B.A., Chello, P.L. and Bertino, J.R. (1972) Cancer Res. 32, 2114-2119.

105. Chabner, B.A., Johns, D.G. and Bertino, J.R. (1972) Nature 239, 395-397.

106. Bertino, J.R., Skeel, R., Makulu, D., McIntosh, S., Uhoch, J. and Chabner, B.A. (1974) Clin. Res. 22, 483A.

Clinical Pharmacology of Anti-Neoplastic Drugs
H. M. Pinedo, editor

CLINICAL INVESTIGATIONS IN THE USE OF THYMIDINE TO REVERSE THE TOXICITY OF METHOTREXATE

GEORGE CANELLOS, M.D.
Sidney Farber Cancer Institute, 44 Binney Street, Boston, Massachusetts 02115.
WILLIAM ENSMINGER, M.D.
Sidney Farber Cancer Institute, 44 Binney Street, Boston, Massachusetts 02115.
STEPHEN HOWELL, M.D.
University of California, Basic Science Building, La Jolla, California 92093.
EMIL FREI, III, M.D.
Sidney Farber Cancer Institute, 44 Binney Street, Boston, Massachusetts 02115

ABSTRACT

High concentrations of thymidine can be achieved in patients without toxicity. These infusions can effectively reverse the toxicity of simultaneous infusions of methotrexate. Thymidine at the dosage of 8 g/m^2 24 hours by continuous infusion can also be used as delayed rescue agent analogous to citrovorum factor. The clearance of thymidine is extremely rapid with T 1/2 approximating 8 to 10 minutes. Thymidine infusions can be an alternative to citrovorum factor (folinic acid) in the rescue of the effects of methotrexate. It may be especially efficacious in those circumstances where persistent high serum levels of methotrexate cannot be rescued by citrovorum factor. A differential anti-tumor effect of methotrexate and thymidine has yet to be defined.

INTRODUCTION

The availability of antidotes to abolish the toxic effects of antineoplastic agents would potentially enhance the therapeutic efficacy of these drugs especially if there was selective reversal of pharmacologic effects of normal tissues. The availability of leukovorin or citrovorum factor has permitted the use of high doses of methotrexate in the treatment of neoplastic disease (1,2). Although a large number of drug schedules have been employed, it is apparent that one can administer leukovorin at intervals, after the cessation of methotrexate, (MTX), up to 36 to 42 hours and reverse the toxic affects of the drug. This has permitted some versatility in the schedule of MTX including the use of high doses for short periods of time. This opportunity is not available with most other neoplastic agents currently in use including other antimetabolites. This is a need to have other methods of reversal MTX toxicity since citrovorum factor may not be effective in those circumstances where very high levels of the drug remain in the circulation such as in renal failure with the resulting competition at the cell membrane between MTX and leukovorin. Further, for transport, it would be potentially useful to have the ability to reverse only one component of the MTX effect at the biochemical level since this might allow for selective rescue of normal tissue but permit the MTX effect at other biochemical levels in tumor tissues that lack the enzymatic apparatus to compensate for the defect. Methotrexate inhibits the synthesis of thymidylic acid (dTMP) as its principal biochemical mechanism of action. In addition purine synthesis inhibition is also well described. Salvage pathways in the cells may allow for the incorporation of performed purines to overcome the anti-purine effect. However, *in vitro* studies and experimental animal studies suggest that thymidine administration can reverse the toxicity of methotrexate on normal and neoplastic cells (3). However, other workers have shown that murine marrow may require both purine and pyrimidines at higher concentrations of methotrexate to maintain cell viability (4). Thymidine in high concentrations can be administered to man without undue toxicity. It is rapidly metabolized and, thus, to maintain blood levels, continuous infusions of high concentrations are required. This report is a summary description of the clinical investigations with MTX and thymidine. Studies of pharmacokinetics of thymidine were required at the onset in order to establish the optimal dose schedule to be used with simultaneous infusions of MTX. The second phase was a study of the use of thymidine in the delayed rescue of MTX and its comparison with leukovorin.

METHODS

All patients were studied either at the Clinical Research Center of the Peter Bent Brigham Hospital or at the Dana Center of the Sidney Farber Cancer Institute.

Thymidine-Methotrexate studies were employed in patients with metastatic cancer refractory to previous therapy or in patients with metastatic cancer for whom no other known effective treatment was available. All patients gave informed consent. The goal of the investigations in patients was to establish an effective dose schedule of thymidine in man that could reverse the effects of methotrexate as a continuous infusion. The second phase attempted to employ thymidine as an agent for delayed rescue of methotrexate analogous to that employed with citrovorum factor. Both methotrexate and TdR were dissolved in 500 ml. of 5% dextrose in water. TdR was supplied by the National Cancer Institute. In the first phase, MTX doses varied over a range of .08 - .6 g/m^2 as a continuous infusion over 24-72 hours. TdR was simultaneously infused at a dose level of 8.0 g/m^2 hours. The dose was an extrapolation from that required for the protection of mice from MTX toxicity. TdR was continuously infused from 72-66 hours. Both drugs were initiated simultaneously. The TdR was continued for 24 hours beyond the cessation of MTX. Serum levels of MTX and TdR were measured by radioimmunoassay. In the second phase TdR was infused at 8 g/m^2/24 hours but beginning after a 24 hours continuous infusion of MTX over a dose range of 0.14 - 8.54 g/m^2.

RESULTS

1. *Simultaneous methotrexate and thymidine.* Either as a result of i.v. pulse doses of 2 g/m^2 of thymidine or following the cessation of a continuous infusion at 8 g/m^2 for 24 hours, the serum clearance of thymidine approximated a T 1/2 of 8 to 10 minutes. The median pretreatment thymidine level was 0.19 micromoles which rose approximately 8 fold to 1.5 micromoles during thymidine infusion (5). Twelve patients were studied in the initial phase of the investigation. Twenty-seven courses of methotrexate infused simultaneously with thymidine were given and only five of these were noted to be associated with toxicity. Only when methotrexate was infused over 72 hours and associated with 96 hour thymidine infusion was significant toxicity seen. The toxicity was consistent with that seen for methotrexate and was characterized by mucositis, myelosuppression, skin eruption, and renal impairment. Thus, it was established that 24 and 48 hour infusions up to 3 g/m^2 were relatively free of methotrexate related side effects during the continuous infusion of thymidine (4). Studies of bone marrow cell labeling indices and cytofluorographic analysis indicated no change in these parameters from pretreatment.

2. *Delayed Rescue.* When methotrexate was infused in the second phase over a 24 hour period in a dosage range of 0.14 to 8.54 g/m^2, 18 out of the 50 courses given to 20 patients were associated with some mucositis (6). Ten out of the 50 courses had myelosuppression. In the latter study, thymidine was initiated at the termination of the 24 hour infusion. Thymidine rescue was initiated with a 1 g/m^2 intravenous bolus injection followed by the constant infusion of 8 g/m^2 per day infused by a continuous infusion pump. Thymidine was infused for three days or until the serum methotrexate level was below 10^{-6} M. Mucositis and myelosuppression were not dose related but were related to the clearance of the serum concentration of methotrexate. Studies of bone marrow deoxyuridine incorporation

and tritiated deoxycytidine incorporation as a measure of DNA synthesis confirm the ability of thymidine to rescue the effects of methotrexate. Like citrovorum factor, thymidine rescue can be delayed and effectively block methotrexate toxicity to normal tissues.

DISCUSSION

A great deal of versatility is available in the scheduling of methotrexate administration since there are a number of methods of rescue from the cytotoxic effects of this agent. The use of leukovorin (folinic acid) is well known and forms the basis for the use of high doses of methotrexate in the treatment of a variety of diseases. It has always been debatable, however, whether folinic acid would allow for selective protection against the toxic effects of methotrexate. Clinical studies, however, have shown that the effectiveness of methotrexate-citrovorum factor is limited to those tumors which are inherently sensitive to folic acid antagonists and appear to have high proliferative activity (7). Thus, the effectiveness of chemotherapy in that setting is related more to the kinetic differences between normal and malignant tissue. In effect, however, malignant tissue is also rescued by the citrovorum factor so that the antitumor effectiveness lasts only for the period that is unrescued. The two other available techniques for the rescue of methotrexate toxicity include the thymidine administration which is discussed in this report, and the possibility of using the enzyme, carboxypeptidase G1, an enzyme which degrades folic acid (8). Two initial clinical investigations in the use of carboxypeptidase G1 have already begun (9). It remains for thymidine to provide the only possible selective biochemical rescue mechanism where differences between normal and malignant cells might be exploited. On a theoretic basis, cells which are deficient in the enzyme, thymidine-uridine kinase, would be unable to convert thymidine to thymidylic acid and might be selectively destroyed by methotrexate while the normal cells would be unaffected in the presence of exogenous thymidine. A comparison of the relative efficacy of thymidine versus citrovorum factor in the rescue of normal human cells has been undertaken following a continuous infusion of MTX at 3.8 g/m^2 for 24 hours (10). The data suggests that high concentrations of thymidine 8 g/m^2 by continuous infusion can initiate DNA synthesis earlier than low doses of citrovorum factor. The relative advantage of thymidine can be matched by the use of high doses of citrovorum factor. However, the latter are not routinely used in most high dose methotrexate protocols. In contrast to murine systems man seems to have adequate levels of circulating purines and does not appear to require an exogenous source to protect against the toxicity of methotrexate. The biochemical basis for the interest of thymidine infusions lies primarily in two areas:

1) the potential for exploiting differences in purine metabolism and nucleoside transport between normal and malignant cells with respect to the affect of methotrexate on them.
2) the availability of an alternative rescue agent which might substitute for citrovorum in those circumstances where there is a persistent high level of methotrexate in the serum which could potentially interfere with the transport of citrovorum factor into cells.

It is known that both methotrexate and citrovorum factor are transported by the same system with approximately equal efficiency. Thus, direct competition between the two could be a significant factor in causing serious toxicity when blood levels of methotrexate are high. Recent investigations suggest that high doses of folinic acid might be able to compensate for these circumstances. However, most rescue programs usually employ low doses of citrovorum factor.

ACKNOWLEDGMENTS

These investigations were supported in part by NIH Grants CA-17979, CA-200 08, CA-19589 and CA-06515 to the Sidney Farber Cancer Institute and Grant S M01 RR00888-02 to the Clinical Center of the Peter Bent Brigham Hospital.

REFERENCES

1. Djerassi, I. et al. (1972) Cancer, 30, 22-30.

2. Hyrniuk, W.M. and Bertino, J.R. (1969) The Journal of Clinical Investigation, 48, 2140-2155.

3. Tattersall, M.H.N. et al. (1975) Nature, 253, 198-200.

4. Pinedo, H.M. et al. (1976) Cancer Research, 36, 4418-4424.

5. Ensminger, W.D. and Frei, E., III (1977) Cancer Research, 37, 1857-1863.

6. Howell, S.B. (1978) Cancer Research, 38, 325-330.

7. Skarin, A.T. et al. (1977) Blood, 50, 1039-1047.

8. Chabner, B.A., et al (1972) Nature, 239, 395-397.

9. Howell, S.B., et al (1978) Europ. J. Cancer, 60, 1-6.
10 Howell, S.B., et al. (1978) Clinical Research, 26, 436A.

Clinical Pharmacology of Anti-Neoplastic Drugs
H. M. Pinedo, editor

THYMIDINE PREVENTION OF METHOTREXATE TOXICITY IN HEAD-AND-NECK CANCER

J.H. SCHORNAGEL, A. LEYVA, J.M. BUESA AND H. M. PINEDO.
Oncology Unit, Dept. of Internal Medicine, University Hospital, Utrecht, The Netherlands.

ABSTRACT

Patients with advanced stage of squamous cell carcinoma of the head and neck region were given constant infusions of thymidine in doses of 8 to 24 g/m^2/day for 72 h. During thymidine infusion the concentration of thymidine in plasma ranged between 2 x 10^{-6} M and 2 x 10^{-4} M and was logarithmically proportional to the administered dose. A 24-h infusion of 600 mg/m^2 methotrexate was administered and was accompanied by a 72-h infusion of thymidine at 8 g/m^2/day, started concurrently with or at the end of the methotrexate infusion. No pharmacokinetic interaction was found between methotrexate and thymidine. Methotrexate toxicity was largely prevented with thymidine infusion. No impairment of bone marrow function was encountered, as peripheral white blood cell counts and platelet counts remained normal and as no inhibitory effect on the *in vitro* colony forming potential of bone marrow aspirates was observed. Mucositis was slight and occurred only occasionally. Significant antitumor response with methotrexate plus thymidine treatment was not observed.

INTRODUCTION

The antifolate methotrexate (MTX) is widely used in the treatment of human cancer (1,2). Its potent inhibition of dihydrofolate reductase leads to a depletion of tetrahydrofolates which function as carbon-1 donors in the *de novo* synthesis of thymine and purine nucleotides. Thus, MTX can produce a "*thymineless*" and "*purineless*" intracellular state resulting in impaired nucleic acid synthesis.

The cytotoxic action of MTX can be reversed by either

a) restoring cofactor pools with leucovorin (5-formyltetrahydrofolate) or
b) providing thymidine (TdR) and purine bases or nucleosides, substrates of the *salvage* pathways for nucleotide biosynthesis (3,4).

Pinedo et al. (5) found that *in vitro*, MTX cytotoxicity to the mouse myeloid precursor cells (CFU-C) can be reversed by the presence of TdR and either one of the purines hypoxanthine, adenosine or inosine. TdR alone however was found to be ineffective in the reversal of MTX cytotoxicity.

More recently, Leyva et al. (6) have reported *in vitro* experiments describing advantages of nucleic acid derivatives over leucovorin in the prevention of MTX cytotoxicity and in the selective protection of murine bone marrow cells compared to L1210 leukemia cells with certain concentrations of TdR and inosine. Tattersall et al. (7) found that in L1210 bearing mice TdR could *in vivo* prevent MTX toxicity to normal host tissues without affecting its antitumor action. A possible explanation of the latter findings is that bone marrow cells utilize predominantly preformed purines, derived from the liver, for nucleic acid synthesis and that TdR may rescue normal proliferating host tissues which do not rely totally on *de novo* purine synthesis, but may not rescue tumor cells in which the *de novo* biosynthetic pathway may be the major route of purine biosynthesis.

Recently, TdR also has been shown to be an effective protective or rescue agent in the prevention of MTX toxicity in man (8,9).

The present phase II study was undertaken to investigate further the effectiveness of TdR in the control of MTX toxicity, to provide additional *pharmacokinetic* information and to determine the doses and schedules required for improved antitumor response.

The specific objectives of the present study were:

a) to determine TdR concentrations attained in plasma during *constant infusion* of this nucleoside at various doses over a period of 3 days.
b) to investigate MTX and TdR pharmacokinetics during simultaneous administration of the two drugs.
c) to evaluate the clinical response to TdR alone and to MTX plus TdR combined
d) to examine the influence of purine availability on the effects of TdR, regarding toxicity and antitumor response, in MTX treatment.

Some preliminary data of the initial parts of this study (a, b and c) are presented here.

METHODS

Patients

All patients in this study had confirmed residual or metastatic *squamous cell carcinoma of the head and neck region* and were inoperable. Also, no alternative therapy was found suitable for these patients. Each patient had a measurable lesion and progressive disease. Patients with any previous chemotherapy were excluded.

Each patient had a normal blood count (WBC > 3000/mm^3, platelets > 100,000/mm^3) and a normal renal function (creatinine clearance > 60/ml).

Therapeutic regimen

Each patient started initially on 72-h intravenous infusion of TdR (NSC-21548) at a dose of 8 g/m^2/day. This dose was extrapolated from the amount of TdR necessary for protection in mice (8). After a 2-day interval the TdR infusion was repeated in doses of 10 to 24 g/m^2/day. Simultaneous, continuous intravenous infusion of MTX and TdR was started at least one week after the last TdR infusion. If there was any indication of tumor regression after TdR treatment, the interval was extended until no further response was evident. MTX, obtained from Lederle Laboratories, was administered in a dose of 600 mg/m^2 over 24 h. TdR infusion was continued for 72 h at 8g/m^2/day. These cycles were repeated every 3 weeks. However, if no effect on the tumor was observed after two cycles of TdR prevention the study was continued with TdR rescue, the 72-h TdR infusion being started at the end of the 24-h MTX administration. If still no effect on the tumor was observed after another 2 cycles, the patient was removed from the study.

Before MTX administration patients received sodium bicarbonate orally or intravenously in doses sufficient to attain a urine pH greater than 7.0. Urine output was maintained at 3 liters/24 h for 48 h from the start of MTX infusion.

Complete blood counts were obtained prior to treatment and daily during treatment. Liver function tests including assays for bilirubin, glutamate-oxalacetate transaminase, glutamate-pyruvate transaminase, alkaline phosphatase and lactate dehydrogenase in patient sera were determined weekly. Renal function was monitored by serum creatinine determination twice a week. Blood samples were drawn twice a day for determination of plasma TdR levels. When MTX and TdR were administered concurrently, *plasma MTX levels* were determined daily and *plasma TdR* levels twice a day.

TdR assay.

TdR concentration in plasma was determined by *high performance liquid chromatography (HPLC)* as described by Leyva et al. (6) for mouse samples. Chromatography was modified slightly for better resolution of TdR peaks from unknown plasma peaks. Aminex A29 (particle diameter size of 5-9 microns) was used in stainless-steel columns, 25 cm x 3 mm i.d. The pH of the alcoholic phosphate-citrate buffer was adjusted to 9.2 Elution was performed at a flow rate of 0.3 ml/min and 50 μl of perchloric acid extracts of plasma samples was injected. This provided a sensitivity of 2 x 10^{-7} M TdR in plasma. All other conditions were the same as those described for HPLC determination of TdR in mouse plasma.

MTX assay

Plasma MTX levels were determined by the enzyme-inhibition assay as described by Bertino and Fischer (10).

Bone marrow culture

Bone marrow aspirates, obtained from the iliac crest, were collected with heparin to prevent coagulation. Bone marrow culture *in vitro* was performed by a technique based on that reported by Iscove *et al.* (11).

After centrifugation the buffy coat was isolated and 10^6 nucleated marrow cells were grown in semisolid culture in McCoy's medium containing 0.8% methylcellulose, 1% bovine serum albumin, 10% undialyzed fetal calf serum (in our hands, human CFU-C's could not be grown in a culture medium supplemented with dialyzed fetal calf serum) and leucocyte conditioned medium (colony-stimulating factor). After 13 days incubation at 37° C, colonies consisting of 20 cells or more were counted using light microscopy. The mean number of colonies was expressed relative to the number of colonies in the patient's own control cultures taken prior to MTX-TdR infusion.

From each bone marrow sample Giemsa stained smears were examined and the ratio of dividing and non-dividing meyloid cells was determined.

RESULTS

To date,8 patients with advanced head- and neck cancer have been admitted to this study.

Patient 1, a 36-yr old man, had a recurrent,epipharyngeal squamous cell carcinoma with invasion to the ethmoidal sinus, skull base and orbita following radiotherapy. Because of rapid progression of the tumor, treatment with MTX and concurrent TdR was begun from the start. He showed progression of disease during two courses. No further treatment after the second course was given due to a marked decline in his general condition. He died a few weeks later.

Patient 2, a 55-yr old woman, with a local, recurrent, inoperable squamous cell carcinoma of the left frontal sinus with invasion of the meninges, was initially treated with radiotherapy with only limited control of disease. She received two 72-h courses of TdR, 8 g/m^2/day. After two courses of simultaneous MTX-TdR treatment there was progressive tumor growth. Therapy was changed and TdR was given as a rescue agent at the end of the MTX-infusion. The sequential administration resulted in protection of normal tissues, equally effective as with concurrent infusion of the two agents; however, the lack of antitumor effect was similar. After two additional courses of sequentially administered MTX-TdR she was removed from the study because of tumor progresssion.

Patient 3, a 59-yr old woman, was previously treated with radiotherapy for a mucoepidermoid carcinoma of the tongue base with extensive bilateral cervical lymph node involvement. She was admitted for a recurrent ulcerating tumor in a previously irradiated area. After two 72-h courses of TdR of 10 g/m^2/day and 20 g/m^2/day she was treated with simultaneous MTX and TdR. She remains currently in the study with no apparent change.

Patient 4, a 75-yr old man, had a submandibular metastasis of a carcinoma of the lower lip, for which he received radiotherapy a year earlier. As there were also bone scan abnormalities, indicating possible metastasis, he was referred for chemotherapy. After the administration of two TdR infusions, 8 g/m^2/day followed later by 24 g/m^2/day, the submandibular tumor showed rapid, progressive growth. It was then decided to refer him to radiotherapy. After irradiation of the only measurable lesion he was no longer eligible for further study.

Patient 5, a 86-yr old man in excellent general condition, was treated with radiotherapy for residual disease after a laryngectomy followed by non-radical neck dissection. Treatment of this patient according to the present protocol was begun after the presence of recurrent carcinoma in the supraclavicular region was noted. He has received now two courses of simultaneous MTX and TdR after the TdR pharmacokinetic studies.

Patient 6, a 58-yr old woman, had received radiotherapy for a carcinoma of the left maxillary sinus. One year later recurrent tumor growth was found in the irradiated area. She received two courses of TdR, and is currently showing signs of progressive disease after two courses of concurrent treatment with MTX and TdR.

Patient 7, a 74-yr old man, had undergone a laryngectomy for a laryngeal squamous cell carcinoma in 1976. One year later a right-sided radical neck dissection was performed because of lymph node metastasis. The following year he had recurrent tumor growth in the same region and received radiotherapy. Recently, after the detection of recurrent tumor growth in the previously irradiated area, he entered the study. After two courses of TdR (8 g/m^2/day followed by 16 g/m^2/day) he received one treatment with MTX plus TdR and is currently under observation.

Patient 8, a 60-yr old man, had undergone non-radical neck dissection for lymph node metastasis in 1977 after laryngectomy performed 6 months earlier because of squamous cell carcinoma of the vocal cords. After neck dissection he received radiotherapy. In 1978 he was found to have recurrent tumor growth. After one course of TdR, MTX-TdR was begun. Two weeks after the first course of the latter treatment, slight regression of the tumor was observed. He is currently under continued observation.

Of the 8 patients described above, 7 were evaluable in the TdR studies. Seven patients received a total of 13 concurrent MTX-TdR infusions and two courses with the drugs sequentially administered.

TdR studies.

The pretreatment plasma TdR concentration was 3.5 ± 1.7 (S.D.) x 10^{-7} M. Fig. 1 shows that in 4 patients during the first 24 h of constant infusion of TdR, 8 g/m^2/day, plasma TdR levels increased and afterward reached steady-state levels 5- to 6-fold higher than pretreatment levels. Higher doses of TdR infused over the same time period resulted in a *logarithmic increase* in plasma levels (Fig. 2). Except for frequent phlebitis, no serious side effects have been recorded during and following these infusions. No reduction in tumor size was observed following any of the TdR infusions.

MTX-TdR studies.

Fig. 3 indicates the plasma concentrations of MTX during and following a 24-h infusion of 600 mg/m^2/MTX. During constant infusion an exposure to 7 x 10^{-6} M MTX resulted. In all of the courses of concurrent and sequential MTX-TdR administration the half-life of MTX in the plasma was 3 h immediately following infusion and approximately 10 h after plasma levels fell below 10^{-7} M. These values are similar to the pharmacokinetic data reported for MTX (50 to 200 mg/kg) infusion accompanied by leucovorin rescue (12). Also, TdR plasma levels measured during and following infusion were not found to be different from those measured when TdR was given alone. No *hematological toxicity* was recorded, as serial white blood cell counts and platelet counts during and after TdR or MTX-TdR infusions did not differ from pretreatment values. Two patients suffered from slight mucositis following combined treatment.

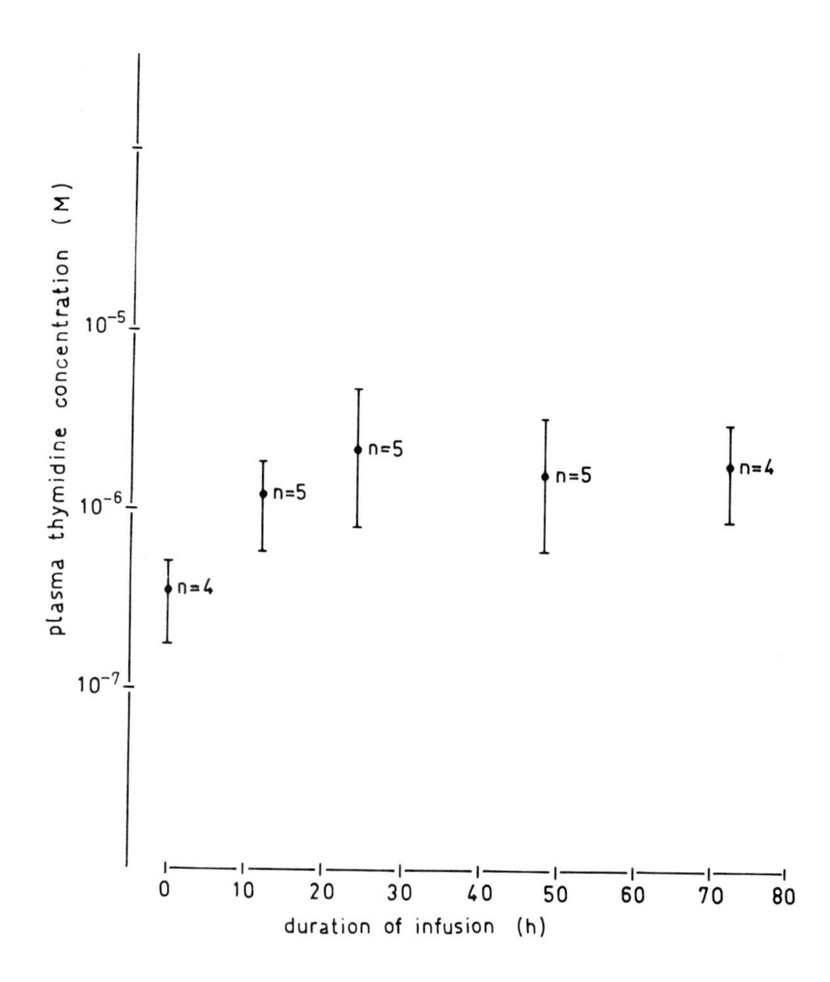

Fig. 1. Mean plasma TdR concentrations (± S.D.) prior to treatment and during constant infusion of TdR 8 g/m^2/day for 72 h.
n = number of determinations. Data were derived from 5 patients.

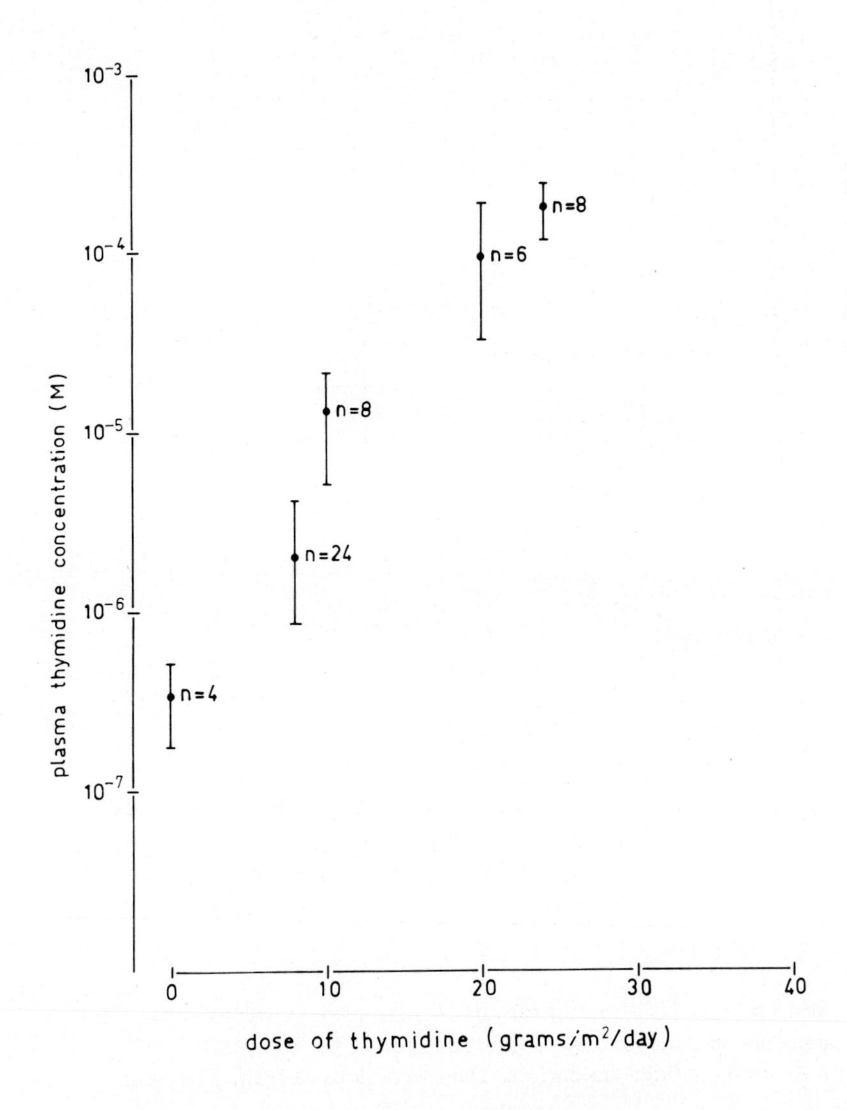

Fig. 2. Plasma TdR concentrations (mean ± S.D.) at steady state levels during constant infusion of various doses of TdR for 72 h.
n = number of determinations.

Effect on myeloid precursor cells.

All patients who received simultaneous MTX-TdR infusions underwent 3 serial bone marrow aspirates, just before infusion (0 h) and 6 and 72 h following initiation of infusion, for examination of colony formation in *in vitro* culture.
Table 1 describes the results obtained for the 5 patients examined. Although control values varied from patient to patient no decrease in *colony forming potential* was observed in the 6- and 72-h bone marrow samples.

TABLE 1
EFFECT OF CONCURRENT MTX-TdR INFUSION ON THE IN VITRO COLONY FORMING POTENTIAL OF BONE MARROW ASPIRATES.

patient no.	number of colonies (mean ± S.D.)		
	0 h from initiation	6 h from initiation	72 h from initiation
2 (E.R.)	56±15	61±15	93±21
3 (E.V.)	92±14	91±13	99±13
5 (G.M.)	36±7	35±3	34±10
6 (W.V.)	55±9	64±9	57±3
7 (J.M.)	55±8	74±9	76±11

Effect on tumor.

In one patient (no. 8) an indication of slight tumor regression was observed after the first concurrent MTX-TdR infusion. As he entered the study only very recently, no further data are available at this time. Another patient (no. 3) showed no change after 3 courses of simultaneous MTX-TdR. All other patients have shown progressive tumor growth.

DISCUSSION

The results of this study show that in seven patients with squamous cell carcinoma of the head and neck region treated with MTX, the *co-administration* of TdR prevented the development of serious toxicity. In all treated cases TdR infusion at a dose of 8 g/m^2/day provided effective protection against the toxic side effects of a 24-h infusion of 600 mg/m^2 MTX, when given during and for 48 h after MTX infusion. There was no indication of MTX-induced myelosuppression as evidenced by the maintenance of normal peripheral white blood cell and platelet

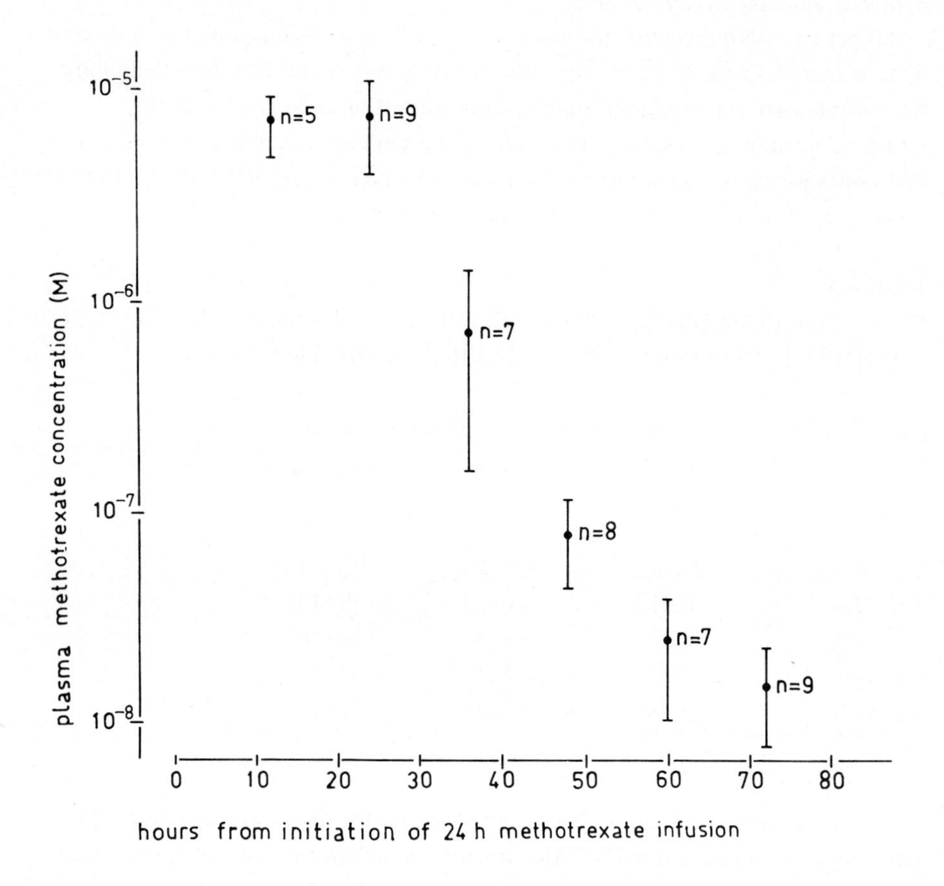

Fig. 3. Plasma MTX levels during and following 24 h MTX infusion. TdR (8 g/m^2/day) was given concurrently and up to 48 h beyond the end of MTX infusion.

counts and the lack of inhibitiory effect on the colony forming potential of bone marrow when cultured *in vitro*. Slight mucositis was observed in two patients during MTX treatment with concurrent TdR infusion. Other potential forms of MTX toxicity were not observed. One patient on two occasions received TdR infusion at the same dose however at the end of the 24-h MTX infusion and also showed no signs of toxicity other than slight mucositis.

The mean TdR concentration in the plasma of the patients studied was found to be 3.5 x 10^{-7} M, similar to that of normal individuals (not reported here). With an infusion of TdR at a dose of 8 g/m^2/day, plasma TdR levels of 2 x 10^{-6} M were achieved and maintained during constant infusion. Increasing the TdR dose resulted in logarithmic increase in plasma TdR levels. Plasma concentrations of TdR as high as 2 x 10^{-4} M were attained with a TdR dose of 24 g/m^2/day. It is important to note that relatively high plasma levels of TdR could be attained despite the known rapid rate of excretion and susceptibility to metabolic degradation of TdR. This latter finding has not been previously observed and suggests that the metabolism and/or the mechanism of excretion of TdR reaches a saturating point.

Our results indicate that MTX elimination from the plasma was not affected by concurrent infusion of TdR. Neither were TdR plasma concentrations during and after MTX infusion found to differ from those during infusion of TdR alone. There does not appear to be any *pharmacokinetic interaction* between these two agents, unlike that reported between TdR and 5-fluorouracil which were found to compete for the same degradation enzyme leading to the prolonged exposure to the pyrimidine analog and to subsequent severe toxicity upon co-administration (13).

The prevention of MTX toxicity by TdR infusion given concurrently with or following MTX has been demonstrated in this study. This finding is consistent with the results reported previously by Ensminger and Frei (8) who observed significant protection with TdR at 8 g/m^2/day against the potential toxicity of a 24-h infusion of MTX at 80 mg/m^2 to 6 g/m^2 when TdR infusion was given simultaneously and continued for 24 or 48 h after MTX. Howell et al. (9) demonstrated that TdR infusion at the same dose and delayed until after the end of the MTX infusion was sufficient to provide *rescue* following exposure to 10^{-5} M MTX for up to 40 h. Effective control of MTX toxicity in experimental animals by the administration of TdR alone however appears to be questionable. Although Tattersall and coworkers demonstrated earlier a protective effect on host tissues plus enhanced antitumor response by TdR in L1210-bearing mice treated with MTX (7), to achieve such results a requirement for both TdR and a purine was reported by others more recently (5). An *antipurine effect* by MTX may occur to a lesser degree in man, due possibly to a greater availability of circulating preformed purines (6).

The observation of *limited response* to MTX plus TdR treatment in the present study is also consistent with the findings of Ensminger and Frei and of Howell and coworkers. Although the latter investigators could achieve prolonged exposure to high concentrations of MTX with subsequent TdR rescue (as mentioned above), no significant selectivity of rescue could be demonstrated. The effectiveness of TdR administration alone in averting clinical MTX toxicity, however without significant antitumor response, suggests that MTX has a limited antipurine effect on both normal and tumor tissues in man. Further studies involving the control of purine availability or the use of lower TdR doses in MTX treatment may prove to be more promising in attempts to modulate metabolic conditions in the patient in order to achieve more *selective* tumor kill.

The primary intention of the escalation of the TdR dose in this study was to determine if plasma levels of 10^{-5} M could be attained. This TdR concentration had been found by Pinedo et al. (5) to be optimal for the prevention of MTX-induced inhibition of mouse CFU-C proliferation. The TdR dose of 8 g/m^2/day with resultant plasma levels of 2×10^{-6} M however was apparently sufficient for the prevention of MTX toxicity. In addition, with doses of TdR as high as 24 g/m^2/day, resulting in an exposure to greater than 10^{-4} M TdR, no toxicity including myelosuppression was observed. Again, *clinical observation* was inconsistent with earlier *in vitro* findings from murine bone marrow culture experiments, indicating an inhibitory effect on CFU-C colony formation by 10^{-4} M TdR (5). An explanation of these discrepancies must await further studies on the effect of TdR on cell growth and MTX cytotoxicity in human bone marrow cultures.

ACKNOWLEDGEMENTS

We wish to thank Dr. E. Frei III of the Sidney Farber Cancer Center (Boston) for making thymidine available to us for this clinical investigation. Ms. E. Italiaander-Kwakkel and Ms. A. Baan-Gout deserve credit for their excellent technical assistance in the performance of plasma thymidine determinations and bone marrow culture studies, respectively. We are also grateful for the secretarial assistance provided by Ms. R.M. van Oldenbeek-Kleef. This work was supported in part by the Netherlands' Cancer Society (The Koningin Wilhelmina Fonds, KWF). (Project number UUKC Int. 77-3).

REFERENCES

1. Bertino, J.R. (1975) in Antineoplastic and Immunosuppressive Agents II, Sartorelli, A.C. and Johns, D.G., eds., Springer-Verlag, Berlin, Heidelberg, New York, 468-483.

2. Bleyer, W.A. (1978) Cancer 41, 36-51.

3. Bertino, J.R. (1977) Seminars in Oncology 4, 203-216.

4. Harrap, K.R. and Renshaw, J. (1978) This Volume.

5. Pinedo, H.M., Zaharko, D.S., Bull, J.M., Chabner, B.A. (1976) Cancer Res. 36, 4418-4424.

6. Levya, A., Van de Grint, L., Pinedo, H.M. (1978) This Volume.

7. Tattersall, M.H.N., Brown, B., Frei, E. III (1975) Nature 253, 198-200.

8. Ensminger, W.D. and Frei, E. III (1977) Cancer Res. 37, 1857-1863.

9. Howell, S.B., Ensminger, W.D., Krishan, A., Frei, E. III (1978) Cancer Res. 35, 325-330.

10. Bertino, J.R. and Fischer, G.A. (1964) Meth. Med. Res., 10, 297-307.

11. Iscove, N.N., Senn, J.S., Till, J.E. and McCulloch, E.A. (1971) Blood 37, 1-5.

12. Stoller, R.G., Jacobs, S.A., Drake, J.C., Lutz, R.J. and Chabner, B.A. (1975) Cancer Chemother. Rep. Part 3, 6, 19-24.

13. Woodlock, Th.M., Martin, D.S., Kemeny, N. and Young, C.W. (1978) Proc. Am. Assoc. Cancer Res. 19, 351.

Clinical Pharmacology of Anti-Neoplastic Drugs
H. M. Pinedo, editor

PHARMACOLOGY AND PHARMACOKINETICS OF HIGH DOSE METHOTREXATE IN MAN

KENNETH R. HANDE, ROSS C. DONEHOWER, AND BRUCE A. CHABNER.
Clinical Pharmacology Branch, Division of Cancer Treatment, National Cancer Institute, Bethesda, Maryland 20014, U.S.A.

ABSTRACT

In order to improve the therapeutic efficacy of methotrexate, recent clinical trials have employed massive doses of methotrexate coupled with citrovorum factor rescue. This chapter outlines the rationale, clinical indications, doses and administration schedules, clinical pharmacokinetics, metabolism, toxicities, and methods for predicting and preventing toxicities of high dose methotrexate therapy.

INTRODUCTION

Methotrexate (4-amino-4-deoxy-N^{10}-methylpteroylglutamic acid) has been in clinical use as a potent anti-neoplastic agent for more than three decades. In recent years, however, major experimental changes have taken place in terms of the dosage of methotrexate administered in hopes of improving the drug's therapeutic efficacy. As has already been mentioned in this symposium, methotrexate traditionally has been given in doses of 0.1 - 1.0 mg/kg on a daily, weekly, or twice weekly basis. Now methotrexate is being employed in very high doses (up to 30 g/m^2) followed by citrovorum factor (leucovorin, folinic acid, 5-formyltetrahydrofolate) to prevent irreparable toxicity to normal tissues. In this chapter we hope to outline the pharmacology of high dose methotrexate as it pertains to its use in the treatment of neoplastic disease.

Mechanism of Action and Rationale

The basic mechanism of action of high dose methotrexate is essentially the same as that already outlined for conventional dose methotrexate therapy. Methotrexate, a folic acid analog, binds to the enzyme dihydrofolate reductase and prevents the conversion of dihydrofolate to tetrahydrofolate. Tetrahydrofolate is an essential cofactor in the synthesis of dTMP, purines, and some amino acids. Citrovorum factor bypasses the metabolic block caused by methotrexate and supplies the reduced folates needed for dTMP, purine, and amino acid synthesis.

High dose methotrexate therapy was first designed as a rational approach for overcoming tumor resistance to methotrexate. Resistance to conventional doses of methotrexate in man has been shown to be due to increased levels of dihydrofolate reductase (1) or to impaired uptake of methotrexate by resistant tumor cells (2). Higher doses of methotrexate might overcome resistance due to increased levels of dihydrofolate reductase. Also, high doses of methotrexate may increase transport into "transport resistant" tumor simply by passive diffusion. In addition, higher doses of methotrexate would have the advantage of better penetration into poorly perfused tissues. Since leucovorin and methotrexate enter cells through the same transport mechanism (3), citrovorum factor, given in doses much lower than methotrexate, would not enter transport resistant cells but would be able to penetrate and rescue normal tissues. Frei, *et al.* (4) have shown evidence that in some instances a selective rescue of normal cells over tumor cells may take place, although this has not been demonstrated clinically.

Further rationale for high dose methotrexate therapy comes from the work of Zaharko, *et al.* (5). They have shown that bone marrow toxicity due to inhibition of thymidylate synthesis occurs at lower free drug concentrations than inhibition of purine synthesis. Thus with high doses of methotrexate, both purine and thymidylate synthesis will be inhibited whereas with lower doses of methotrexate only thymidylate synthesis is inhibited. The purine defect can be tolerated for only 18 hours before lethality occurs, while thymidylate inhibition can be tolerated for over 48 hours (5). Tumor toxicity has been postulated to be primarily dependent on inhibiting purine synthesis while normal bone marrow toxicity is more a function of thymidylate inhibition. This differential is the basis for trials of high dose methotrexate with thymidine rescue discussed later in this symposium. With high doses of methotrexate, both purine and pyrimidine synthesis would be inhibited. Citrovorum factor rescue given after 18 hours but before 48 hours of methotrexate exposure would rescue normal cells dependent upon thymidylate with purine-dependent tumor cells already having been killed. However, some experimental studies (5) have indicated that bone marrow cells may be subject to purine as well as thymidylate deprivation, and Pinedo, *et al.* (6) have shown that marrow toxicity is a function of both drug dosage and duration of drug exposure.

Clinical Indications for High Dose Methotrexate Therapy

Although several exciting and suggestive reports regarding the clinical efficacy of high dose methotrexate have been published over the past few years, high dose methotrexate therapy must still be regarded as an experimental treatment with no definite clinical indications for its use. The first trials with high dose methotrexate therapy were conducted on patients with acute lymphocytic leukemia who had relapsed on maintenance methotrexate therapy. With high dose methotrexate therapy, roughly 50% of these patients achieved either a complete or partial remission (7). Since that time, responses have been reported in osteogenic sarcoma, head and neck carcinoma, CNS tumors, soft tissue sarcomas, carcinoma of the lung, and melanoma (8). Confirmation of these responses has not yet been reported for most of these tumors. In addition, few studies have compared the efficacy of high dose methotrexate therapy with that of conventional doses of methotrexate. Levitt, *et al.* (9) reported an improved therapeutic ratio for high dose methotrexate - citrovorum factor rescue compared with conventional dose methotrexate alone in the treatment of head and neck cancer. However, the results of this study were not confirmed in two subsequent trials (10). The most compelling data regarding the clinical efficacy of high dose methotrexate has been that reported for the treatment of non-Hodgkin's lymphoma, including patients with central nervous system (CNS) disease (11), and for the adjuvant treatment of osteogenic sarcoma (12). However, even these studies have limitations. The response duration was relatively short in most patients with non-Hodgkin's lymphoma treated with high dose methotrexate, and the osteogenic sarcoma trial was based on a small number of patients followed for a relatively short time period, and their response compared to historical controls. Until confirmative studies of these initial encouraging trials are reported, high dose methotrexate therapy cannot be recommended as the standard therapy of any disease.

Drug Doses and Modes of Administration

All high dose methotrexate therapy has been given by intravenous infusion. High dose methotrexate regimens have varied from investigator to investigator in terms of the dose of drug administered and the duration of drug administration. Doses of as little as 250 mg/m^2 up to 650 mg/kg have been given as a bolus or as infusions of from 4 to 42 hours in duration (Table 1). No clear therapeutic advantage has yet been demonstrated for any dose of methotrexate or any infusion period, although several authors have claimed that patients resistant to lower doses may show responses after continuous dose escalation. The best studied and most widely used regimen has probably been that of Jaffe (12) where 50-250 mg/kg of methotrexate are infused over a 4-6 hour period.

TABLE 1

DOSES OF METHOTREXATE AND ADMINISTRATION SCHEDULES USED IN HIGH DOSE METHOTREXATE THERAPY

Methotrexate Dose	*Infusion Period*	*Reference*
250 - 500 mg/m^2	36-42 hours	9
50 - 500 mg/kg	6 hours	12,15
1 - 15 g/m^2	bolus	14
50 - 200 mg/kg	4 hours	16
1550 mg/m^2	36 hours	13
1 - 15 g/m^2	20 hours	14
1 - 7.5 g/m^2	20-40 min.	11
690 mg/m^2	42 hours	8

In addition to variation in the dose and infusion duration of methotrexate, the doses and administration schedule for citrovorum factor rescue have varied widely. Doses of citrovorum factor from 3 to 40 mg/m^2 have been given intravenously, intramuscularly, or orally every 6 hours beginning at any time from 6 to 72 hours following the start of the methotrexate infusion (7). The use of oral citrovorum is based on the clinical studies of Nixon, *et al.* (17) who demonstrated that orally administered leucovorin was well absorbed. Whether the enterohepatic circulation of methotrexate interferes with this absorption is not known. Most researchers prefer the use of intravenous or intramuscular leucovorin, at least for the initial rescue doses. Again, the best citrovorum factor regimen in terms of anti-tumor activity is not well defined.

Clinical Pharmacokinetics

The exact plasma pharmacokinetics of high dose methotrexate therapy vary according to the dose of drug administered and the duration of drug infusion. For a given dose of methotrexate, shorter infusion periods produce high peak plasma levels. Infusions of 50 -250 mg/kg of methotrexate infused over a 4-6 hour period produce peak plasma levels of 0.1 to 1.0 mM with peak plasma levels being roughly proportional to the dose of drug administered. At the end of the infusion, plasma methotrexate disappearance curves fit a biexponential model with half lives of 2 and 10 hours respectively (15,16). The relatively slow terminal half life is believed to be responsible for the toxic effects seen on the gastrointestinal tract and bone marrow if leucovorin rescue is not given. The normal plasma methotrexate decay results in plasma levels shown in Table 2. In general, higher doses of methotrexate are associated with higher plasma levels at any time point.

TABLE 2

AVERAGE RANGE OF PLASMA METHOTREXATE LEVELS FOLLOWING THE INFUSION OF HIGH DOSE METHOTREXATE BY VARIOUS REGIMENS

		Serum MTX Level (μM) After Start of Infusion					
Dose	*Infusion Period*	*Peak*	*12 h*	*24 h*	*48 h*	*72 h*	*Ref.*
1 - 15 g/m^2	bolus	50 1000	5-50	0.1-20	.01-1	.015-.3	14
50 - 200 mg/kg	4 hours	50-1000	5-100	0.5-20	.01-1	.005-.3	16
50 - 250 mg/kg	6 hours	50-1000	1-100	0.5-20	.01-1	.005-.3	18
1500 mg/m^2	36 hours	10-100	10-100	10-100	.5 -5	.01-.5	13

However, there is considerable range of plasma levels from patient to patient (generally ± 1 log) for any dose or any time point.

Infusions of equivalent amounts of methotrexate (1 - 7.5 g/m^2) but given over a more prolonged infusion period (24 to 42 hours) produce lower peak plasma levels (generally 1-100 μM) but these toxic concentrations of drug are maintained for a longer duration of time. Fig. 1 contrasts the plasma pharmacokinetics of a 6-hour infusion of methotrexate with that of a 36-hour infusion. Shorter infusion periods have the advantage of higher peak plasma levels for potentially better tumor penetration, while with long infusions toxic drug concentrations are maintained for a longer time in hopes of treating a higher percentage of tumor cells during the vulnerable S-phase of the cell cycle. With either regimen, plasma methotrexate disappearance is identical once the infusion has been stopped.

About 50% of methotrexate is bound to protein in plasma. Sulfa drugs and salicylates may partially displace this bound drug resulting in higher free drug levels (19). However, even if all bound methotrexate were released, this would raise free drug concentrations only 2-fold, probably an insignificant rise considering the log higher doses of drug employed with high dose as compared with conventional dose methotrexate. Methotrexate's volume of distribution is essentially that of total body water (76% of body weight). The drug diffuses into the cerebral spinal fluid (CSF) in significant amounts although the peak CSF methotrexate levels are 10-50 fold lower than peak plasma levels attained with high dose infusions (11,20).

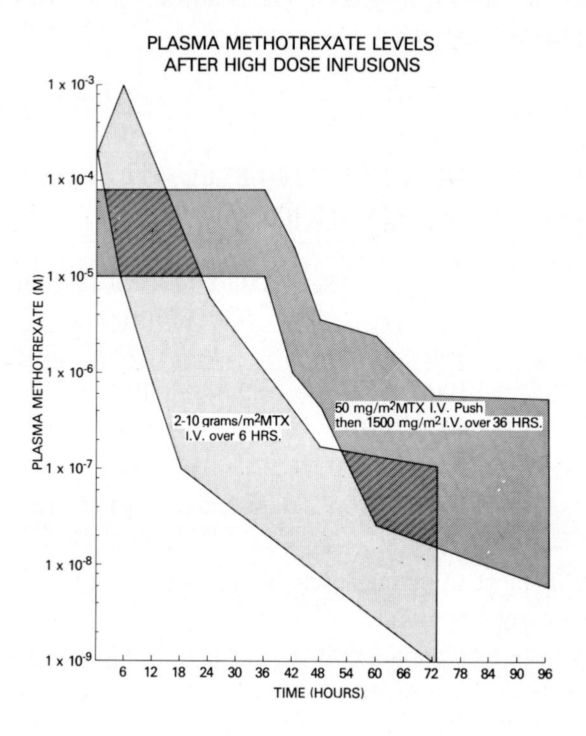

Fig. 1. Range of plasma methotrexate levels following a 6-hour infusion of 2-10 g/m^2 compared with those found following a bolus injection of 50 mg/m^2 and a 36-hour infusion of 1500 mg/m^2.

The CSF levels attained (1-10 μM) are slightly lower than the intraventricular levels achieved with intrathecal administration of 12.5 mg/m^2 methotrexate (21) but are still cytotoxic for "sensitive" tumor cells. The half life of methotrexate in the CSF is roughly twice that of the plasma (20).

In addition to entering normal body compartments such as the CSF, methotrexate also distributes into abnormal "third spaces" such as ascites, pleural effusions, and edematous tissue, probably by simple passive diffusion. Clearance of methotrexate from these "third spaces" is generally considerably slower than methotrexate plasma clearance (5-10 ml/min from ascites fluid versus a renal clearance of 150- 200 ml/min) (22). These "third spaces" will therefore act as a reservoir for methotrexate and delay the rate of methotrexate excretion from the body. This delayed methotrexate clearance places patients with large pleural effusions or ascites at higher risk for developing myelosuppression following high dose methotrexate therapy.

The primary route of methotrexate excretion is through the kidney. Over 50% of a 4-6 hour infusion of high dose methotrexate is excreted through the kidney within 12 hours. Renal clearance of methotrexate has been measured at roughly 180 ml/min (19), indicating that the drug is both filtered and secreted. Urinary concentrations of methotrexate exceed 1 mM during high dose methotrexate infusions and these high urinary concentrations of drug are believed to account for the renal toxicity seen with this form of treatment due to precipitation of insoluble concentrations of methotrexate in the renal tubule. Weak acids such as aspirin, sulfonamides, and some penicillins, interfere with the renal secretion of methotrexate (19). Concomitant use of these drugs during high dose methotrexate therapy may delay methotrexate excretion and lead to the subsequent development of myelosuppression. Methotrexate is also excreted through the biliary system, but most of the drug is reabsorbed through the enterohepatic circulation and only 2% of an administered drug appears in the feces (23). Methotrexate is concentrated in the bile and bile levels of drug may approach at least 1 mM following high dose therapy.

Metabolism

Following the administration of conventional doses of methotrexate, most (>90%) of intravenously administered methotrexate is excreted unchanged in the urine and drug metabolites are found in insignificant quantities. However, with high dose methotrexate therapy it is now becoming apparent that significant quantities of metabolites are formed and that these may account for a large percentage of circulating drug, particularly at later time points following methotrexate infusion. Fig. 2 outlines some of the metabolites of methotrexate which have been demonstrated in tissues, plasma, or urine of patients following high dose methotrexate therapy. Kimelberg (24) has noted that four hours after the injection of high doses of [^{3}H]-labeled methotrexate to monkeys more than 50% of the labeled material appearing in the urine was not parent drug. In addition, the renal clearance of some of these metabolites does not appear to be as rapid as that of methotrexate. Thus, the percentage of metabolite as compared to parent drug in plasma increases with time following methotrexate infusion. Watson and co-workers (25) have recently shown that 7-hydroxy methotrexate concentrations exceed those of methotrexate in plasma samples taken 24 hours after drug administration.

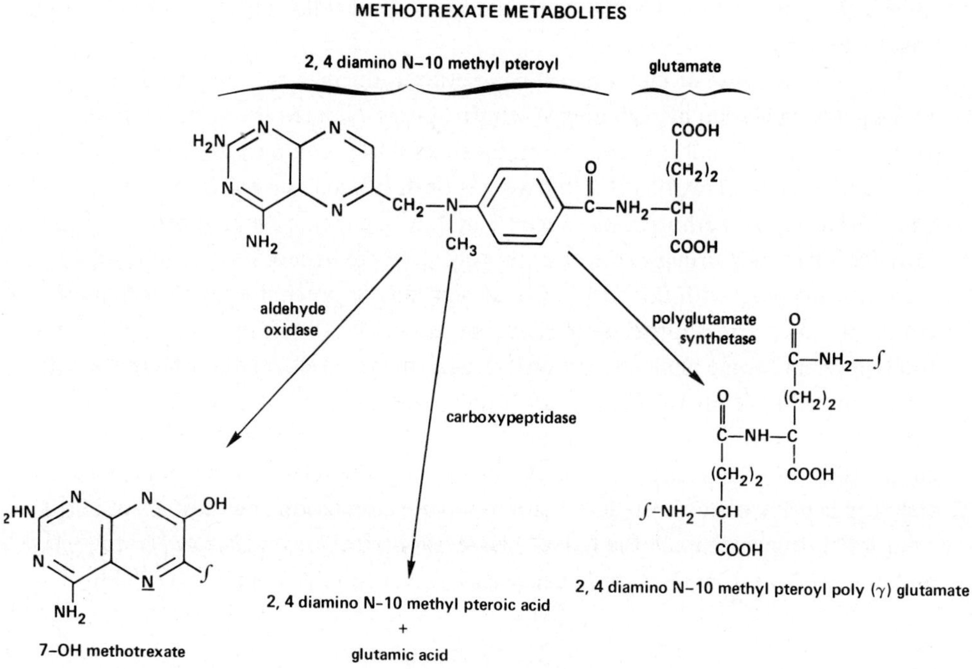

Fig. 2. Formation of methotrexate metabolites in man. Methotrexate is converted to

(a) 7-hydroxymethotrexate through the action of hepatic aldehyde oxidase,
(b) 2,4 diamino, N-10 methyl pteroic acid through the action of the enzyme carboxypeptidase found in gut bacteria, and
(c) polyglutamates through the action of polyglutamate synthetase.

Jacobs *et al.* (26) have documented the excretion of significant (7-33% of total drug) quantities of 7-hydroxymethotrexate in the urine of patients 18-24 hours following high dose methotrexate therapy. 7-Hydroxymethotrexate is presumably formed from methotrexate through conversion by the enzyme hepatic aldehyde oxidase (Fig. 2). The Km for this enzyme is roughly 1 mM, and it has been difficult to demonstrate this reaction with homogenates of human liver, although the aldehyde oxidase conversion of methotrexate to 7-hydroxymethotrexate is known to occur readily in other species. Plasma concentration of methotrexate approaching this Km are found only following high dose methotrexate therapy. With conventional doses of methotrexate, this concentration of drug is not achieved and the rate of metabolite formation would be expected to be much less. 7-Hydroxymethotrexate is 3-4 fold less soluble than methotrexate and formation of this metabolite may be a possible cause for the renal toxicity seen with high dose methotrexate therapy.

Metabolites other than 7-hydroxymethotrexate have also been identified. Significant quantities of polyglutamate derivatives of methotrexate have been found in human liver (27). These polyglutamates represent only a small fraction of methotrexate administered but are stored in the liver for long periods and become a predominant form of methotrexate in the liver months after drug administration. Peripheral tissues, including tumor cells, also form polyglutamates at a slow rate. Methotrexate is also converted to 2,4 diamino, N-10 methyl pteroic acid (DAMPA) through the action of the enzyme carboxypeptidase which is found in gut bacteria (Fig. 2). Methotrexate is presumably excreted into the bile, converted to DAMPA by gut bacteria, and then DAMPA is reabsorbed in the intestine (28). Administration of non-absorbable antibiotics to sterilize the gut in rodents has decreased the formation of metabolites (29). Recent evidence suggests this same phenomena may occur in man (23,30).

Not only are metabolites of methotrexate formed *in vivo* but significant quantities of drug contaminants are infused with high dose methotrexate therapy. In the past, commercially synthesized methotrexate has contained 7 to 8 percent of the material as non-methotrexate contaminants (31). Since high dose therapy may involve the administration of up to 20 grams of methotrexate, patients receiving this form of therapy may receive up to 1.5 grams of contaminant material. These contaminants have been identified as 2,4 diamino, N-10 methyl pteroic acid, N-10 methyl pteroylglutamic acid, and at least five other impurities. The clinical importance of the contaminants and metabolites in terms of anti-tumor effect and in terms of toxicity is not well understood. Some of these agents, such as 7-hydroxymethotrexate and DAMPA, bind to dihydrofolate reductase although to a lesser extent than methotrexate (32). They will, therefore, be detected to some extent by competitive protein binding assays or enzyme inhibition assays which have been discussed earlier in this symposium and may act as folic acid antagonists. The agents are also detected by the radioimmunoassay for methotrexate. In one investigation

(32), DAMPA was detected equally well by radioimmunoassay as methotrexate itself. Since these assays for methotrexate are important in predicting and preventing methotrexate toxicity, one should be aware of the specificity and sensitivity of the assay technique being used when interpreting results of methotrexate levels.

Toxicity

High dose methotrexate therapy has the potential for life threatening toxicity; in one series (33), 6% of patients treated with this form of therapy died from drug-related toxicity. Although with careful attention to hydration and alkalinization of urine during drug administration and with pharmacologic monitoring, this mortality incidence has been reduced, high dose methotrexate therapy is still clearly a potentially lethal form of treatment. Many of the toxicities seen with high dose methotrexate therapy are similar to those described for conventional doses of methotrexate, including nausea and vomiting, myelosuppression, and mucositis. Nausea and vomiting occur during the methotrexate infusion in approximately 10-50% of patients (11,34). The nausea and vomiting usually stop with the end of the infusion and are often controlled with antiemetics.

Myelosuppression (WBC $< 2000/mm^3$; platelets $< 75{,}000/mm^3$) and mucositis occur during 2-11% of all infusions. The development of myelosuppression has been clearly related to delayed clearance of methotrexate from the body (18,20,34, 35). This slow clearance of methotrexate from the body is related to the presence of pleural effusions, ascites, acidosis, and renal dysfunction (18,35).

Renal failure has been a major toxicity resulting from high dose methotrexate therapy which is rarely seen following conventional doses of methotrexate. Studies by Jacobs *et al.* (26) have indicated that this toxicity is due to the precipitation of methotrexate or methotrexate-derived material in the renal tubules. As mentioned earlier in this chapter, urinary concentrations of methotrexate approach 1-10 μM during high dose infusions. In addition, significant quantities of 7-hydroxymethotrexate are also found in urine. Table 3 shows the solubility of methotrexate and 7-hydroxymethotrexate at pH 5 and 7.

As can be seen from the table, urinary concentrations of methotrexate exceed the maximum solubility of the drug at pH 5 leading to precipitation of crystals of methotrexate material in the renal tubule. Since 7-hydroxymethotrexate is 3-5 fold less soluble than methotrexate, formation of this metabolite may be an important factor in the development of renal toxicity. The development of renal toxicity leads to delayed excretion of methotrexate with subsequent development of myelosuppression and mucositis if unrecognized and untreated.

TABLE 3
SOLUBILITY OF METHOTREXATE AND 7-HYDROXYMETHOTREXATE IN URINE

	Methotrexate	*7-Hydroxymethotrexate*
pH 5	1.0 mM	0.3 mM
pH 7	20.0 mM	3.4 mM

A rise in hepatic transaminases to greater than 1.5 x normal is seen in roughly 30-50% of patients following high dose methotrexate infusions. These elevations are transient and have not as yet been associated with significant clinical toxicity. However, the repeated use of conventional doses of methotrexate has led to the development of hepatic cirrhosis in psoriasis patients. The risk of severe liver disease is greater with continuous therapy as opposed to intermittent treatment. The basis for hepatic toxicity may be due to interference with choline synthesis, since this compound has been shown to prevent histological changes in the liver due to methotrexate therapy (36).

Other less frequent toxicities have been reported with high dose methotrexate treatment. Anaphylactic reactions have been seen in patients presumably allergic to methotrexate or to a methotrexate contaminant (37). Seizures, vasculitis, and reactivation of radiation or solar dermatitis have all been reported but are rare. Mild conjunctivitis occurs frequently but is usually not a major patient complaint.

Prediction and Prevention of Toxicity

Although high dose methotrexate therapy has the potential for life-threatening toxicity, with careful preventive measures and pharmacologic monitoring of the individual patient, this toxicity can be kept to a minimum. One key aspect in preventing myelosuppression is the prevention of renal toxicity. As is shown in Table 3, the solubility of methotrexate increases dramatically as the pH changes from 5 to 7. To prevent renal toxicity, adequate hydration (generally greater than 3 l/ 24 hours) along with alkalinization with either sodium bicarbonate or acetazolamide to maintain a urinary pH >7 should be accomplished in all patients before, during, and for 48 hours following high dose methotrexate infusions. This hydration and alkalinization has been shown to dramatically decrease the incidence of renal toxicity and the subsequent development of myelosuppression (20,34). Hydration does not alter the clearance of methotrexate from the body but does change the urinary methotrexate concentration (38). The effect of alkalinization on the renal clearance of methotrexate has not been investigated, although most major pharmacologic studies (15,16,18) have been done using urinary alkalinization. Drugs such as aspirin, sulfonamides, some penicillins or other weak acids should be avoided during high dose methotrexate therapy as these drugs compete for renal tubular excretion with methotexate and delay the clearance of methotrexate from the body (8,19). In patients with renal failure or extensive pleural effusions or ascites, methotrexate therapy should be withheld altogether or doses reduced drastically because of the increased likelihood of toxicity in this group of patients due to delayed clearance of drug.

In addition to pretreatment hydration and urinary alkalinization of the patient, close monitoring of methotrexate disappearance in the individual patient is required. As mentioned earlier, delayed excretion of methotrexate is associated with a high incidence of the development of myelosuppression. Studies correlating plasma methotrexate levels as a guide to toxicity have been done following the high dose methotrexate regimen of Jaffe (12) (50-250 mg/kg infused over 4-6 hours with citrovorum given 15 mg/m^2 q6h x 8 doses started 2 hours after the end of the infusion). The development of myelosuppression has clearly been related to elevated plasma methotrexate levels at 24 or 48 hours following the administration of methotrexate by this regimen.

In the National Cancer Institute series (18), no patients with plasma methotrexate levels below 0.4 μM at 48 hours following the 6-hour infusion of 50-250 mg/kg methotrexate developed myelosuppression with the standard leucovorin rescue (Table 4). However, 6 of 13 patients (42%) with plasma levels above 0.9 μM at 48 hours developed significant myelosuppression. Similar results have been reported in other series (20,34,39). Elevations of serum creatinine are seen in many patients who eventually develop myelosuppression; however, in the NC 1 series 50% of patients who developed myelosuppression did not show a rise in serum creatinine. Therefore, a change in serum creatinine following treatment is an unreliable guide to the development of myelosuppression, and a plasma methotrexate level determined within 48 hours of the start of the infusion is a much better predictor of toxicity. As mentioned earlier, some variation exists for various assay techniques in regard to their specificity and sensitivity of various metabolites. Therefore, the exact plasma levels used for predicting toxicity may vary slightly depending on the assay technique used. In addition, all investigations using plasma methotrexate levels as a guide to toxicity have been done using the Jaffe regimen. Plasma levels predicting toxicity for other infusion schemes of other leucovorin rescue schedules

TABLE 4

CORRELATION OF 48-HOUR PLASMA METHOTREXATE LEVELS WITH TOXICITY FOLLOWING THE INFUSION OF 50-250 MG/KG METHOTREXATE OVER 48 HOURS

Number of Infusions	*48-Hour Plasma MTX Level*	*Supplemental Leucovorin Dose*	*Myelosuppression*
375	<0.4 μM	none	none
7	>0.4 μM but <0.9 μM	15 mg/m^2 i.v. q6h for 48-96 hrs	none
8	>0.9 μM	15-30 mg/m^2 i.v. q6h for 2-20 days	6 of 8
5	>0.9 μM	75 100 mg/m^2 i.v. q4h for 2-20 days	none

have not been determined.

For patients with 48-hour plasma methotrexate levels less than 0.4 μM, no further citrovorum factor is necessary other than that given in the standard rescue regimen. For patients with 48-hour plasma methotrexate values between 0.4 to 0.9 μM, additional citrovorum at a dose of 15 mg/m^2 q6h appears adequate to prevent toxicity (Table 4). For patients with 48-hour values greater than 0.9 μM, continued standard (15 mg/m^2 q6h) citrovorum rescue does not appear adequate to prevent the subsequent development of myelosuppression (18, 39). Our results suggest that higher doses of citrovorum (>75-100 mg/m^2 i.v. q6h) may prevent the development of myelosuppression in patients with high 48-hour plasma levels (Table 4). In an earlier section of this symposium, Dr. Pinedo has indicated that at least equimolar concentrations of leucovorin were needed to rescue from methotrexate toxicity in tissue culture. Standard doses of leucovorin (15 mg/m^2 i.v.) achieve plasma levels of roughly 1 μM. We try to adjust our citrovorum rescue to produce equimolar concentrations of citrovorum in the presence of high plasma methotrexate levels. Citrovorum rescue should be continued until plasma methotrexate levels fall below 0.05 μM.

The renal toxicity seen with high dose methotrexate therapy is generally reversible over a 1-2 week period. However, more rapid clearance of methotrexate from the body in the face of renal failure would be beneficial. Removal of methotrexate through peritoneal or hemodialysis appears to be of little benefit in patients with drug-induced renal failure (40). Two other approaches–inactivation of methotrexate through the use of the enzyme carboxypeptidase (41) and removal of methotrexate by hemoperfusion through charcoal filters (42)—are still investigational procedures but may have potential therapeutic use.

Although high dose methotrexate therapy has shown promise for the treatment of several malignancies, it should still be regarded as an investigational treatment modality. Because of its investigational status in clinical practice, the potential toxicities of this regimen, and the facilities necessary for monitoring plasma levels, high dose methotrexate therapy should be restricted to those centers familiar with its use and with the facilities available to closely monitor patients and to treat complications that may result.

REFERENCES

1. Bertino, J.R., Donahue, D.R., Gabrio, B.W., Silber, R., Alenty, A., Meyer, M. and Huennekens, F.M. (1962). Increased levels of dihydrofolic reductase in leucocytes of patients treated with amethopterin. Nature, 193, 140-142.

2. Kessel, D., Hall, T.C. and Roberts, D.W. (1968). Modes of uptake of methotrexate by normal and leukemic human leukocytes *in vitro* and their relation to drug response. Cancer Res., 28, 564-570.

3. White, J.C., Bailey, B.D. and Goldman, I.D. (1978). Lack of stereospecificity at carbon 6 of methyltetrahydrofolate transport in Ehlich ascites tumor cells. J. Biol. Chem., 253, 242-245.

4. Frei, E. III, Jaffe, N., Tattersall, M.H.N., Pitman, S. and Parker, L.(1975). New approaches to cancer chemotherapy with methotrexate. N. Engl. J. Med., 292, 846-851.

5. Zaharko, D.S., Fung, W-P. and Yang, K-H. (1977). Relative biochemical aspects of low and high doses of methotrexate in mice. Cancer Res., 37, 1602-1607.

6. Pinedo, H.M. and Chabner, B.A. (1977). The role of drug concentration, duration of exposure, and endogenous metabolites in determining MTX cytotoxicity. Cancer Treat. Reports, 61, 709-715.

7. Bender, R.A. (1975). Anti-folate resistance in leukemia: Treatment with "high-dose" methotrexate and citrovorum factor. Cancer Treat. Reviews, 2, 215-224.

8. Bleyer, W.A. (1978). The clinical pharmacology of methotrexate. Cancer, 41, 36-51.

9. Levitt, M., Mosher, M., DeConti, R.C., et al. (1973). Improved therapeutic index of methotrexate with "leucovorin rescue". Cancer Res., 33, 1729-1734.

10. Catane, R., Bono, V., Louie, A. and Muggia, F. (1978). High-dose methotrexate, not a conventional treatment. Cancer Treat. Reports, 62, 178-180. (letter).

11. Skarin, A.T., Zuckerman, K.S., Pitman, S.W., Rosenthal, D.S., Maloney, W., Frei, E. and Canellos, G.P. (1977). High-dose methotrexate with folinic acid in the treatment of advanced non-Hodgkin's lymphoma including CNS involvement. Blood, 50, 1039-1047.

12. Jaffe, N., Frei, E., et al. (1974). Adjuvant methotrexate and citrovorum factor treatment of osteogenic sarcoma. N. Engl. J. Med., 291, 994-1000.

13. Goldberg, N.H., Chretian, P.B., Elias, E.G., Hande, K.R., Chabner, B.A. and Myers, C.E. (1977). Preoperative high dose methotrexate–a well tolerated regimen in head and neck cancer. Proc. Am. Assoc. Cancer Res., 18, 292. (abstract).

14. Tattersall, M.H.N., Parker, L.M., Pitman, S.W. and Frei, E. III. (1975). Clinical pharmacology of high-dose methotrexate (NSC-740). Cancer Chemother. Rep., 6, 25-29.

15. Stoller, R.G., Jacobs, S.A., Drake, J.C., et al. (1975). Pharmacokinetics of high-dose methotrexate (NSC-740). Cancer Chemother. Rep., 6, 19-24.

16. Isacoff, W.H., Morrison, P.F., Aroesty, J., Willis, K.L., Block, J.B. and Lincoln, T.L. (1977). Pharmacokinetics of high-dose methotrexate with citrovorum factor rescue. Cancer Treat. Rep., 61, 1665-1674.

17. Nixon, P.F. and Bertino, J.R. (1970). Absorption and utilization of oral 5-formyl-tetrahydrofolate. Fed. Proc., 29, 610. (abstract).

18. Stoller, R.G., Hande, K.R., Jacobs, S.A., et al. (1977). Use of plasma pharmacokinetics to predict and prevent methotrexate toxicity. N. Engl. J. Med., 297, 630-634.

19. Liegler, D.G., Henderson, E.S., Hahn, M.A., et al. (1969). The effect of organic acids on renal clearance of methotrexate in man. Clin. Pharmacol. and

Therapeut., 10, 849-857.

20. Pitman, S.W. and Frei, E. (1977). Weekly methotrexate-calcium leucovorin rescue: Effect of alkalinization on nephrotoxicity; pharmacokinetics in the CNS; and use in CNS non-Hodgkin's lymphoma. Cancer Treat. Rep., 61, 695-701.

21. Shapiro, W.R., Young, D.F. and Mehta, B.M. (1975). Methotrexate: Distribution in cerebrospinal fluid and intravenous, ventricular, and lumbar injections. N. Engl. J. Med., 293, 161-166.

22. Chabner, B.A., Jacobs, S., Stoller, R.G., Hande, K.R. and Young, R.C. Methotrexate disposition in humans: Case studies in ovarian cancer and following high-dose infusions. Drug Metab. Reviews, in press.

23. Calvert, A.H., Bondy, P.K. and Harrap, K.R. (1977). Some observations on the human pharmacology of methotrexate. Cancer Treat. Rep., 61, 1647-1656.

24. Kimelberg, H.K., Biddlecombe, S.M. and Bourke, R.S. (1977). Distribution and degradation of [^{3}H] methotrexate after intravenous and cerebral intraventricular injection in primates. Cancer Res., 37, 157-165.

25. Watson, E., Cohen, J.L. and Chan, K.K. High-pressure liquid chromatographic determination of methotrexate and its major metabolite, 7-hydroxymethotrexate, in human plasma. Cancer Treat. Rep., in press.

26. Jacobs, S.A., Stoller, R.G., Chabner, B.A., et al. (1976). 7-Hydroxymethotrexate as a urinary metabolite in human subjects and rhesus monkeys receiving high-dose methotrexate. J. Clin. Invest., 57, 534-538.

27. Jacobs, S.A., Derr, C.J. and Johns, D.G. (1977). Accumulation of methotrexate diglutamate in human liver during methotrexate therapy. Biochem. Pharmacol., 26, 2310-2313.

28. Valerino, D.M., Johns, D.G., Zaharko, D.S. and Oliverio, V.T. (1972). Studies on the metabolism of methotrexate by intestinal flora. Biochem. Pharmacol., 21, 821-831.

29. Zaharko, D.S., Bruchner, H. and Oliverio, V.T. (1969). Antibiotics alter methotrexate metabolism and excretion. Science, 166, 887-888.

30. Creaven, P.J., Cohen, M.H. and Allen, L.M. (1976). Methotrexate plasma decay kinetics: Possible alteration in patients undergoing gut sterilization. Brit. J. of Cancer, 34, 571-575.

31. Hignite, C.E., Shen, D.D. and Azarnoff, D.L. (1978). Separation and identification of impurities in parenteral methotrexate dosage forms. Cancer Treat. Rep., 13-18.

32. Donehower, R., Myers, C., Drake, J., Gallelli, J., Chabner, B. and Engle, R. (1978). Comparison of radioimmunoassay and competitive reductase binding assay. Proc. Am. Assoc. Cancer Res., 19, 687. (abstract).

33. VonHoff, D.D., Penta, J.S., Helman, L. and Slavik, M. (1977). Incidence of drug-related deaths secondary to high-dose methotrexate and citrovorum factor administration. Cancer Treat. Rep., 61, 745-748.

34. Isacoff, W.H., Townsend, C.M., Eilber, F.R., Forster, T., Morten, D.L. and Block, J.B. (1976). High dose methotrexate therapy of solid tumors. Observations relating to clinical toxicity. Med. Pediatr. Oncol., 2, 227-241.

35. Chan, H., Evans, W. and Pratt, C.B. (1977). Recovery from toxicity associated with high-dose methotrexate: Prognostic factors. Cancer Treat. Rep., 61, 797-804.

36. Freeman-Narrod, M., Narrod, S. and Custer, R.P. (1977) Chronic toxicity of methotrexate in rats: Partial to complete protection of the liver by choline. J. Natl. Cancer Inst., 59, 1013-1016.

37. Goldberg, N.H., Romolo, J.L., et al. (1978). Anaphylactoid type reactions in two patients receiving high dose intravenous methotrexate. Cancer, 41, 52-55.

38. Romolo, J.L., Goldberg, N.H., Hande, K.R. and Rosenberg, S.A. (1977). Effect of hydration on plasma methotrexate levels. Cancer Treat. Rep., 61, 1395-1396.

39. Nirenberg, A., Mosende, C., Mehta, B., et al. (1977). High-dose methotrexate with citrovorum rescue: Predictive value of serum methotrexate concentrations and corrective measures to avert toxicity. Cancer Treat. Rep., 61, 779-783.

40. Hande, K.R., Balow, J.E., Drake, J.C., Rosenberg, S.A. and Chabner, B.A.

(1977). Methotrexate and hemodialysis. Ann. Intern. Med., 87, 495-496. (letter).

41. Chabner, B.A., Johns, D.G. and Bertino, J.R. (1972). Enzymatic cleavage of methotrexate provides a method for prevention of drug toxicity. Nature, 239, 395-397.

42. Djerassi, I., Ciesielka, W. and Kim, J.S. (1977). Removal of methotrexate by filtration-adsorption using charcoal filters or by hemodialysis. Cancer Treat. Rep., 61, 751-752.

Clinical Pharmacology of Anti-Neoplastic Drugs
H. M. Pinedo, editor

CLINICAL STUDIES ON THE CENTRAL-NERVOUS-SYSTEM PHARMACOLOGY OF METHOTREXATE

W. ARCHIE BLEYER and DAVID G. POPLACK
Children's Orthopedic Hospital and Medical Center, University of Washington Department of Pediatrics, and the Fred Hutchinson Cancer Research Center, P.O. Box C-5371, Seattle, Washington, 98105 and the Pediatric Oncology Branch, National Cancer Institute, Bethesda, Maryland 20014 (United States).

ABSTRACT

This article presents an overview of the authors' studies on the central-nervous-system (CNS) pharmacology of methotrexate (MTX). The routes of administration studied included intrathecal (IT) injection (120 patients), intraventricular injection (18 patients) and intravenous infusion (26 patients). After intralumbar injection of 12 mg/m^2, MTX disappearance from lumbar cerebrospinal fluid (CSF) was triphasic, with concentrations of 10^{-5}, 10^{-7} and 10^{-9} M at 0.5, 2 and 6.5 days respectively.

Elevated levels of lumbar MTX occurred with

1) administration to adults and adolescents
2) overt meningeal leukemia
3) lumbar puncture syndrome
4) communicating hydrocephalus
5) clinical neurotoxicity.

Decreased levels of lumbar MTX were associated with

1) decreased therapeutic effect
2) administration to young children

The latter was attributed to the use of body surface area for dosage determination in that young children have a smaller body surface area relative to CNS volume. Ventricular MTX concentrations after lumbar administration were invariably lower than lumbar drug levels. Intraventricular injection resulted consistently in higher antifolate concentrations in both ventricular and lumbar CSF. Plasma MTX peaked 3 hours after IT injection and remained above 10^{-8} M for 16-36 hours, as compared to 6-18 hours after systemic administration of the same dose, indicating that IT MTX is potentially more cytotoxic to systemic target organs than an equimolar dose administered systemically.

With high-dose intravenous infusions, the mean CSF: plasma MTX ratio, at steady state, was 1:33. The ratio was independent of plasma MTX concentrations up to 10^{-4} M and there was no difference between ventricular and lumbar antifolate concentrations. These observations suggest that intravenous MTX can be as effective as IT MTX if given in a high enough dose (one that provides plasma drug levels approximately 33-fold greater than the desired steady-state CSF level), for a sufficiently long interval (e.g. the tumor cell cycle time), and in conjunction with a systemically-administered MTX-neutralizing agent which does not enter the CNS.

INTRODUCTION

After a drug is injected into the CSF, a number of processes may affect its subsequent distribution within and removal from the CNS. These include:

1) bulk flow of entrained drug via the normal pathways of CSF flow
2) diffusion into and through the extracellular space of the brain parenchyma and spinal cord
3) back diffusion from the extracellular fluid of brain parenchyma into the CSF
4) removal from the CNS by the normal pathways of CSF absorption
5) removal by diffusion from the extracellular fluid into the capillaries of the brain and spinal cord.

Other processes may include:

6) diffusion into the arachnoid and dural membranes and removal via the circulating blood of the meninges
7) absorption from ventricular fluid by an active transport mechanism located in the choroid plexus
8) uptake by certain cells in the brain and spinal cord.

To achieve a high concentration at the site of a CNS tumor there must be little loss of drug as it moves along the CSF pathways and then diffuses into the CNS parenchyma towards the tumor. Thus, the ideal agent is one that is cleared slowly from the CSF, diffuses rapidly through the extracellular space, and undergoes little, if any, uptake by the glial cells, neurons and capillaries within the CNS. The drug must also be tumoricidal at the concentrations achieved and it should have no significant neurotoxic side effects.

Information on the degree to which MTX satisfies these criteria should suggest ways in which to improve IT chemotherapy in man. The studies to be described were undertaken with this objective, notwithstanding the limitations of obtaining adequate data in human subjects, particularly children. A six-year effort is summarized, beginning with a description of the drug's disappearance kinetics in human CSF and including attempts to identify those factors which influence the distribution of the drug into and within the human CNS.

PATIENTS AND METHODS

All patients were under care of the Division of Hematology/Oncology, Children's Orthopedic Hospital and Medical Center, Seattle or the Pediatric Oncology Branch, National Cancer Institute, Bethesda. The patients ranged in age from 6 months to 64 years. CSF samples were obtained in 120 patients administered MTX via lumbar puncture, 18 patients administered MTX intraventricularly via an Ommaya reservoir, and 26 patients given 42-hour high-dose intravenous infusions. Forty-four patients had signs or symptoms related to overt CNS leukemia, lumbar puncture syndrome, or IT MTX neurotoxicity. Seventy-six patients who received intralumbar MTX for prevention of CNS leukemia did not develop symptoms of lumbar puncture syndrome or IT MTX neurotoxicity. In 14 patients, serial plasma samples were also obtained after IT injection.

Except where specified, intralumbar MTX was given at a dose of 12 mg/m^2 diluted in Elliott's B solution to a concentration of 1.0 to 1.5 mg/ml. The volume of injection was 12 ml/m^2, with a maximum volume of 18 ml. Intraventricular MTX was given at a dose of 6-12 mg/m^2 in 5 ml Elliott's B solution. All injections were administered over 1-2 minutes without barbotage, after isovolumetric removal of CSF.

In general, lumbar CSF samples for MTX determination were obtained only at the time of lumbar puncture for the second and third scheduled doses of IT chemotherapy. The interval between injections varied from 2 to 8 days depending on the clinical protocol. Since the residual MTX in the CSF 2 days after injection represented 0.1% of the administered dose and since accumulation of the drug with successive doses was not noted, concentrations measured after consecutive doses of MTX in the same patients were included in the analysis. Ventricular samples were obtained after pumping the reservoir chamber 6 times; the last 0.5 ml aliquot of fluid removed was used for MTX determination.

Intravenous MTX was given as high-dose 42-hour infusions. A primary infusion was given over 1 hour followed immediately by a sustaining maintenance infusion for 41 hours. In the initial studies, the priming dose was 75 mg/m^2 and the maintenance dose was 15 mg/m^2/h. Citrovorum factor was commenced immediately at the end of the infusion at a dose of 12 mg/m^2 every 6 hours until the plasma MTX concentration was below 8 x 10^{-8} M. In subsequent groups of patients, the priming and maintenance MTX doses, and the first citrovorum dose, were doubled. Subsequent citrovorum doses were held constant at 12 mg/m^2/dose and continued until the plasma MTX level fell below 8 x 10^{-8} M. In general, simultaneous plasma and CSF samples were obtained only once during each infusion.

One-half ml of each patient specimen was kept in the dark at 4°C until antifolate measurement was performed, usually within 3 days after collection. MTX concentration was determined in triplicate by the dihydrofolate reductase inhibition method (description available upon request). The assay has a lower limit of sensitivity of 5 x 10^{-10} M in CSF and 10^{-9} M in plasma.

Sodium MTX was obtained from Lederle Laboratories, Pearl River, New York, U.S.A., as 5 mg and 50 mg vials containing other methyl- and propylparabenz preservatives (in early studies) or benzyl alcohol (in later studies) and from the National Cancer Institute, U.S.A., as 1000 mg vials containing lyophylized sodium MTX without preservatives. Citrovorum factor (Calcium Leukovorin), 3 and 50 mg vials, were obtained from Lederle Laboratories.

RESULTS

Pharmacokinetics of IT MTX in nontoxic patients after lumbar injection. CSF and plasma MTX concentrations were analyzed in 76 patients who received prophylactic IT MTX, 12 mg/m^2, without developing signs or symptoms of lumbar puncture syndrome or drug-induced neurotoxicity (1). The mean patient age was 11 years and the mean body surface area was 1 m^2. After an initial CSF distribution phase (not depicted), MTX disappearance from lumbar CSF was biphasic (Fig. 1), with half-disappearance times of 4.5 and 14 h, respectively. Since the average patient had a 1 m^2 surface area and a dose of 12 mg, the volumes of distributions were estimated to be 0.5 and 15.7 l/m^2, respectively. Drug clearance from CSF, calculated from the formula (0.693) (volume of distribution)/(half-disappearance time), was 1.2 and 13 ml/m^2/min, respectively. To determine whether or not the kinetics of disappearance were concentration dependent, the dosage was varied in some patients from 1 to 12 mg/m^2, and serial CSF samples were obtained. The half-life of the first phase of disappearance remained constant and the concentration was linearly proportional to dose, consistent with first-order kinetics (1). MTX concentrations in plasma reached a peak of 2 x 10^{-7} M 3 h after injection and then fell biexponentially with half-lives of 5.5 and 24 h (Fig. 1). The plasma half-lives were greater than the corresponding half-lives of the CSF disappearance curve, such that the CSF:plasma MTX ratio fell continuously from 100:1 at 12 h to 30:1 at 72 h.

Plasma MTX concentrations after IT and systemic administration. Plasma MTX fell below 10^{-8} M 16-36 hours after IT injection of 12 mg/m^2 and

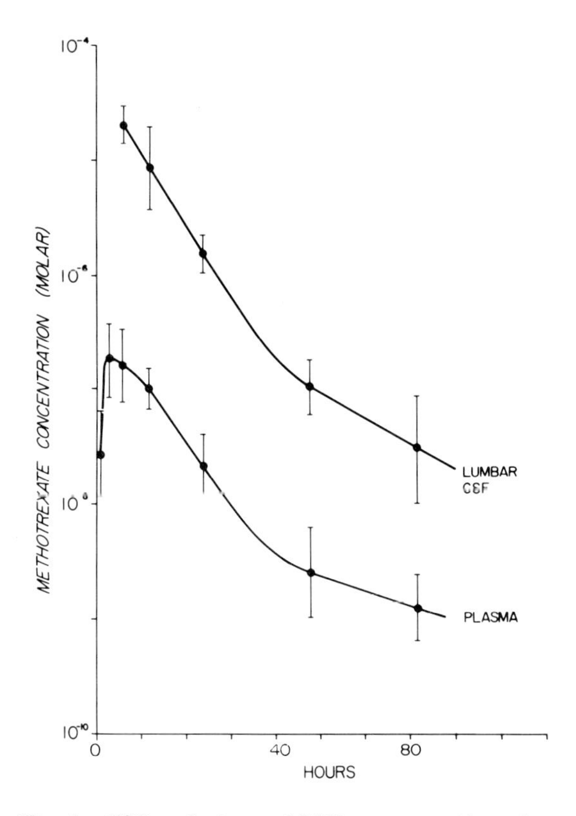

Fig. 1. CSF and plasma MTX concentrations (geometric mean ± 1 SD) in patients treated with intralumbar MTX, 12 mg/m^2.

6-18 hours after systemic administration (oral, intramuscular, intravenous) of the same dosage. A direct comparison of oral and IT administration in two patients revealed that the plasma half-lives were 2.6 and 5.2 times greater, and the area under the curve 1.7 times greater, with the IT route than with the oral route of administration (2). Fig. 2 illustrates these differences in one patient.

Entry into the cerebral ventricles after intralumbar administration. Ventricular CSF samples were obtained in 18 patients with indwelling Ommaya reservoirs. Ventricular MTX after intralumbar administration (12 mg/m^2 in 12 ml/m^2 Elliott's B solution) averaged 2.1 x 10^{-6}, 4.1 x 10^{-7} and 1.2 x 10^{-7} M at 6, 12 and 24 h after injection, respectively. The mean antifolate concentrations were 1 log lower in ventricular CSF than in lumbar CSF, confirming limited entry of the drug into the ventricular compartment after spinal injection. A representative patient is shown in Fig. 3.

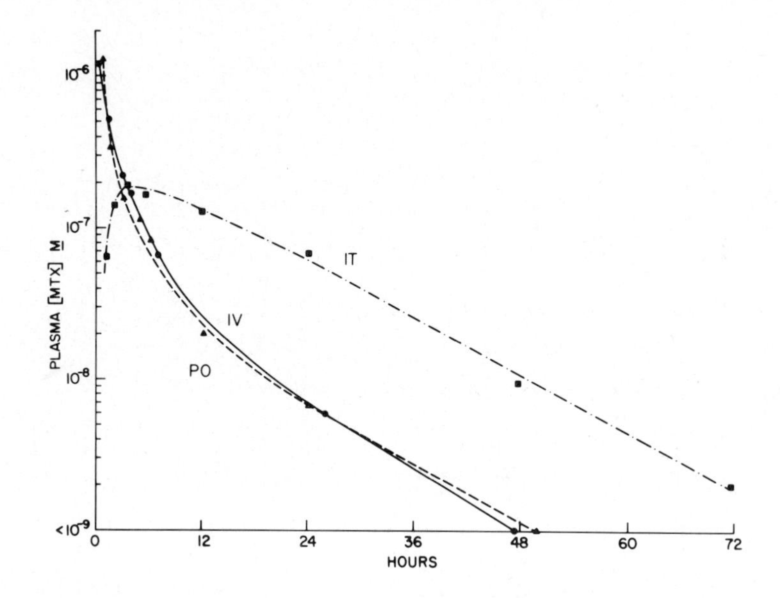

Fig. 2. Plasma MTX concentrations after oral (PO), intravenous (IV) and IT administration of 20 mg (12 mg/m^2) in the same patient.

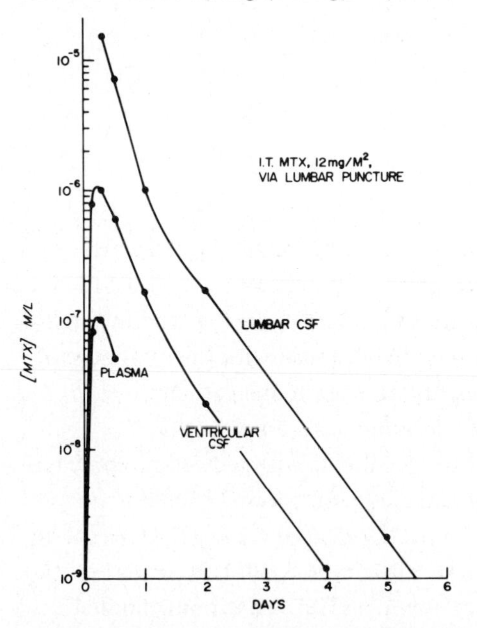

Fig. 3. MTX concentrations in plasma, lumbar CSF and ventricular CSF after intralumbar injection of 12 mg/m^2.

Intraventricular administration. Injection of MTX, 12 mg/m^2, via the Ommaya reservoir resulted in mean (± 1 SD) ventricular antifolate levels of 2.0 (± 2.7) x 10^{-4} M at 3 h, 1.8 (± 1.6) x 10^{-5} M at 6 h, 0.9 (± 1.4) x 10^{-5} M at 12 h, 4.6 (± 4.3) x 10^{-7} M at 24 h and 2.7 (± 3.0) x 10^{-7} M at 48 h after injection. Intraventricular injection provided consistently higher ventricular MTX concentrations than intralumbar injection (3), as previously shown by Shapiro and his colleagues (4). Within 6 h after intraventricular injection, lumbar levels exceeded ventricular levels and remained 4.7 (range 1.5-13.0) times greater thereafter (Fig. 4).

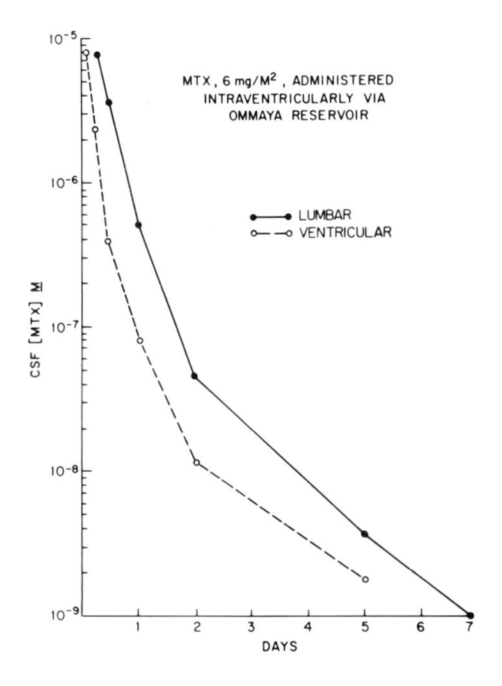

Fig. 4. MTX concentrations in lumbar and ventricular CSF after intraventricular injection of 6 mg/m^2 (same patient as in Fig. 3).

Interestingly, the lumbar levels 2-8 days after injection were also higher with intraventricular injection than with direct intralumbar administration, although this difference was not statistically significant.

Clinical Determinants of CSF MTX. Five conditions were found to be associated with elevated CSF MTX concentrations

1) administration to adults and adolescents
2) overt meningeal leukemia

3) lumbar puncture syndrome
4) communicating hydrocephalus
5) clinical neurotoxicity.

Two conditions were associated with decreased levels of lumbar MTX
1) administration to children and
2) decreased therapeutic effect.

The correlation of age and lumbar CSF MTX levels was first recognized when body surface area was tested as a determinant of CSF MTX concentration (Fig. 5). Patients with surface areas greater than 1 m^2 (adolescents and adults) had significantly higher antifolate levels than patients with surface areas less than 1 m^2 (children) ($p < .01$). Further analysis demonstrated that CSF MTX was directly proportional to age, adults having higher levels than adolescents and adolescents having higher levels than children (5). This pattern appeared to be due, at least in part, to the use of body surface area as a basis for dosage calculation (12 mg/m^2 surface area). Since CNS volume is essentially constant after 3 years of age (5), we subsequently administered a constant dose of 12 mg (not 12 mg/m^2) to 24 patients between 3 and 40 years of age.This group was compared with 25 patients treated with 12 mg/m^2 body surface area. The groups were matched for age and body surface area and all patients in this study received IT MTX for prophylaxis of CNS leukemia. The mean (± 1 SD) molar concentrations for 3, 4 and 7 days were 2.8 (± 1.60) x 10^{-8}, 1.4 (± 0.80) x 10^{-8}, and 3.2 (± 2.50) x 10^{-9} respectively for the 12 mg/m^2 dose group, and 2.5 (± 0.95) x 10^{-8}, 1.0 (± 0.15) x 10^{-8} and 1.5 (± 0.50) x 10^{-9} respectively for the 12 mg dose group. This comparison revealed that the SDs were 1.7 - 5.3 times greater in the group whose dosage was based on body surface area than in the constant-dose group.

We also observed that overt CNS leukemia (presence of leukemia cells in the CSF) resulted in higher CSF MTX concentrations (Fig. 6) (3,5). Correction for surface area did not eliminate this difference. Communicating hydrocephalus, a not uncommon complication of CNS leukemia, may contribute to this effect (Fig. 7). However, we have observed elevated CSF MTX levels with overt meningeal leukemia in the absence of communicating hydrocephalus as demonstrated by normal subarachnoid scintigraphs and computed tomograms.

CSF MTX concentrations were also evaluated in 7 patients with lumbar-puncture syndrome, identified by orthostatic symptomatology and low opening CSF pressure. The mean (± 1 SD) lumbar CSF MTX levels were 1.45 ± 0.17 SDs above the mean values of the 76 nontoxic patients.

Clinical response and CSF MTX concentrations. We previously reported that neurotoxicity of IT MTX is associated with elevated concentrations of the drug

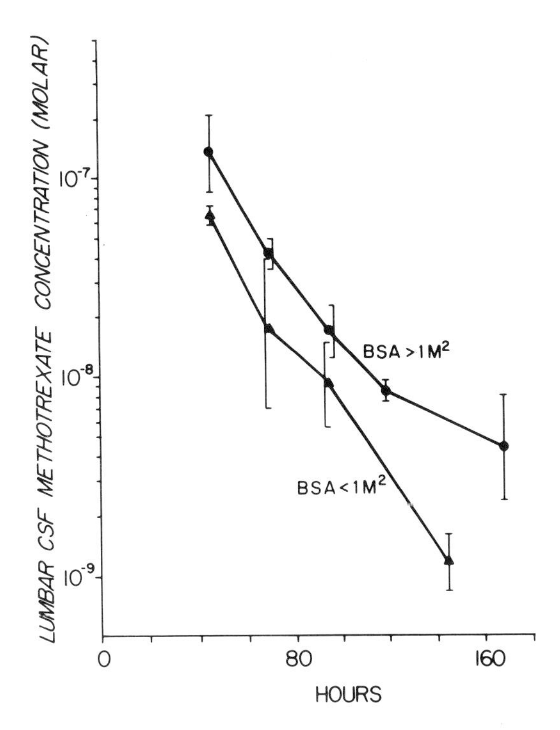

Fig. 5. Lumbar CSF MTX (geometric mean ± 1 SD) after intralumbar MTX, 12 mg/m^2 of body surface area (BSA).

in the CSF (5,6). These findings suggested that the neurotoxicity of IT MTX could be reduced by adjusting each patient's dosage relative to the concentration of the drug in his CSF. We applied this approach to 50 patients, increasing or decreasing the dosage depending on the drug level. Three of these patients (6%) had neurotoxic reactions, in comparison to 21 (38%) of the 56 patients treated similarly but without dosage modification during the two previous years ($p < .05$) (7). Of the three patients with neurotoxicity despite dosage modification, two had arachnoiditis with the first dose and one developed a reversible encephalopathy three months after induction therapy (8).

Another observation was that the lowest CSF MTX levels were observed in patients with the least therapeutic benefit from IT therapy (5). Two of the 3 patients with the lowest concentrations developed CNS leukemia within 1 month and the other patient failed to achieve remission from CNS leukemia. There seemed to be a difference of approximately one log between ineffective levels and potentially toxic concentrations of the drug in CSF (5).

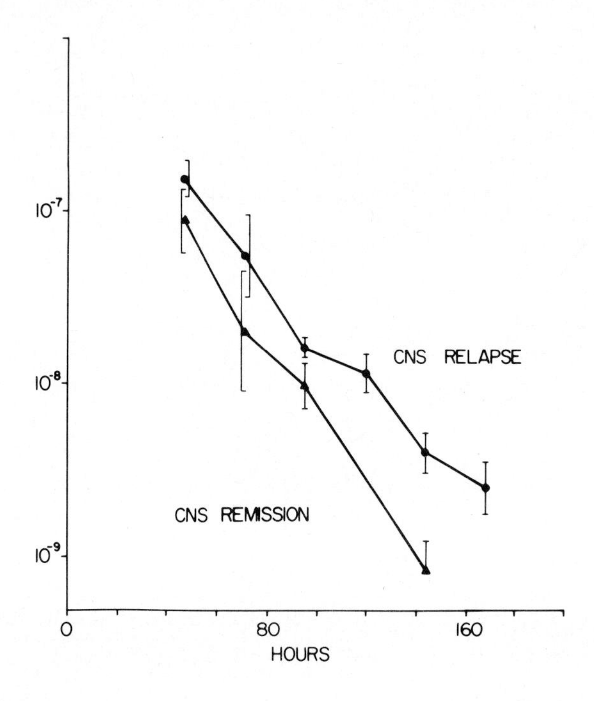

Fig. 6. Lumbar CSF MTX (geometric mean ± 1 SD) after intralumbar MTX, 12 mg/m^2.

Improved anti-leukemia therapy with intraventricular administration. Although primarily characterized by meningeal involvement, CNS leukemia not infrequently invades the ventricular compartment. We found leukemia cells in 7 of 9 ventricular CSF samples obtained at the time of Ommaya reservoir surgery (3). Because of this observation and the apparent pharmacologic advantages of direct intraventricular administration, we began using the Ommaya reservoir routinely for overt CNS leukemia. Ten patients had a previous CNS relapse treated with intralumbar MTX which could be compared with a subsequent relapse treated with intraventricular MTX. Seven patients had a longer, and one a shorter, CNS remission with intraventricular MTX ($p < .05$) (9). The CNS relapse rate per 1000 patient days at risk was 3.02 with intralumbar therapy and less than 1.02 with intraventricular therapy.

Diminished neurotoxicity of intraventricular MTX with a fractionated dosage schedule. Unfortunately, intraventricular MTX, 12 mg/m^2, appears to be excessively neurotoxic (11). Nineteen patients undergoing intraventricular MTX therapy

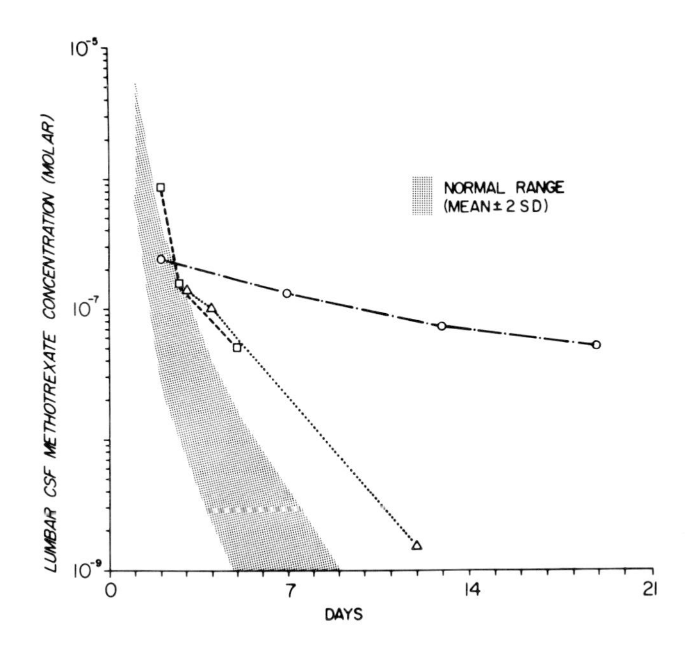

Fig. 7. Lumbar CSF MTX concentrations in three patients with communicating hydrocephalus (○—— - ——○, △................△, □--------------□).

for CNS leukemia were randomized to receive either standard-dose single injections of MTX, 12 mg/m^2, or a low-dose fractionated schedule of 1 mg q 12 h x 6 (12). The mean (± 1 SD) cumulative MTX dose was 149 (± 47) mg/m^2 in the standard-dose group and 54 (± 42) mg/m^2 in the low-dose group ($p < .005$). Neurotoxicity during remission occurred in 7 of 10 patients in the standard-dose group and in 1 of 8 patients in the low-dose group ($p < .05$). These results suggest that the fractionated dosage schedule is equally effective against CNS leukemia with less MTX and with a lower risk of toxicity. Whether a lower single dose (e.g. 6 mg) would have the same effect is under study.

Intravenous administration. We have also explored the possibility of replacing IT chemotherapy with effective systemic therapy. Our approach was to infuse large amounts of MTX intravenously at a rate sufficient to overcome those processes which ordinarily limit the penetration of MTX into the CNS, and to use delayed citrovorum factor rescue to prevent excessive systemic toxicity. A relatively constant plasma drug level was maintained for 42 hours, after which citrovorum fac-

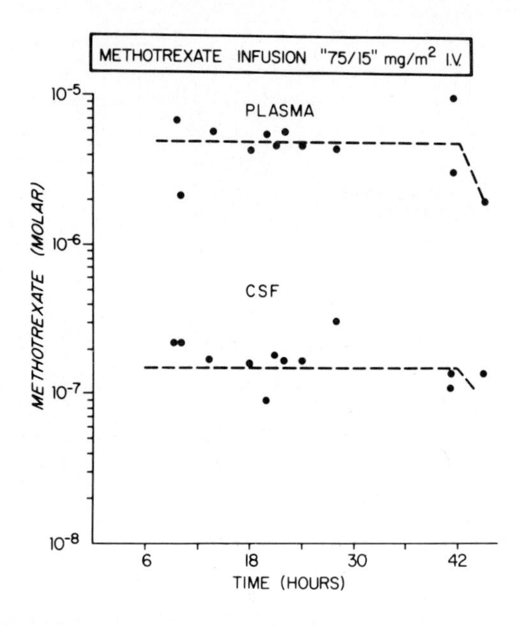

Fig. 8. Plasma and CSF MTX concentrations in 10 patients treated with the "75/15" mg/m^2 high-dose intravenous MTX regimen.

tor rescue was initiated. A 1-h priming intravenous infusion was administered at a dose (mg/m^2) of 1.5 x 10^{-7} times the desired plasma MTX concentration, in M/1, followed immediately by a 41-h maintenance infusion at an hourly rate of one-fifth the priming dose. For example, a plasma MTX level of 5 x 10^{-6} M required a dose of "75/15" mg/m^2, the "75" referring to the priming dose and the "15" to the hourly maintenance dose. Twelve simultaneous CSF and plasma MTX levels in 10 patients treated with such a regimen are depicted in Fig. 8. Note that both CSF and plasma levels were relatively constant after the first 8 hours of the infusions, and that the mean CSF:plasma drug ratio was 1:33.

Subsequent groups of patients were treated at higher doses by doubling the priming and maintenance doses to 150/30, 300/60 and 600/120 mg/m^2. The results of 56 infusions in 26 patients are shown in Fig. 9. The mean CSF:plasma MTX ratio was 1:32.7. CSF MTX was linearly proportional to plasma MTX over a 100-fold range of plasma drug concentrations (10^{-6} to 10^{-4} M). In two patients, the dose was escalated serially at two to three week intervals. The steady-state CSF: plasma determinations in these patients are depicted in Fig. 10. The results show that individual patients demonstrate the same CSF:plasma drug relationships ob-

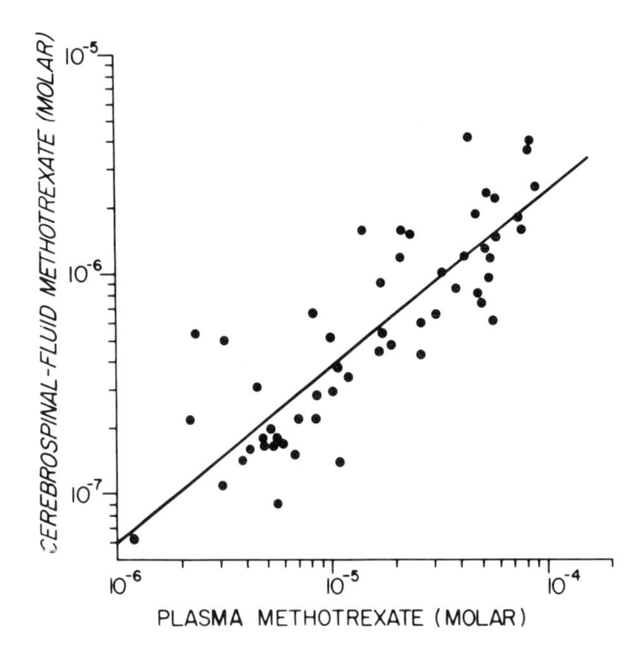

Fig. 9. "Steady-state" CSF vs. plasma MTX concentrations in 26 patients treated with intravenous MTX administered by constant infusion (N=56; r=0.85, $p < 0.01$).

served in the composite group. Whether these relationships occur at higher plasma drug concentrations ($> 10^{-4}$ M) is under study.

Of the 56 CSF determinations in the composite group, 19 were ventricular samples obtained via indwelling Ommaya reservoirs and 37 were lumbar samples. The mean CSF:plasma ratio was 1:33.2 for the ventricular specimens and 1:32.5 for the lumbar samples, indicating no differences between the two sampling sites.

DISCUSSION

The assay used in these studies measures dihydrofolate-reductase inhibition activity. At the concentrations of MTX measured it does not detect citrovorum factor, N^{10}-methyl folic acid, 7-hydroxy MTX or 2,4-diamino-N^{10}-methyl pteroic acid (13). Additionally, there is no evidence that MTX is metabolized within the CNS (14). Hence, the studies reported here should reflect the actual distribution of MTX within the human CNS.

Several studies were summarized. First, the pharmacokinetics of intralumbar

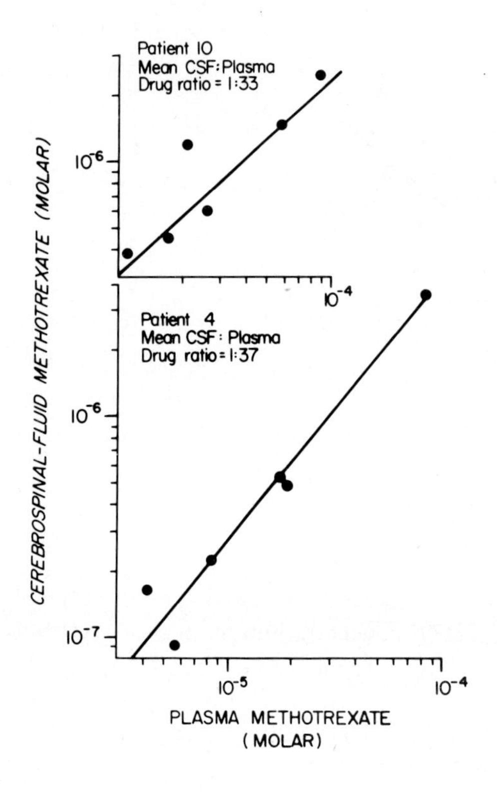

Fig. 10. CSF vs. plasma MTX concentrations in 2 patients treated at varying plasma antifolate levels. (Patient 10: N=6, r= 0.94, $p < 0.01$; patient 4: N=6, r= 0.99, $p < 0.01$).

MTX was assessed in patients who were treated prophylactically and did not develop therapy-related neurologic toxicity. The results of this group is thought to represent the "normal" pharmacology of IT MTX in asymptomatic patients. They demonstrate that disappearance of MTX from lumbar CSF is normally affected by several different physiologic processes and anatomic compartments. A triphasic disappearance curve (the intermediate and terminal phases were shown in Fig. 1) suggests a minimum of three compartments. The initial phase occurs during the first 3 hours and probably represents bulk flow distribution within subarachnoid CSF, and to some extent within ventricular CSF. The limited entry of MTX into the cerebral ventricles after subarachnoid injection was previously demonstrated by Shapiro and his associates (5). Our studies confirm this finding and indicate that under conditions of normal CSF dynamics, ventricular MTX levels average less than 10% of subarachnoid levels. The fact that plasma MTX peaks about 3 hours after injection (Fig. 1) indicates that those processes which remove MTX from the CNS are also operant during the initial phase.

The next phase is manifest between 4 and 36 hours. It has a volume of distribution approximating the extracellular fluid volume of the CNS and presumably reflects distribution within the extracellular fluid of the brain and spinal cord, as well as translocation of drug across the CSF-blood interfaces. The terminal phase (48-96 h) has a long half-life (14 h) and probably represents the net effect of multiple processes, including back-diffusion of drug from brain parenchyma into CSF and translocation across the brain-blood barrier. The respective CSF clearance rates of 1.2 and 13 ml/m^2/min are more rapid than the rate of CSF production (approximately 0.4 ml/min) and suggests that bulk-flow reabsorption of CSF accounts for only a portion of MTX removal from CSF. The extent to which total CSF clearance may be determined by active transport processes is under study.

A subsequent study showed that plasma MTX is prolonged by IT administration when compared to systemic administration of the same dose (Fig. 2). This difference can be attributed to a reservoir effect of the CNS compartment(s). Since 10^{-8} M is toxic to human bone marrow (15), the persistence of plasma MTX after IT administration suggests that IT MTX is, mg for mg, potentially more toxic to systemic target organs. An example of this effect may have been observed in one of the patients we studied who developed fatal interstitial pneumonitis during IT MTX therapy (16). It suggests that IT MTX cannot be given without concern for systemic effects and that frequent IT MTX therapy may require a systemically administered methotrexate-neutralizing drug, preferably one which does not enter the CNS (e.g. carboxypeptidase-G_1).

A search for factors which may influence CSF MTX concentrations identified several conditions which appear to alter the disappearance kinetics. Severe communicating hydrocephalus had the most dramatic effect on retarding clearance of MTX from the CSF (Fig. 7), suggesting that normal CSF production and resorption is essential for normal MTX clearance. Active CNS leukemia (as defined by the presence of leukemia cells in the CSF) and low CSF pressure (lumbar puncture syndrome) also were associated with delayed clearance although to lesser degree. Although clinical neurotoxicity was also correlated with elevated CSF MTX concentration, the mechanism of action of MTX-induced neurologic dysfunction is not understood.

The correlation of CSF MTX concentration with patient age appears to be due, at least in part, to relative differences in the initial volume of distribution and body surface area upon which dosage was based. CNS volume approaches the adult level years before body growth ceases (4). Consistent with this explanation is the observation that the initial volume of distribution approximates the extracellular-fluid volume of the CNS. When CSF drug levels were adjusted retrospectively for differences in CNS volume, the variability in CSF MTX concentrations was reduced (5). When studied prospectively, a constant dose (12 mg) produced more consistent CSF MTX levels than a surface-area derived dose (12 mg/m^2) (5). The latter observation suggests that variability in CSF drug concentration can be significantly decreased in patients between 3 and 40 years (the age range studied) if they receive the same IT dose rather than varying doses adjusted for body surface area.

In children with overt CNS leukemia who served as their own controls, intraventricular administration was shown to be superior to lumbar injection. Shapiro *et al.* obtained similar results in nine children with meningeal leukemia (10). These results confirm that intraventricular chemotherapy is significantly more effective against overt CNS leukemia than the same therapy given by lumbar puncture.

The kinetics of translocation across the "blood-brain barrier", in terms of entry into CSF after high-dose intravenous infusion, were also studied. The results show that the CSF:plasma drug ratio, at steady-state, is independent of plasma MTX concentration up to 10^{-4} M, and that a specified CSF antifolate level below 10^{-5} M can in general be achieved with a 33-fold greater plasma drug level. The similarity in ventricular and lumbar MTX levels with intravenous infusions suggests that systemic therapy also has the advantage of providing consistent drug concentrations throughout the CSF axis. Whether high-dose intravenous therapy can provide higher CNS parenchymal levels than IT administration requires further study. If the "blood-brain barrier" can be overcome, IT chemotherapy could eventually be replaced by systemic drug therapy. This objective may be facilitated either by altering the "blood-brain barrier" such that more drug enters the CNS, as for example by simultaneous intracarotid hyperosmolar mannitol (17) or by pretreatment with microwave (18) or X-irradiation (19), or by inhibiting the drug's exit from the CNS. Since MTX appears to be partially removed from the CNS by bulk flow reabsorption of CSF, inhibitors of CSF production (acetazolamide, digitalis, ouabain, isosorbide, etc.) may help trap the drug in the CNS. To the extent that MTX is actively transported out of the CSF, probenicid or other competitors for the transport carrier may have the same effect (20). These possibilities should first be tested in an animal model, preferably one that resembles the physiologic and pharmacokinetic characteristics in man.

REFERENCES

1. Bleyer, W.A. and Dedrick, R.L. (1977) Cancer Treat. Rep., 61, 703-708.
2. Jacobs, S.A., et al. (1975) Lancet, I, 455-456.
3. Bleyer, W.A., et al. (1975) N. Engl. J. Med., 293, 1152.
4. Shapiro, W.R. (1975) N. Engl. J. Med., 239, 161-166.
5. Bleyer, W.A. (1977) Cancer Treat. Rep., 61, 1419-1425.
6. Bleyer, W.A., et al. (1973) N. Engl. J. Med., 289, 770-773.
7. Bleyer, W.A. (1977) Natl. Cancer Inst. Monogr., 46, 171-178.
8. Pizzo, P.A., et al. (1976) J. Pediat. 88, 131-133.
9. Bleyer, W.A. and Poplack, D.G. (1977) Proc. Amer. Assoc. Cancer Res. 18, 103.
10. Shapiro, W.R. (1977) Cancer Treat. Rep. 61, 733-744.
11. Bleyer, W.A. et al. (1976) Proc. Am. Assoc. Canc. Res. & Am. Soc. Clin. Onc., 17, 253.
12. Bleyer, W.A., et al. (1978) Blood 51:835-842.
13. Donehower, R., et al. (1978) Proc. Amer. Assoc. Cancer Res., 19, 172.
14. Kimelberg, H.K., et al. (1977) Cancer Res., 37, 157-165.
15. Young, R.C. and Chabner, B.A. (1973) J. Clin. Invest., 52, 92a.
16. Gutin, P.H., et al. (1976) Cancer, 38, 1529-1534.
17. Allen, J.C., et al. (1978) Neurology, 28, 351.
18. Chang, B.K. and Huang, A.T. (1976) Amer. Soc. Hemat. 19th Ann. Mtg. Abst. #107.
19. Griffin, T.W., et al. (1977) Cancer, 40, 1109-1111.
20. Domer, F.R. and Kaiser, L.R. (1977) Arch. Int. Pharmacodyn., 225, 17-24.

Clinical Pharmacology of Anti-Neoplastic Drugs
H. M. Pinedo, editor

Summary of discussions on the papers presented on methotrexate

ASSAYS (papers Bertino, Wilkinson, Hande)

Radioassay: the methotrexate metabolite DAMPA (2,4-diamino-N-methyl pteroic acid) is a contaminant of the commercial kits and the commercial preparations. It probably accounts for 2 to 3% of what is given to patients as methotrexate. The greater deviations (Fig. 2, Hande) from the expected graph for methotrexate plasma concentrations after 48 h, as compared to those after 24 h infusions, may be explained by either

1) an increase in DAMPA formation with time or
2) a lower rate of excretion of DAMPA by the kidney, relative to the parent drug.

Significant differences can also be found with respect to the animal species generating antibody. This may well be the reason for the slight differences between Bertino's and Hande's results. There is no difference between the use of [^{125}I]- or [^{131}I]- labelled antibody.

False high values of methotrexate will be measured in patients treated with carboxypeptidase (the enzyme which catalyses the conversion of methotrexate to DAMPA) in cases where methotrexate is assayed by the radioimmunoassay, since both the parent drug and its metabolites are measured with this method.

COMPARTMENT MODELS (papers Lankelma, Wilkinson)

Based on calculations according to the method as presented, Lankelma concluded that the peripheral compartment has a smaller volume than the central compartment. On the contrary, Wilkinson, applying accepted equations, found a much higher value (100 litres) for the volume of the peripheral compartment. This figure is close to published data.
This discrepancy could not be explained.

TOXICITY (papers Bertino, Lankelma, Wilkinson, Hande)

Patients can tolerate infusions with high doses quite well up to 42 h. If infusions are continued longer than 48 h toxicity becomes irreversible.
However, even with precautions like hydration and alkalinisation, there is still a small segment of the patients who develop renal toxicity. Some patients with myelosuppression, however, do not show renal toxicity. These differences without any difference in filtration rate (creatinine clearance) may be caused - as some studies indicate - by methotrexate not only being filtered but also being secreted.

The 7-hydroxy-metabolite, detectable with HPLC, may compete with methotrexate for uptake into the cell. As it can thus influence methotrexate toxicity, induction of 7-hydroxy-methotrexate formation in the patient may reduce toxicity.
The 7-OH methotrexate was found in the various drug regimens, also with low dose methotrexate. It has also been detected in the CSF.

REVERSAL OF TOXICITY (papers Leyva/Pinedo, Harrap, Canellos and Schornagel/ Pinedo)
In the *in vitro* experiments the drug and the reversal agents were added simultaneously. Sequential exposure of the cells is not very well possible with the semisolid cell culture medium used. It is also not possible to expose the cells prior to culture as the plating efficiency of the CFU-C decreases too rapidly when the cells are kept in suspension during incubation with methotrexate.

A difference of thymidine toxicity to CFU-C and L1210 cells may be due to their different thymidine kinase levels. This is difficult to confirm as enzyme studies are not easily performed with CFU-C, and fresh bone marrow consists of a nonhomogenous cell population.
It is unlikely that cell death in the initial phase of cell culture, which is higher for CFU-C causes a significant increase in the concentration of nucleosides. The cells are rescued at a high concentration (10^{-5} M); consumption of the added nucleosides has not been measured after rescue.

If, in the future patients can, on a routine basis, be rescued from methotrexate toxicity with nucleosides, the achievement of selectivity will probably depend on the clinical situation. It was thought that, when methotrexate would be used to treat lymphatic leukemia, this would lead to release of nucleosides because of the massive cell kill; hyperuricemia in this situation is observed. Obviously, this kind of effect of methotrexate is not anticipated in osteosarcoma. However, in leukemia patients on methotrexate, purine levels are below the level of sensitivity of the assay method. In the mouse the purine plasma levels are also low. The level of thymidine in plasma appears to be too low for rescue.

In the animal experiments a methotrexate-dose dependency of the antipyrimidine and the antipurine effects were confirmed. Low dose methotrexate yields an antipyrimidine effect, whereas a high dose results in an antipyrimidine and an antipurine effect as well.
A purine deficiency is tolerated by cells for a time period of 18 h, a pyrimidine deficiency for longer periods. However, rescue 24 h after administration of me-

thotrexate gives essentially the same result as rescue 12 h after the drug has been given.

GENERAL DISCUSSION ON METHOTREXATE, particularly on the use of high dose versus low dose methotrexate

Bertino

Summary of the papers that were presented on methotrexate:
There have been described four methods to assay methotrexate. The high pressure liquid chromatography (HPLC) method is new. It has some advantages in terms of rapidity and studying drug metabolism. We heard about the rescue of methotrexate in the experimental system both in tissue culture and *in vivo.* In general the L1210 has been used as a tumor model and the bone marrow as normal tissue to study methotrexate cytotoxicity. Both systems have their problems. One is that the mouse bone marrow data has to be extrapolated to the human bone marrow. There are new techniques to grow human marrow in experimental animals in chambers. It might be interesting to use these *in vivo* models as well. The L1210 system is, as we know, a highly experimental tumor with a very rapid growth and it is interesting to investigate other tumor tissues as well in terms of purine death and thymidine rescue by nucleosides. Both Dr. Pinedo and Dr. Harrap have pointed out the possibility that such differential rescue may be justified not only with thymidine but also with a combination of thymidine with a purine. This purine could be both hypoxanthine and inosine. It would be interesting to test this situation *in vivo* in man. Then, we come to the point of the pharmacology and the kinetics of high dose methotrexate. This brings us to the very important problem that has not been answered: what is the value of this high dose regimen? As we know high dose methotrexate is being used in industrial quantities and there are many private doctors in the U.S.A. who feel that their patients are not getting the best treatment possible because they are denied the use of high dose methotrexate, and if they want to use high dose methotrexate they have to resort to the use of 50 mg vials which contain preservatives and are tremendously expensive. We estimated for example one time that it would cost a couple of thousand dollars to treat a patient with high dose methotrexate in the U.S.A. In addition,the drug has to be monitored carefully and it costs money to assay, the serum level of the drug. Moreover, it takes much of the nurses time. There is another very pertinent question to ask: in what disease state is high dose methotrexate really justified? Is it an experimental model of treatment? When is it experimental and when is it really good clinical practice?
Bertino opened the discussion about high dose methotrexate versus low dose methotrexate.

ACUTE LYMPHATIC LEUKAEMIA (Bertino, Canellos, Hande, Harrap, Van Putten)

If it is accepted that all that is needed is, that methotrexate inhibit the enzyme dehydrofolate reductase in human cells containing this enzyme, then why not use this in the leukemias as major test parameter to see whether inhibition is achieved with the low dose or not. If not so, see whether the high dose is effectively inhibiting the enzyme.
This is something that has not been extensively investigated. Only some limited data are available in that regard. The leukemias would be suitable to use for such a study. The intracellular concentration of methotrexate should be measured in relation to the concentration of the reductase and in relation to the Ki of that enzyme. The affinity of the enzyme for methotrexate can vary from one cell to the other and this affinity has been determined to be the major cause of the sensitivity of the cell. However, it might be simplier than that. All that would have to be done really, is to measure the free methotrexate in the cell and if it is in excess of dihydrofolate reductase, it is probable that the cell's DNA synthesis has been inhibited.
This will only work if the population of cells is homogeneous. But if there is say one percent resistant cells and the average concentration of methotrexate in all cells is measured, this very important group of cells would go unnoticed.

In acute lymphocytic leukemia one of the major advantages of high dose methotrexate is that methotrexate does get into the cerebrospinal fluid and maybe in other sanctuaries, such as testicular sanctuaries, which have never been measured. Secondly, it is clear from some studies in patients who are resistant to conventional doses of methotrexate, that high dose methotrexate really works. So far high dose methotrexate has not been used routinely in the management of ALL.
The common practice in the U.S.A. is to use the St. Judes regimen or one of its variations in which induction is performed with vincristine and prednisone. A brain radiation program with intrathecal methotrexate is followed by treatment with conventional doses of methotrexate in combination with 6-mercaptopurine. Some studies, such as the one at Roswell Memorial Park, are going on with high dose methotrexate plus intrathecal methotrexate, instead of whole brain radiation therapy. In the Roswell Park study the intracerebral calcifications that have been described in patients treated with whole brain radiation plus intrathecal methotrexate are not seen. Secondly, the long term survivors of the St. Judes type regimen have learning disabilities. The programs which do not use whole brain radiation therapy, may not cause that kind of problem.

What the long term complications may be in terms of brain tumors with radiation plus intrathecal methotrexate is another area. What will happen in a few years from now if the incidence of gliomas in these children suddenly starts rising? Now is probably the time to do a prospective trial comparing high dose methotrexate alone versus intrathecal methotrexate plus cranial radiation.
The usual dose of methotrexate for this purpose is 500 mg/m^2 over 24 hours and patients are rescued 36 or 48 hours later with a minimal dose of leucovorin. It is not a very toxic regimen. About 500 mg/m^2 is needed to obtain a minimal sufficient concentration of 10^{-7} M in the CSF. It is agreed that the comparative study needs to be done in ALL.
Another point is, that high dose methotrexate in certain cases of ALL is more effective than low dose methotrexate. High dose methotrexate is effective in many patients who are or have become resistant to conventional doses. There is some reason to believe that at least moderately high doses of methotrexate are useful in this disease over and above the conventional way of administering methotrexate.

Methotrexate followed by asparaginase is a unique drug combination. Capizzi studied this combination and his results have now been verified in various other centers. It is a unique combination because asparaginase not only rescues normal tissues from methotrexate toxicity, but it in fact kills leukemia cells in addition. So, there is a double kill in the leukemia cell population and a rescue of normal cells from methotrexate toxicity as well.
The mechanism is not known except for the fact that asparaginase inhibits protein synthesis and might thus be putting the normal cells out of cycle so that there is a peak in the G1 phase where the cells are not affected by methotrexate.
In some of the other studies that were done with the methotrexate-asparaginase program many of the patients who were previously treated with asparaginase were responsive to asparaginase itself, and so one of the possibilities is that there is actually no additive effect of the methotrexate.
This might be an answer to the question as to how methotrexate could work if the tumour cells are also being set out of cycle and are not synthesizing DNA.
However, many responses were long term, which would be very unusual for asparaginase alone.
The explanation of the favourable working of the asparaginase-methotrexate combination is certainly much more complicated.
Asparaginase rescues only partially; the kinds of doses of methotrexate that can be ad-

ministered with leucovorin or thymidine cannot be given. Most patients tolerate up to 600 mg/m^2, maybe a little higher, but with higher doses one starts to get toxicity due to methotrexate. The schedule is an every-10 day schedule. One of the remarkable things about the first 11 patients treated at Yale was that all patients were resistant to conventional doses of methotrexate, yet 9/11 had a complete remission with this programme. Some patients had even been given asparaginase before. The programme deserves to be considered earlier in the treatment of ALL as well.

LYMPHOMA (Bertino, Canellos, Colvin, Hande, Schein, Smyth, Wilkinson)

The other tumor group in which high dose methotrexate has some value is the lymphoma group.

Many years ago Djerassi showed that a childhood lymphoma was at least responsive to high dose methotrexate. He was able to obtain very significant responses in a few patients and transient responses have been seen in a few patients recently. At the Sidney Farber Cancer Institute studies with high dose methotrexate in lymphoma indicate that perhaps antimetabolites, especially methotrexate, have a role in the treatment of diffuse histiocytic lymphoma and perhaps in other bad histologies as well.

Canellos:

These were all patients who had failed on their previous therapies. High dose methotrexate was used in this population of poorly differentiated lymphocytic and histiocytic lymphoma. Twenty-two patients have been treated and 2/3 had some response. It is a transient response that is seen, but again, the patients have been resistant to everything else and had very proliferative lesions at the time of treatment. It can even be a dramatic response in this patient population, but it lasts only 1-3 months. The tumors have the tendency to become resistant very quickly. We are focusing on patients referred to us who have failed all the other conventional drugs.

We really don't advocate high dose methotrexate as standard therapy. The schedule used for that population the lymphoma group is an i.v. push of methotrexate with rescue at 24 hours. Most patients object to the bicarbonate, which they hate. Hydration is no problem. The methotrexate itself is almost no problem. The patients have transient nausea and vomiting. Most patients were adequately rescued. The spinal fluid concentrations of methotrexate at 24 hours hover in an area that is cytotoxic and is adequate for the very sensitive cell populations, certainly for tumor cells floating in the spinal fluid. In our group of 22 patients, 8 had positive spinal fluid cytology, clinical manifestations of CNS involvement and high CSF protein levels. Again, the response to methotrexate as a single agent and without any other CNS drugs, in this group of patients pretreated with radiation etc., was quite impressive. We saw complete regressions. There was a partial clearing of the spinal fluid and space occupying lesions regressed.

The best case was a patient with a very rare disease; primary histiocytic lymphoma of the brain was the second location. She had a posterior fossa tumor before, which was resected, followed by radiotherapy (4500 rad) of the skull. She relapsed shortly afterwards and developed a large frontal tumor. She was not a renal transplant patient;

usually this disease, which is actually a tumor of the microglial system, is seen in renal transplants. She had not had a disease that would indicate that she had a high predilection. She got the treatment and remains free of disease at the moment with a Cat-scan which has returned to normal on high dose methotrexate alone.
Initially, she was treated weekly with methotrexate. After a while the treatment was stretched out to every 3 weeks. We have seen her recently and she is in good shape. We just stopped the methotrexate treatment. This is a disease that has a high incidence of multifocality; so she will probably have a new lesion somewhere else.

Methotrexate used with other cytotoxic drugs can cause serious toxicity when patients have been treated previously, especially with radiation to the pelvis. Currently we are treating lymphomas with a very busy program called MBCOD, which includes many drugs, among them methotrexate given on day 14. This is an attempt to give the drug at a time when the bone marrow is covered by other drugs and when other cytostatic drugs which are toxic to the bone marrow cannot be given.
Previously we appreciated the recurrences between the cycles, and Dr. Schein will remember well in the BACOP program in Bethesda where we used bleomycin and prednisone at that phase of the chemotherapy to try to arrest the regrowth of lymphoma between cycles.
Here we used methotrexate because
a) we felt the drug has some activity and
b) we could rescue from toxic side effects.
And then we start chemotherapy again on day 21. The patients receive 10 cycles. We have only so treated previously untreated patients. We are almost religious about giving methotrexate on day 14 to try to overcome the kinetic situation with presumably recurring lymphoma. This is an on-going trial. We really have not had any serious problems. We give the methotrexate with a platelet level of 30.000/mm^3 and with a blood count of 500/mm^3. When the patients have had heavy previous therapy, then one may meet with trouble.

It was stressed that lymphomas become almost immediately resistant to high dose methotrexate. One has to tighten and tighten the doses, maybe to an every 5-day administration, because by day 7 the lumps reappear. This is a very important, though disappointing, observation in the face that one of the major justifications for giving high doses of methotrexate had been to overcome either transport resistance or induced high levels of dihydrofolate reductase. Biopsies to assay the tumor tissue for dihydrofolate reductase before and after were not taken. Since if one is looking for resistant cell populations, only serial biopsies of this tumor will be of value.

Bertino:

We have to remember though, that we are dealing with far advanced disease in these circumstances where there is a high tumor burden. Kinetically, this stage of disease is unfavourable for methotrexate because plateau phase disease is being treated. Actually, it can be shown very nicely in the L1210 system that even with high concentrations of methotrexate once plateau phase disease is treated, the drug is fairly ineffective. That is the reason why we treat with methotrexate as part of the second cycle. We also have a second generation program called ACOMA now, which consists of adriamycin plus cyclophosphamide in the first part of the cycle; the second part of the cycle has high dose methotrexate plus Ara-C. Again, this seems to be working quite well. The frequency of CNS relapse is very high in these poor histology lymphomas, maybe as high as 30%. It is interesting that the COMA program of Ultman and our data show very few CNS relapses. It could be that not only methotrexate but also Ara-C is preventing CNS relapses. Thus, this is an area where maybe high dose methotrexate has some value and probably should be considered more seriously in the programs.

In regard to the effectiveness of intrathecal methotrexate, most patients have very good control of their CNS histiocytic lymphoma with just intrathecal drug, and usually CNS relapse is not the cause of death. The predominant factor is bone marrow involvement. Maybe these bone marrow positive patients are the high risk ones. High dose methotrexate is very effective when given intrathecally in terms of clearing the cells and controlling the CNS symptoms.

OSTEOSARCOMA, SOFT TISSUE SARCOMA (Bertino, Canellos, Cleton, Colvin, Hande, Pinedo, Van der Kleijn, Wilkinson, Schein)

Wilkinson has a limited experience with treating osteogenic sarcoma. No difference in response was found between high dose methotrexate and conventional doses of the drug. Actually, high dose methotrexate did not appear to be effective in advanced osteogenic sarcoma. It has been applied in 10 patients. Similar results were obtained in soft tissue sarcoma.
Isakow recently presented data on high dose methotrexate in soft tissue sarcoma. Only the rhabdomyosarcoma seemed to respond well.
Wilkshaw published her recent results with conventional doses of methotrexate in patients with soft tissue sarcoma. She found a high response rate in sarcomas in general, but again, particularly in rhabdomyosarcoma. So, a study of high dose versus low dose methotrexate seems to be worthwhile. Historical controls of osteogenic sarcoma did not show responses to low dose methotrexate either.
In the adult (over 16 years) population Canellos did not find high dose methotrexate terribly useful for metastatized osteogenic sarcoma. One out of 9 patients had a good response. Fifty-three protocols including high dose methotrexate are registered at the NCI. There is not one study comparing low or moderate doses to high dose. This should be done in the advanced disease. One of the problems with which we are faced in the advanced situation is that some reports are very positive for the use of high dose methotrexate as an adjuvant, and it is very difficult for physicians to enter now their patients in a trial which has one arm with no-treatment. The Mayo Clinic is doing such a trial.
If such a study is performed in patients with advanced disease there is always the argument that kinetically different models are being treated and that high dose methotrexate may be useful in situations with low tumor burden where more cells are in log-phase, while it may not be useful in advanced disease.
If done in the advanced situation with no success, it may never be able to do it in the situation where it might work.

The data of Jaffe have been obtained in a pediatric population. Basically there are now about 40 patients at risk. When the data were reported, they were reported as free of disease. This does not mean that the patients have not developed pulmonary metastases. A patient may have had a resection of a metastasis and is still included in this group of disease-free patients. Thus, there is a large group, now close to about 56%, achieving disease-free, metastasis-free survival. But again, when they appear with pulmonary metastases they are having them resected. What is being done in this childhood population, which tends to have a very aggressive disease, is that the first phase of pulmonary metastases is probably being eliminated or somehow affected and fewer pulmonary metastases and slower growing ones are being seen. A kinetically different population is selected out. The children are not dying of what they used to.

The other kind of positive feeling we have about osteogenic sarcoma comes from the data observed with pretreatment of patients with high dose methotrexate before surgery. At the Farber Institute definite tumor regressions have been observed; the follow-up for many of these patients is, however, short. The Memorial group has pretreated 20 patients with a combination of drugs including high dose methotrexate; 16 out of these patients appeared to have histology free disease at surgery. You may even do local resections on those patients.

As far as a positive study is concerned, the St. Judes appears to be borderline. There are other studies, like the NCI study, which are not at all confirmatory. However, the mean age of the NCI patients was 18 years; so, a little older population may make a difference.

The pediatricians in the Netherlands' Cancer Institute have treated 20, all very young, patients with postoperative radiotherapy on the lungs. They report a 60-70% 4 year survival without any adjuvant chemotherapy. Most of the metastases appear within the first two years. In untreated patients there seems to be a burst in metastases in this period. Later on, these are not seen any more.

One of the very positive things that the methotrexate report of Jaffe does is to point our attention to the variability in osteogenic sarcoma. Nobody would have bothered to look for prognostic factors unless there was some provocative report like Jaffe's. He has clearly shown that his treatment has delayed metastases and has changed the biology of the disease to a certain extent. Whether ultimately all these patients will be cured is difficult to tell. There will be a long time to wait for late appearing metastases that are not accounted for yet, because the biology of the disease has changed.

The patients all died in the past, about 80% usually within a year. The Mayo Clinic's historical experience has been a little bit variable. Their best 5-year segment was 40% survival indeed. But their worst is clearly worse than that; the pattern of referral to the Mayo Clinic may vary from time to time. Jaffe's historical experience has been very bad (20% survival) with very few long term survivals. Except for the Mayo Clinic, no one has had a historical experience much better than 20%.

MD Anderson first reported their entire historical experience with osteogenic sarcoma up to the point where they start using the adjuvant protocol called CONPADRI. The long term surgical cure was 20%. So, the biology of the tumor may be changing and time will have to pass before we can talk about cures. The biology may have changed with methotrexate as well.

The drug is being administered in different ways. Essentially, there are two ways of administering the drug, either by push or by infusion for some period of time. Now, for the drug to reach a tissue which is poorly perfused it would seem likely that infusion would be the best way to administer the drug. There are more than 50 protocols, but not any data to favor one regimen over another.
Ideally, one wants to reach a maximum exposure of the tumor cells. The maximum tolerable time is probably 36 to 48 hours. Beyond this, toxicity becomes irreversible. In brain tumors this maximum exposure time is being tested. It is known that dihydrofolate reductase is present in brain tumors, which was not thought to be the case in the past. Whether or not methotrexate in high doses for prolonged periods of time, maybe even longer than 42 hours when using carboxypeptidase to rescue general toxicity, will work is still not known.
The best way of administering the drug may depend entirely on the tumor in question. If it is a rapidly proliferating tumor, like diffuse histiocytic lymphoma, perhaps once a week is the way to give methotrexate. In that case the interval between drug and rescue may have to be decreased to 24 hours. That is what is done in the second phase of treatment of diffuse histiocytic lymphoma. In the case of head and neck cancer perhaps the one-gram infusion over 36 hours + rescue is good.
With a bolus a good plasma level cannot be maintained. A considerable amount of drug would be already lost during the first phase. Thus, four or five times the amount of drug infused, would have to be injected. "Economics" favor the infusion of high dose methotrexate over the administration of a bolus.

PART II: FLUOROPYRIMIDINES, ADRIAMYCINS, BLEOMYCIN, CYCLOPHOSPHAMIDE, NITROSUREAS, VINCA ALKALOIDS AND CIS-PLATINUM

© 1978 Elsevier/North-Holland Biomedical Press
Clinical Pharmacology of Anti-Neoplastic Drugs
H. M. Pinedo, editor

ASSAY OF 5-FLUOROURACIL

O.M.J. DRIESSEN, P.J.A. TIMMERMANS and D. DE VOS
Leiden University Medical Centre, Department of Pharmacology, Wassenaarseweg 72, 2333 AL Leyden, The Netherlands.

INTRODUCTION

The antimetabolite 5-fluorouracil (5-FU) has been in clinical use for about 20 years. Like of many other cytostatic agents, the dose-effect relationship is difficult to establish in the individual patient. The application in regimens of combinations with other cytostatic agents makes it even more difficult to define this relationship. There is a clear lack of knowledge of the pharmacokinetics of the drug; assays for the drug and its metabolites are being developed. The biological availability of 5-FU to the tumour varies from patient to patient. This can be ascribed to variable resorption after oral administration and also to huge first-pass effect. Therefore, intravenous administration of 5-FU has been advocated in recent years. Yet, it should be mentioned that oral administration of 5-FU can be effective and that routine determinations of 5-FU and its metabolites may lead to more adequate dose regimens for the individual patient. Two factors have hampered such routine application hitherto. Most important are the technical difficulties of a 5-FU assay. The second problem is the short half-life of 5-FU in plasma; it is rapidly transformed intracellularly into its true antineoplastic form. Besides 5-FU, metabolites as 5-fluorouridine, 5-fluorodeoxyuridine and alpha-fluoro-beta-alanine are important in the study of the pharmacokinetic profile of 5-FU in individual patients. In this contribution the assay of 5-fluorouracil with the aid of gas liquid chromotography will be outlined. Separation of drug and metabolites became possible through high performance liquid chromatography.

MATERIALS AND METHODS

Methods for the determination of 5-FU

5-Fluorouracil can be determined in plasma by the methods as referred to in Table 1.

We chose to develop a gas liquid chromatography (GLC) method, as such a method is rapid, fairly sensitive and practicable. For GLC analyses, 5-FU has to be deriva-

TABLE 1
ANALYTICAL METHODS

- Radioactivity measurements (1).
- Microbiological assay (2,3).
- Spectrophotometry (2,4).
- High performance liquid chromatography (5,6).
- Gas chromatography/mass spectrophotometry (7,8,9,10).
- Gas liquid chromatography (11,12,13).

tized, as the native compound is polar and hence separation from other plasma compounds on columns, which are not deactivated, would not very well be possible. Fig. 1 shows two derivatization reactions, in which the active nitrogens are shielded.

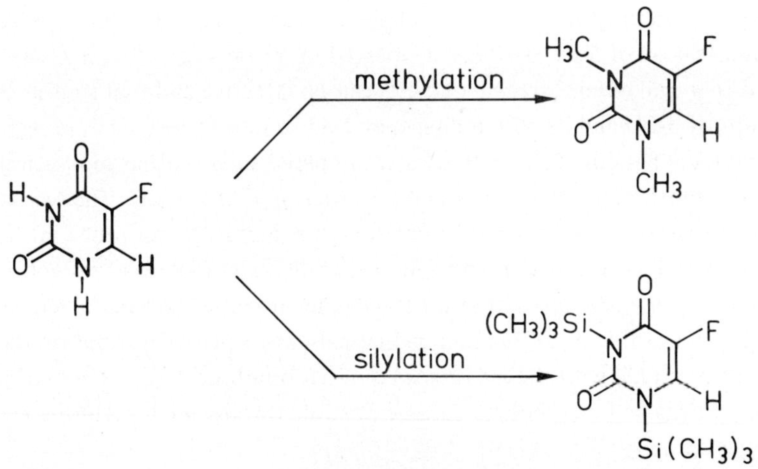

Fig.1. Derivatization reactions of 5-FU.

For many reasons we avoided derivatization, and wanted to determine the original compound. The importance of this approach became clear during the development of the method.

The assay of non-derivatized 5-FU; adherence of 5-FU to glass

Preparation of the column

Columns were deactivated to a level that would permit the determination of small quantities (nanograms) of 5-FU. This was performed by deactivation procedures of the glass column and its contents, lest active sites could not irreversibly adsorb 5-FU. Short columns were always used. We observed that 5-FU after evaporation of the solvent strongly adhered to the glass surface of the vials used. This was observed by GLC-measurements, as well as by measurements with radioactive 5-FU. This phenomenon, not described in the literature hitherto, may also influence the extraction and derivatization techniques as currently in use. Fig. 2 shows a calibration curve of 5-FU, together with the recoveries of the same standards after evaporation of the solvent from glass and from plastic vials.

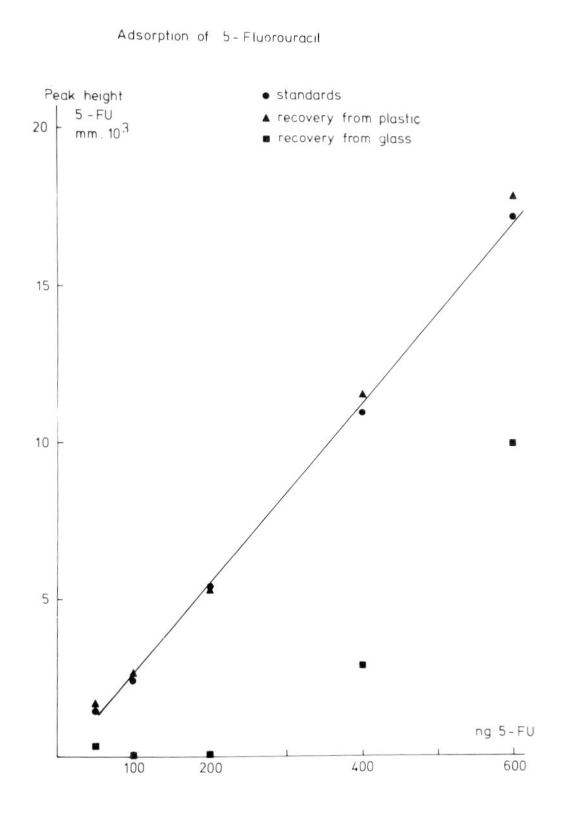

Fig. 2. Different behaviour of glass and plastic towards 5-FU.

Fig. 3 shows the recovery of samples of 5-FU in the range of 50 - 600 μg; 5-FU was dissolved in methanol, transferred into vials of different material, evaporated under nitrogen and redissolved in methanol.

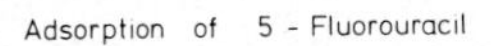

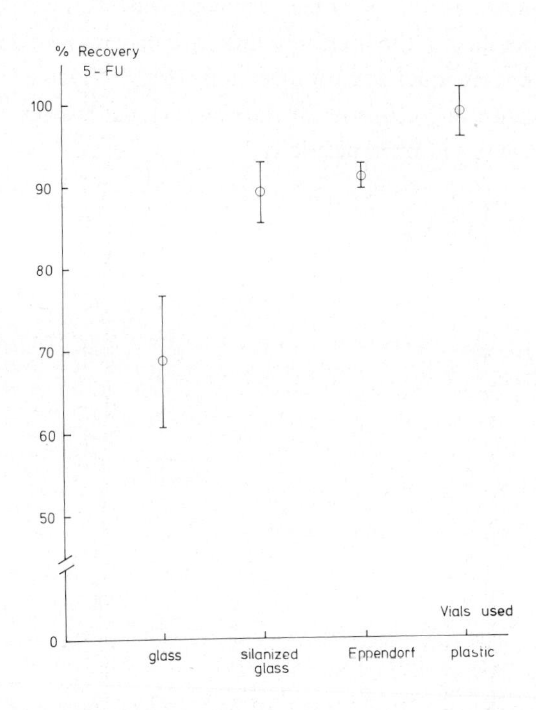

Fig. 3. Recovery of 5-FU from vials made of different material.

The recoveries from glass were always lower than from other materials, the standard deviation of the recoveries from glass was considerably larger than that for the other materials. We have no indications that 5-FU is adsorbed to a large extent by glass surfaces from solutions.

Technical details of the GLC-procedure
Equipment and material as used for GLC:

- a glass column 0,45 m x 0,8 mm I.D.
- 3% Versamid 930 as adsorbent
- Gaschrom Q (140 - 160 μ) as column support material
- 5-chlorouracil as internal standard
- a solid phase injector
- a nitrogen and phosphorus sensitive detection system.

Measures taken to prepare inert GLC columns:

- the silanization of glassware
- resilanization of the column support material Gaschrom Q
- deactivation of the glass column with 1% Carbowax 20 m dissolved in methanol
- the use of micropacked 3% Versamid as adsorbent.

Column technique: the support material is sifted carefully and the batch of 140 - 160 microns is resilanized afterwards. With the coated support a short micropacked column is prepared. As we do not need the full separation capacity of the column, the column is only packed to one half or one third of the length with the coated support material. The column is never sealed with glass wool; if necessary, a small glass plug is used instead.
Injection technique: a solid phase injection system is used. The injection side of the column reaches the level of the piston in the sluice system (14,15).
Detection technique: the very short column makes the separation capacity small; in order to exclude the effect of interfering compounds, a nitrogen and phosphorus sensitive detection system is used.
Internal standardization: 5-chlorouracil (5-CU) appeared to be a good internal standard in the gaschromatographic procedure.
Technical details of the extraction procedure
Several extraction procedures, as described in the literature, have been tried out. Eventually the following procedure was adopted:

- 0,2 ml plasma is transferred into a plastic vial containing 100 ng of 5-chlorouracil. The solution is shaken vigorously and is extracted twice with 3 ml ethyl acetate.
- after separation and evaporation of the organic layer the residue is dissolved in 100 μl water;

- 10 μl of the solution is used for injection.

The recovery of the extraction procedure is approx. 80%. This was determined by means of radioactive 5-FU.

Injection technique

10 μl of the afore mentioned solution is applied on the tip of the rod of the solid state injector and evaporated there.

RESULTS

Fig. 4 shows three chromatograms of extraction experiments.

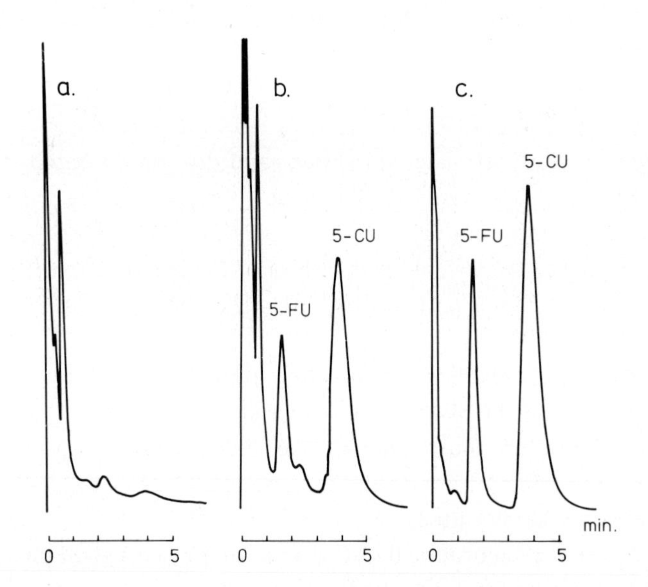

Fig. 4. Chromatograms of extraction experiments.

a. extract from control plasma.

b. extract from plasma to which 5-FU was added (500 ng 5-FU to 0,2 ml plasma; 10% of the extract is injected onto the column).

c. standard solution containing 50 ng 5-FU and 100 ng 5-CU.

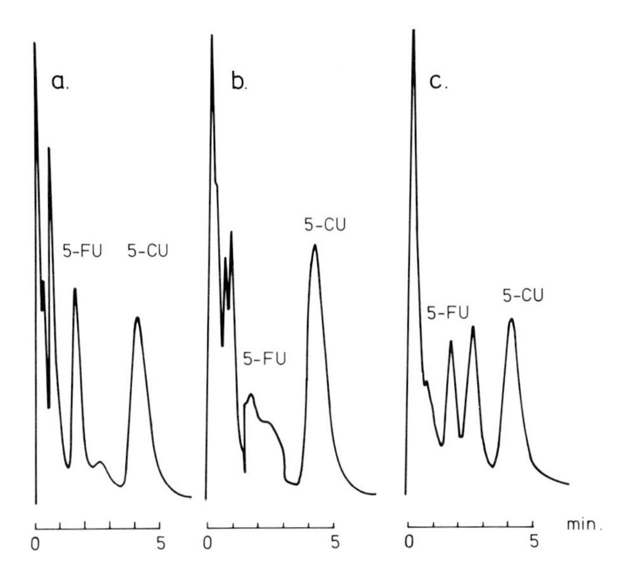

Fig. 5. Examples of routine chromatograms.

a. chromatogram of a known amount of 5-FU added to plasma, used as standard.

b. patient sample, with an amount of 5-FU close to the limit of sensitivity (less than 1 ng per injection).

c. a quantity of approx. 50 ng 5-FU; a large peak of unknown origin in between the 5-FU and 5-CU peak (rarely observed).

Close examination of the chromatogram of control plasma (a) reveals small peaks at the position where 5-FU and 5-CU are to be expected. These ghost or injection memory peaks are due to the use of a glass syringe for the application of the extract to the rod tip.

Fig. 5 shows three examples of routine chromatograms.

In Fig. 6 a standard curve of 5-FU is given; the absolute peak height and the amount of 5-FU are plotted.

Fig. 7 compares the recoveries of 5-FU and 5-CU, as measured by absolute peak heights observed in the glass adherence experiments as described before. The behaviour of 5-CU towards glass is comparable to that of 5-FU, showing that also in this respect 5-CU is a good internal standard.

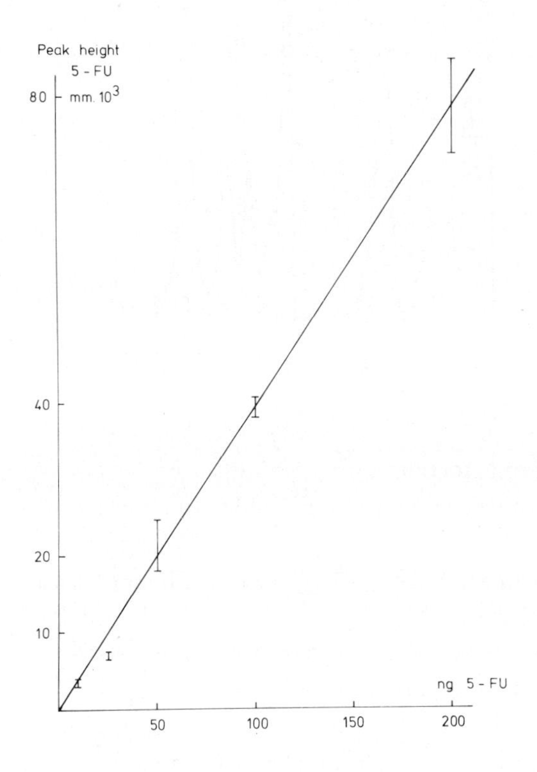

Fig.6. Standard curve of 5-FU; absolute peak height on the ordinate, amount of 5-FU on the abscissa.

In Fig. 8 the ratios of peak heights of 5-FU and 5-CU in standards containing the same amount of 5-CU and the quantity of 5-FU in these standards are plotted. Such a reference line, when obtained from extracts of plasma to which the standard solutions were added, is equal to the line as shown in Fig. 8 with an analytical error of 5%. The reference from plasma extracts is always measured together with patients samples. From the standard line the sensitivity can be estimated as to be less than 10 ng.

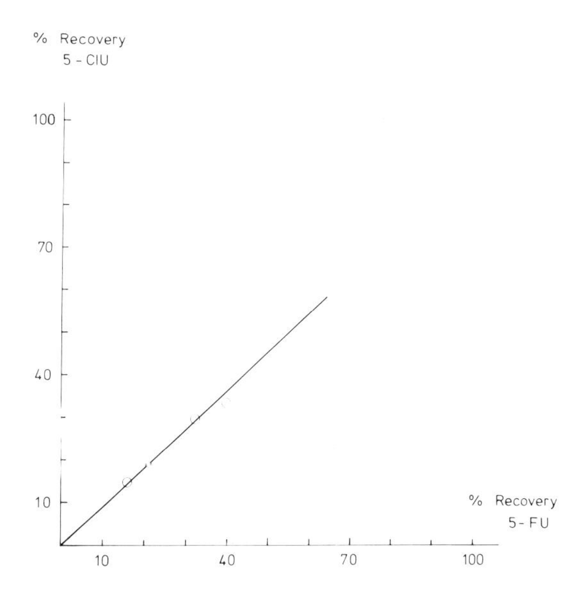

Fig. 7. Percentage recovery of 5-FU and 5-CU from glass.

Two examples of clinical applications

Routine analyses of patients samples are being carried out in co-operation with the Department of Oncology of the Leiden University Medical Centre; two examples of clinical applications will be shown (Fig. 9 and 10). The studies aim at

- an estimation of the biological availability of 5-FU in patients. This implies that plasma concentrations are measured after intravenous and after oral administration,
- management of therapy of patients with liver metastases, receiving 5-FU in the hepatic artery.

Fig. 9 illustrates the plasma decay of 5-FU after an intravenous bolus injection of 1 g 5-FU. When plotted on a logscale the graph is a straight line. The calculated half-life of seven minutes is in accordance with values mentioned in the literature. Fig. 10 shows plasma 5-FU concentrations achieved in a patient during perfusion of the hepatic artery for three weeks. The doses as administered are indicated on the abscissa.

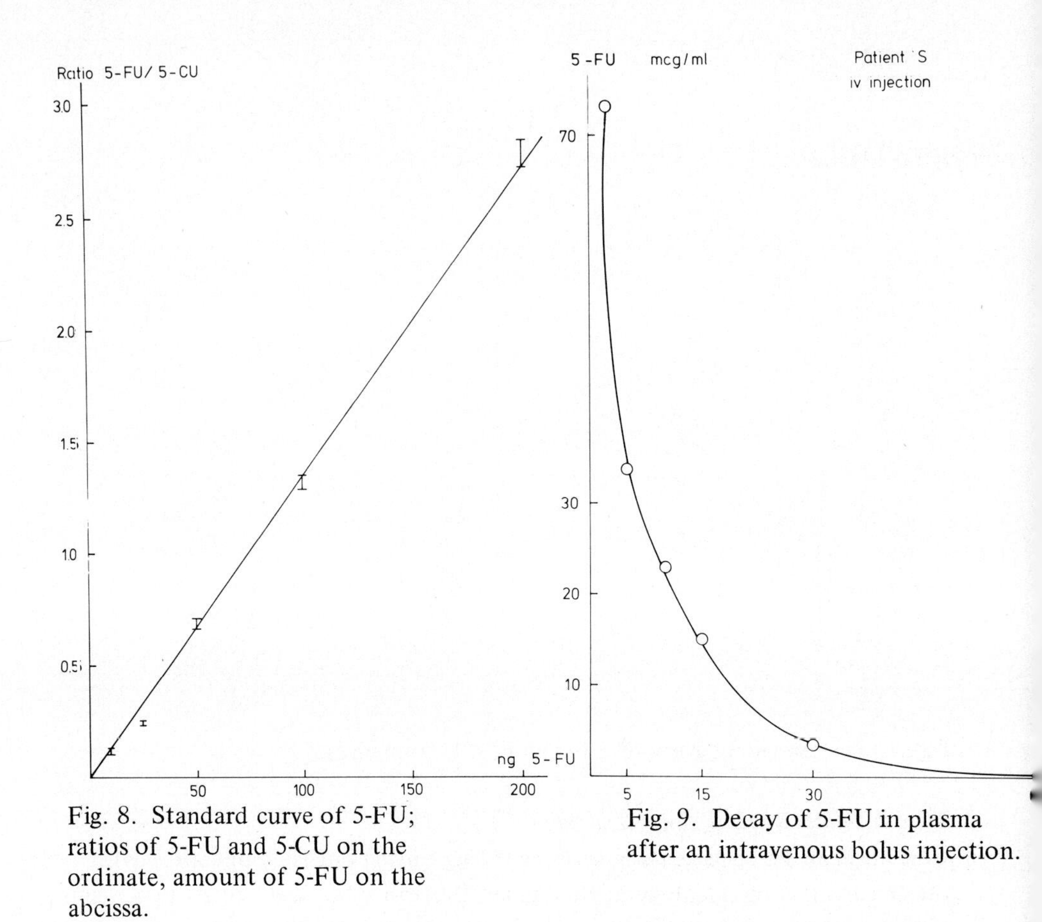

Fig. 8. Standard curve of 5-FU; ratios of 5-FU and 5-CU on the ordinate, amount of 5-FU on the abcissa.

Fig. 9. Decay of 5-FU in plasma after an intravenous bolus injection.

The very low 5-FU plasma concentrations were anticipated, as 5-FU is metabolized in the liver and similar results were already known, e.g. from radioactive measurements of 5-FU. On the last day of the perfusion the clinical situation deteriorated and the perfusion was terminated. An increase of the 5-FU plasma concentration was observed; this was presumably due to a trombus in the hepatic artery and consequently hepatic metabolism of 5-FU was cut off.

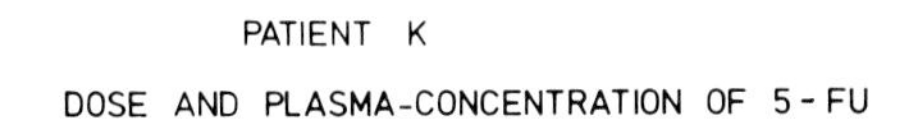

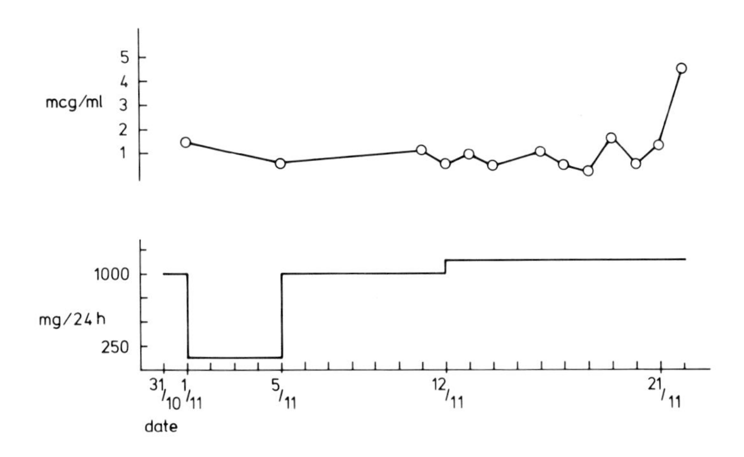

Fig. 10. Administered dose and measured concentration of 5-FU in plasma during perfusion of the hepatic artery.

Preview of clinical studies.

The assay as described will be used in clinical studies:

- determination of the biological availability of 5-FU in individual patients;
- the relation of 5-FU plasma curves to the pathophysiological state of the patient;
- the use of determination of 5-FU and of other cytostatic drugs for individual dosage prescriptions.

CONCLUSION

A reliable and rather simple GLC-method for the determination of 5-FU in plasma has been developed. As shown in table 4, 40 samples can be assayed in 8 hours, provided that extractions have been performed the previous day. The limit of sensitivity of 1 ng per injection seems to be satisfactory. The assay with the improved sensitivity of 40 picograms per injection is less accurate and is not routinely used. However, it shows that the analytical method may yield additional sensitivity.

TABLE 4
CONCLUSIONS ABOUT THE PRACTICABILITY AND THE SENSITIVITY OF THE GLC-ASSAY OF 5-FU IN PLASMA

Number of GLC measurements per working day
- a standard extraction curve is determined twice: 2 x 5 GLC's;
- a number of 15 plasma samples can be measured in duplo: 2 x 15 GLC's.

Sensitivity
1 ng/injection from 50 ng/ml plasma: analytical error 5%
0,04 ng/injection from 2 ng/ml plasma: less accurate.

Acknowledgements
We are indebted to Dr. M.G. Herben and Dr. A.T. van Oosterom of the Department of Oncology of the Leiden University Medical Centre for their co-operation in this study.
We are grateful to Hoffman-La Roche B.V., for furnishing the 5-FU.
The investigations were financially supported by the Netherlands' Cancer Society (The Koningin Wilhelmina Fonds, KWF).

REFERENCES

1. Chaudhuri, N.K., Montag, B.J., and Heidelberger, C. (1958) Studies on fluorinated pyrimidines III. The metabolism of 5-fluorouracil-2-C^{14} and 5-fluoroorotic 2-C^{14} acid in vivo, Cancer Research, 18: 318-328.

2. Clarkson, B., O'Connor, A., LaReine, W., and Hutchinson, D. (1964) The physiologic disposition of 5-fluorouracil and 5-fluoro-2'-deoxyuridine in man, Clin. Pharmacol. Ther., 5: 581-610.

3. Garrett, E.R., Hurst, G.H., and Green, J.R. Jr. (1977) Kinetics and mechanism of drug action on microorganisms XXIII. Microbial kinetic assay for fluorouracil in biological fluids and its application to human pharmacokinetics, J. Pharm. Sci., 66: 1422-1429.

4. De Leenheer, A.P., Cosyns-Duyck, M.C. and Van Vaerenberg, P.M. (1977) Application of ion-pair methods to extraction of fluorouracil from aqueous fluids, J. Pharm. Sci., 66: 1390-1393.

5. Benvenuto, J.A., Lu, K., and Loo, T.L. (1977) High-pressure liquid chromatographic analysis of ftorafur and its metabolites in biological fluids, J. Chro-

matogr., 134: 219-222.

6. Sitar, D.S., Shaw, D.H. Jr., Thirlwell, M.P., and Ruedy, J.R. (1977) Disposition of 5-fluorouracil after intravenous bolus doses of a commercial formulation to cancer patients, Cancer Research, 37: 3981-3984.

7. Pantarotto, C., Martini, A., Belvedere, G., Bossi, A., Donelli, M.G., and Frigerio, A. (1974) Application of gas chromatography-chemical ionization mass fragmentography in the evaluation of bases and nucleoside analogues used in cancer chemotherapy, J. Chromatogr., 99: 519-527.

8. Finn, C., and Sadée, W. (1975) Determination of 5-fluorouracil plasma levels in rats and man by isotope dilution-mass fragmentography, Cancer Chemother. Rep., 59: 279-286.

9. Hillcoat, B.L., Kawai, M., McCulloch, P.B., Rosenfeld, J., and Williams, C.K.O. (1976) A sensitive assay of 5-fluorouracil in plasma by gas chromatography-mass spectrometry, Br. J. Clin. Pharmac., 3: 135-143.

10. Wu, A.T., Schwandt, H.J., Finn, C., and Sadée, W. (1976) Determination of ftorafur and 5-fluorouracil levels in plasma and urine, Res. Comm. Chem. Path. Pharmacol., 14: 89-102.

11. Windheuser, J.J., Sutter, J.L., and Auen, E. (1972) 5-Fluorouracil and derivatives in cancer chemotherapy. Determination of 5-fluorouracil in blood, J. Pharm. Sci., 61: 301-303.

12. Cohen, J.L., and Brennan, P.B. (1973) GLC assay for 5-fluorouracil in biological fluids, J. Pharm. Sci. 62: 572-575.

13. Rao, K.V., Killion, K., and Tanrikut, Y. (1974) GLC determination of fluorouracil, J. Pharm. Sci. 63: 1328-1330.

14. Driessen, O.M.J. (1974) Proc. Kon. Ned. Akad. Wet. C77, 171-181.

15. Driessen, O.M.J. (1975) Proc. Kon. Ned. Akad. Wet. C78, 449-460.

Clinical Pharmacology of Anti-Neoplastic Drugs
H. M. Pinedo, editor

THE CLINICAL PHARMACOLOGY OF THE FLUOROPYRIMIDINES

DONALD MURINSON AND CHARLES MYERS
Medicine Branch and Clinical Pharmacology Branch, National Cancer Institute, Bethesda, MD 20014, U.S.A.

ABSTRACT

Since the initial synthesis of 5-fluorouracil over 20 years ago, fluoropyrimidines have found wide application as antitumor and antifungal agents. This paper will review our current knowledge of fluoropyrimidine pharmacology and attempt to point out major existing gaps in that knowledge.

After 20 years of clinical experience, 5-fluorouracil (5 FU) continues to be widely used both as a single agent and, more recently, with other chemotherapeutic agents against cancers of the gastrointestinal tract (1,2), breast (3,4), ovary (5), and skin (6). 5-FU is one of the few antineoplastic drugs whose mechanism of action and metabolism are relatively well understood, thus making feasible the use of biochemical and pharmacological principles to develop more discriminating therapy.

Like most base and nucleoside antimetabolites, 5-FU must be converted to

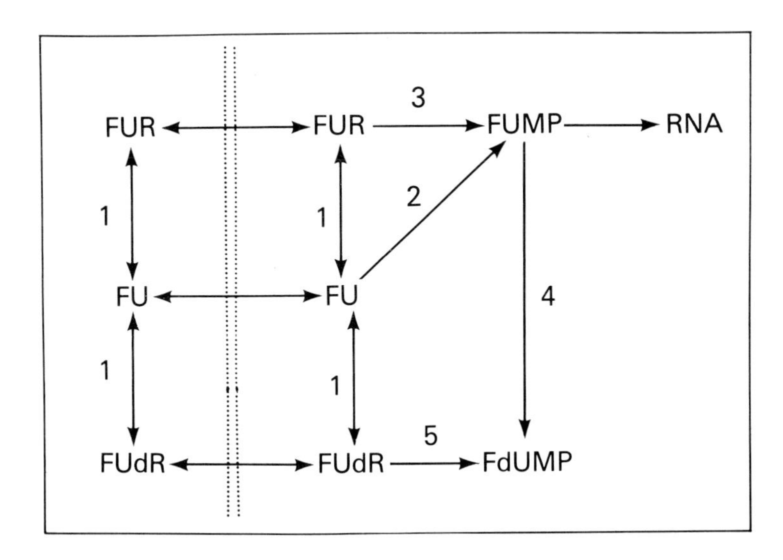

Fig. 1.

its respective nucleotide before it can be active. Since cell membranes are impermeable to nucleotides, this activation process must occur in the target cell itself. With one important exception, both the anabolic and catabolic reactions of 5-FU are identical to those of uracil. As depicted in Fig.1, 5-FU enters cells by passive diffusion (7) and is then converted to the nucleosides fluorouridine (FUR) and fluorodeoxyuridine (FUdR) by nucleoside phosphorylase (8). Both FUR and FUdR are metabolized to their respective nucleotides FUMP and FdUMP by specific kinases (9,10). Alternatively, 5-FU may be converted directly to FUMP by the action of a pyrimidine phosphoribosyltransferase (11).

FUMP can be incorporated into RNA or it can be converted to FdUMP in a series of reactions which include ribonucleotide reductase (12). It is well established that FdUMP is a tight binding inhibitor of the enzyme thymidylate synthetase, which catalyzes the formation of thymidylate from deoxyuridylate and, as a result, plays a crucial role in DNA synthesis (13,14).

The nature of the interaction between FdUMP and thymidylate synthetase has been a subject of intense current interest. Thymidylate synthetase has a molecular weight of 70,000 and is composed of two 35,000 molecular weight subunits. There appear to be two enzyme active sites per molecule, one per subunit. Santi *et al.*(15) and Heidelberger *et al.* (16) have shown that this binding is covalent in the presence of the cofactor 5,10-methylene tetrahydrofolic acid. As a result, the trivalent enzyme 5,10-methylene tetrahydrofolic acid complex will survive acid precipitation or SDS-gel chromatography. In addition, pronase digestion yields small polypeptide fragments with FdUMP still firmly attached. Recently, evidence has accumulated that the two enzymatic sites may not possess equal affinity for FdUMP. One site appears to have a very high affinity for FdUMP with an apparent K_i in the order of 10^{-11}M. The second site binds with much lower affinity and, in practice, never is saturable. At present, it is not clear whether this results from a per primum nonequivalence of the two enzymatic sites or represents negative cooperatively. In practice, this means that only one of the enzymatic sites is likely to be occupied by FdUMP at levels attained *in vivo.*

The consequences of 5-FU incorporation into RNA have been extensively reviewed by Heidelberger (17). Up to 6% of the uracil in Ehrlich ascites carcinoma cells is replaced by 5-FU; however, this replacement is much higher in bacteria and viruses. Although errors in translation have been demonstrated, under most circumstances these events are rare and often have few biological sequelae. An analysis of thymidine and uridine rescue experiments following fluorinated pyrimidine administration has suggested that for at least some mammalian cells, the incorporation of 5-FU into RNA may be biologically significant (18,19). By regulating the conversion of FUMP into RNA and FdUMP, the enzymes which activate 5-FU can determine whether interference with RNA or DNA will prevail in a specific cell. The precise consequences resulting from 5-FU alteration of RNA remain ill-defined, whereas the inhibition of DNA synthesis is better understood and is generally felt to be more important biologically (17).

Studies of murine tumor extracts for uridine phosphorylase (20), uridine kinase (21), thymidine kinase (22), and phosphosibosyltransferase (23,24) has helped elucidate resistance mechanisms to the fluorinated pyrimidines. In murine tumors, the level of phosphosibosyltransferase appears to be the major determinant of response. Unfortunately, few investigations of this type have been carried out in human tumor tissue. A study of enzymatic activity in human colon tumors does not include enough 5-FU treated patients to evaluate this approach in predicting tumor responsiveness (25). Nevertheless, biochemical parameters associated with 5-FU response in human tumors do have therapeutic significance, especially for patients being considered for adjuvant therapy, and should be diligently pursued.

It is important to note that these salvage pathways are not essential for the synthesis of nucleic acids since most mammalian cells can generate pyrimidine nucleotides via the *de novo* pathway. Thus, deletion of the salvage pathway enzymes is a particularly succesful form of FU resistance.

Whereas the activation of 5-FU occurs in the target cell, the major documented site of FU inactivation occurs in the liver (26,27). The pyrimidine ring is initially reduced by the rate limiting enzyme dihydrouracil dehydrogenase and is subsequently cleaved nonenzymatically. The final products formed are α-fluoro-β-analine, urea, ammonia, and carbon dioxide, which are primarily excreted in the urine and lack antitumor activity. Earlier observations had suggested that the inability of certain tumors, including human breast and colon carcinomas to degrade 5-FU was an important factor in the selective antitumor activity against these tumors(28,29), however, inhibition of the catabolic pathway in rats did not support to this theory(27).

Knowledge of pyrimidine catabolism has provided an understanding of the cerebellar toxicity which occurs in 2% of patients receiving 5-FU and in 10-20% of those receiving ftorafur(30,31). It has been proposed that some α-fluoro-β-alanine may be metabolized to fluoroacetate which is converted to fluorocitrate, an inhibitor of aconitase, a key enzyme of the Krebs Cycle. Fluorocitrate produces neuronal lesions in cats similar to those produced by 5-FU (30).

The most common toxicities of 5-FU relate to the bone marrow and gastrointestinal tract. Mucositis and diarrhoea tend to occur more commonly with 5-FU than most chemotherapeutic agents.

Following a single 15 mg/kg dose of 5-FU intravenously, the drug rapidly diffuses into all body compartments and is distributed in a volume equivalent to the total body water (9). Peak plasma levels of 10^{-4} - 10^{-3}M occur immediately and the drug is cleared rapidly from plasma with a half-time of 10-20 minutes. After 2-3 hours plasma levels are below 10^{-8}M and are no longer detectable (32, 33,34). Finn and Sadee using a highly sensitive mass fragmentography assay were able to define a second phase of elimination in rats and in patients receiving oral 5-FU. The half-life for this phase was 20 hours (33). Approximately 20% of the parent durg is excreted unchanged in the urine, most of this during the first hour (28,34). The remaining 80% of the administered dose is metabolized primarily in the liver. The inactive metabolites formed are excreted in the urine over the next 3-4 hours with 90% of the dose being accounted for during the first 24 hours (28,34).

Oral administration of 5-FU produces widely variable plasma levels (29,32,33, 35,36). Peak plasma concentrations are usually lower and occur later than similar doses given intravenously. In addition, clearance is prolonged. An explanation for these observations is found in the unreliable absorption of the drug, especially when it is given in a low pH solution such as orange juice (32). Furthermore, a prominent first pass effect through the liver or recycling of the drug via the enterohepatic circulation may also account for the variability noted (32,33). In spite of greater patient convenience, most studies have shown that the oral route has been associated with either lower clinical responses (37,38) or shorter durations of remission (36).

The optimal dosage and method of administering 5-FU have been debated for some time. The original 5-day loading course of Curreri and Ansfield (39) produced unacceptable toxicity. A modification of this regimen has recently been compared with weekly intravenous 5-FU and an oral loading schedule in a randomized clinical trial. The modified intravenous schedule was found superior, particularly in patients with cancer of the colon and rectum (38). Single intravenous doses of 5-FU in excess of 20-30 mg/kg have produced a disproportionate increase in toxicity (40,41).

It is generally agreed that the five-day continuous infusion produced considerably less hematologic suppression, allowing higher doses to be given with safety (42,43,44). Whether this gives better responses remains unclear. In one study, infusion of 5-FU failed to produce any objective responses in 14 patients with gastrointestinal malignancy unresponsive to weekly 5-FU (43).

The ineffectiveness of 5-FU in the treatment of patients with hepatic metastases has led to trials of hepatic arterey infusion in the hope that high drug concentrations would be obtained in the hepatic parenchyma, while at the same time reducing systemic toxicity. This approach has been particularly appealing in patients with gastrointestinal malignancy whose disease is often confined to the liver. Although a randomized clinical trial evaluating systemic and intrahepatic 5-FU has not been published, several reports have noted response rates of 35-85%. Some of these responses have endured for several years (45,46). In some cases responses were noted in patients who had previously failed systemic 5-FU (47). The possible value of this therapy is offset by complications related to the indwelling catheter; however, intermittent courses by repeated percutaneous catheterizations appears to be a suitable alternative with minimal risk.

5-FU enters both malignant peritoneal and pleural effusions where it may persist for up to 12-24 hours, while it is gradually released into the circulation (34). The use of FUdR in patients with effusions might cause unexpected toxicity since prolonged infusions of this drug, in contrast to infusions of 5-FU, are approximately twenty times more toxic than daily single dose therapy(48). Intra-cavitary administration of 5-FU produces levels in the effusion several hundred times higher than that obtained after systemic administration. Furthermore, plasma concentrations are 100-1000 times less than those in the effusion giving a wide margin of safety from adverse system effects (34).

In spite of its limited lipid solubility, 5-FU diffuses readily across the blood-brain barrier and distributes in cerebrospinal fluid (CSF) and brain (49). Following 15 mg/kg intravenously, maximum levels in the CSF occur within 1-2 hours and persist at greater than 10^{-8}M for 12 hours (34,49). A rapid rate of injection maximizes brain and CSF levels.

The pharmacokinetics of drug elimination have not been defined in patients with either severe renal or liver impairment. Since most of an administered dose is normally inactivated in the liver, 5 -FU dosage may need to be modified in those patients with liver dysfunction. Severe renal disease may also require dosage modification, but is probably less critical. Ideally, such patients should be monitored by plasma drug levels to insure optimal activity and lessen the likelihood of toxicity.

In contrast to the rapid extracellular clearance of the parent drug and its nucleosides, the active inhibitor FdUMP has a much slower rate of disappearance from normal murine tissues and tumor (50,51). More information about FdUMP pharmacokinetics is needed to enhance our understanding of 5-FU action and toxicity. Progress in the areas cited will hopefully provide the clinician with a more rational approach to therapy with this useful agent.

The nucleoside thymidine has recently been used in an attempt to increase the efficacy of 5-FU. Although thymidine can reverse the cytotoxicity of 5-FU in cell culture systems (18), studies in both mice and humans have consistently shown a potentiation of 5-FU action when thymidine is co-administered. In 1959, Burchenal *et al.* reported enhanced toxicity in mice when either 5-FU or FUdR was combined with thymidine (52). This observation was recently extended by reports of greater antitumor effect against murine breast cancer (53) and AKR leukemia (54) by 5-FU-thymidine than by 5-FU alone. Other deoxynucleosides appear to have similar effects. Co-administration of deoxyuridine with either 5-FU or FUdR in mice with sarcoma 180 produced more tumor inhibition than identical doses of the antimetabolite alone. However, any therapeutic benefit achieved with the combination therapy could be achieved by using 5-FU or FUdR at a higher dose; thus, the therapeutic ratio for each of the drugs was not improved by deoxyuridine (55). During the past year at least three Phase I trials of 5-FU-thymidine therapy have been initiated. Although the studies differ in the method of administering the two agents, enhanced toxicity was a universal finding and included 3 deaths in 21 patients (56,57,58). Both gastrointestinal and hematologic toxicity were pronounced with myelosuppression being dose-limiting in two of the three studies. When 15 g of thymidine was administered as a 30-minute infusion 30 minutes prior to a rapid injection of 5-FU, the second phase half-life of the antimetabolite was prolonged from less than 30 minutes to 6 hours (57). In addition, there was increased urinary clearance of intact 5-FU and decreased $^{14}CO_2$ production from the labelled 2-position of the pyrimidine ring suggesting a profound inhibition of the catabolic pathway. 5-FU incorporation into nuclear RNA was markedly increased and the conversion of 5-FU to FUdR, normally undetectable in plasma, was enhanced.

These dramatic alterations of 5-FU pharmacology have stimulated much speculation into the biochemical events involved. A thymidine infusion may have at least four biochemical consequences:

1. Competitive inhibition of dihydrouracil dehydrogenase by thymidine leading to delayed plasma clearance of 5-FU.
2. Enhanced formation of FUdR in plasma by thymidine phosphoraylase due to the plentiful availability of a deoxyribose donor, TdR.
3. Thymidine triphosphate-induced allosteric inhibition of ribonucleotide reductase resulting in greater incorporation of FUMP into RNA rather than conversion in FdUMP.

4. Finally, thymidine may rescue cells from the consequences of FdUMP dependant inhibition of thymidylate synthetase.

Martin *et al.* have shown a coincidental relationship between the enhanced therapeutic effect in some murine tumors with increased 5-FU incorporation into nuclear RNA (59). However, increased FdUMP formation is also likely in view of the increased FUdR levels and slow clearance of FU thus providing an alternate explanation for the increased impact of FU plus thymidine. Thus, these authors have failed to provide convincing evidence that this incorporation of 5-FU into RNA explains the biologic effects observed.

After a 30-minute infusion of thymidine plasma levels fall from 10^{-3}M to less than 10^{-5}M in 5 hours with a half-life of 40 minutes. In contrast, Myers *et al.* (51) and Chadwich and Rogers (50) have demonstrated that FdUMP may persist in sensitive tumors and in murine bone marrow cells for as long as 7 days. Thus, the delayed plasma clearance of 5-FU combined with the slow metabolism of the potent inhibitor FdUMP might lead to progressive FdUMP accumulation in both tumor and host tissues. Intermittent thymidine infusions would not be expected to produce a sustained reversal of DNA inhibition in view of both the relatively rapid degradation of thymidine and the rapid turnover of the TTP pools.

It is unfortunate that the published work on the FU-thymidine interaction have not examined in a more comprehensive fashion the four effects mentioned earlier.

Since the introduction of 5-FU in 1957, several other fluorinated pyrimidines have attracted clinical interest, but none has seriously challenged the parent compound for its position in cancer treatment. 5-fluoro-2'-deoxyuridine (FUdR) has superior activity against several murine tumors (60), but does not seem to be more effective than 5-FU against human tumors (61,62), probably because of its rapid conversion to 5-FU by nucleoside phosphorylase, which exists in a wide variety of tissues (26,63).

Ftorafur, a relatively new drug developed in the U.S.S.R., is currently undergoing Phase II evaluation, the preliminary results of which suggest a spectrum of activity similar to that of 5-FU (31). However, ftorafur is less toxic for mice and clinical trials in humans have noted less hematologic suppression (31,64,65); a feature which is especially advantageous for combination therapy with myelosuppressive agents. Gastrointestinal and neurological toxicities are most frequently dose limiting. Cohen has suggested that ftorafur may act as a depot form of 5-FU and that the liver is the primary site for the conversion (66). The slow release of 5-FU *in vivo* could explain ftorafur's lessened bone marrow toxicity since continuous infusions of 5-FU produce a similar effect (42,44).

The third fluoropyrimidine of clinical value is fluorocytosine. Because humans lack cytosine deaminase, the administration of FC to man is not associated with significant conversion of FC to FU. In addition, FC is itself not incorporated to a significant extent in either RNA or DNA. As a result, FC has little toxicity for human tissues. Certain pathogenic fungi such as *Candida albicans* or *Cryptococcus neoformans* have cytosine deaminase and do, as a result, convert FC to FU (67). The therapeutic efficacy of FC in the treatment of *Candida albicans* or *Cryptococcus neoformans* is thought to be dependent on this conversion. In sensitive fungi, it is possible to show incorporation of FC into the FUMP of RNA. In addition, FdUMP is rapidly synthesized leading to nearly complete disappearance of fungal thymidylate synthetase and an immediate cessation of fungal cell growth. The impact of FdUMP upon these cells may be potentiated by the absence of any mechanism for thymidine uptake in *Candida albicans.*

REFERENCES

1. Moertel, C.G. (1975) Clinical Management of Advanced Gastrointestinal Cancer, Cancer 36:675-682.

2. Moertel, C.G. (1976) Gastrointestinal Cancer: Treatment with Fluorouracil-Nitrosourea Combinations, JAMA 235:2135-2136.

3. Carter, S.K. (1972) Single and Combination Nonhormonal Chemotherapy in Breast Cancer, Cancer 30:1543-1555.

4. Canellos, G.P., DeVita, V.T., Gold, G.L., Chabner, B.A., Schein, P.S., and Young, R.C. (1976) Combination Chemotherapy for Advanced Breast Cancer: Response and Effect on Survival, Ann. Int. Med. 84:389-392.

5. Young, R.C. (1975) Chemotherapy of Ovarian Cancer: Past and Present, Seminars in Oncology 2:267-276.

6. Klein, E., Burgess, G.H., and Helm, F. (1974) Neoplasms of the Skin, in Cancer Medicine, Holland, J.F., and Frei III, E. eds., Philadelphia, Lea and Febiger, pp. 1789-1822.

7. Jacquez, J.A. (1962) Permeability of Ehrlich cells to Uracil, Thymine and Fluorouracil, Proceedings of the Society of Experimental Biology and Medicine 109:132-135.

8. Sköld, O. (1958) Enzymatic Ribosidation and Ribotidation of 5-Fluorouracil by Extracts of the Ehrlich Ascites Tumor, Biochimica et Biophysica Acta 29:651.

9. Chaudhuri, N.K., Montag, B.J., and Heidelberger, C. (1958) Studies on Fluorinated Pyrimidines, III. The Metabolism of 5-Fluorouracil-2-^{14}C and 5-Fluorourotic acid-2-^{14}C *in vivo*. Cancer Research 18:318-328.

10. Harbors, E., Chaudhuri, N.K., and Heidelberger, C. (1959) Studies of Fluorinated Pyrimidines. VIII. Further Biochemical and Metabolic Investigations. Journal of Biological Chemistry 234:1255-1262.

11. Reyes, P. (1969) The Synthesis of 5-Fluorouridine-5'-Phosphate by a Pyrimidine Phosphoribosyltransferase of Mammalian Origin. I. Some Properties of the Enzyme from P1534J Mouse Leukemic Cells. Biochemistry 8:2057-2062.

12. Kent, R.J. and Heidelberger, C. (1972) Fluorinated Pyrimidines. XL. The Reduction of 5-Fluorouridine-5'-Diphosphate by Ribonucleotide Reductase. Molecular Pharmacology 8:465-475.

13. Cohen, S.S., Flaks, J.G., Barner, H.D., et al. (1958) The Mode of Action of 5-Fluorouracil and its Derivatives, Proceedings of the National Academy of Science U.S.A. 44:1004-1012.

14. Reyes, P. and Heidelberger, C. (1965) Fluorinated Pyrimidines. XXVI. Mammalian Thymidylate Synthetase: Its Mechanism of Action and Inhibition by Fluorinated Nucleotides. Molecular Pharmacology 1:14-30.

15. Santi, D.V., McHenry, C.S., and Sommer, H. (1974) Mechanism of Interaction of Thymidylate Synthetase with 5-Fluorodeoxyuridylate, Biochemistry 13: 471-481.

16. Danenberg, P.V., Langenbach, R.J., and Heidelberger, C. (1974) Structures of Reversible and Irreversible Complexes of Thymidylate Synthetase and Fluorinated Pyrimidine Nucleotides, Biochemistry 13:926-933.

17. Heidelberger, C. (1974) Fluorinated Pyrimidines and Their Nucleosides, in Sartorelli and Johns Handbook of Experimental Pharmacology, pp. 193-231.

18. Umeda M. and Heidelberger, C. (1968) Comparative Studies of Fluorinated Pyrimidines with Various Cell Lines, Cancer Research 28:2529-2538.

19. Wilkinson, D.S., and Crumley, J. (1977) Metabolism of 5-Fluorouracil in Sensitive and Resistant Novikoff Hepatoma Cells, The Journal of Biological Chemistry 252:1051-1056.

20. Kessel, D., Bruns, R., and Hall, T.C. (1971) Determinants of Responsiveness to 5-Fluorouracil in Transplantable Murine Leukemias, Molecular Pharmacology 7:177-121.

21. Sköld, O., Magnusson, P.H., and Revesz, L. (1962) Studies on Resistance Against 5-Fluorouracil. III. Selective Value of Resistant, Uridine Kinase-Deficient Tumor Cells, Cancer Research 22:1226-1229.

22. Kessel, D. and Wodinsky, I. (1970) Thymidine Kinase as a Determinant of the Response to 5-Fluoro-2'-Deoxyuridine in Transplantable Murine Leukemias, Molecular Pharmacology 6:251-254.

23. Reyes, P. and Hall, T.C. (1969) Synthesis of 5-Fluorouridine-5'-Phosphate by a Pyrimidine Phosphoribosyltransferase of Mammalian Origin. II. Correlation Between the Tumor Levels of the Enzyme and the 5-Fluorouracil Promoted Increase in Survival of Tumor-Bearing Mice, Biochemical Pharmacology 18:2587-2590.

24. Kasbekar, D.K. and Greenberg, D.M. (1963) Studies on Tumor Resistance to 5-Fluorouracil, Cancer Research 23:818-824.

25. Nahas,A., Savlov, E.D., and Hall, T.C. (1974) Phosphoribosyl Transferase in Colon Tumor and Normal Mucosa as an Aid in Adjuvant Chemotherapy with 5-Fluorouracil, Cancer Chemotherapy Reports 58:909-912.

26. Chaudhuri, N.K., Mukherjee, K.L., and Heidelberger, C. (1958) Studies on Fluorinated Pyrimidines. VII. The Degradative Pathway, Biochemical Pharmacology 1:328-341.

27. Cooper, G.M., Dunning, W.F., and Greer, S. (1972) Role of Catabolism in Pyrimidine Utilization for Nucleic Acid Synthesis *in vivo,* Cancer Research 32:390-397.

28. Mukherjee, K.L. and Heidelberger, C. (1960) Studies on Fluorinated Pyrimidines. IX. The Degradation of 5-Fluorouracil-6-C^{14}, Journal of Biological Chemistry 235:433-437.

29. Mukherjee, K.L., Curreri, A.R., Javid, M., et al (1963) Studies on Fluorinated Pyrimidines. XVII, Tissue Distribution of 5-Fluorouracil-2-C^{14} and 5-Fluoro-2'-Deoxyuridine in Cancer Patients, Cancer Research 23:67-77.

30. Koenig, H. and Patel, A. (1970) Biochemical Basis for Fluorouracil Neurotocicity. The Role of Krebs Cycle Inhibition by Fluoroacetate, Archives of Neurology 23:155-160.

31. Valdivieso, M., Bodey, G.P., Gottlieb, J.A., et al (1976) Clinical Evaluation of Ftorafur (Pyrimidine-Deoxyribose N_1-2'-Furanidyl-5-Fluorouracil) Cancer Research 36:1821-1824.

32. Cohen, J.L., Irwin, L.E., Marshall, G.J., et al (1974) Clinical Pharmacology of Oral and Intravenous 5-Fluorouracil, Cancer Chemotherapy Reports 58:723-731.

33. Finn, C. and Sadee,W. (1975) Determination of 5-Fluorouracil Plasma Levels in Rats and Man by Isotope Dilution-Mass Fragmentography, Cancer Chemotherapy Reports 59:279-286.

34. Clarkson, B., O'Connor, A., Winston, L., et al (1965) The Physiologic Disposition of 5-Fluorouracil and 5-Fluoro-2'-Deoxyuridine in Man, Clinical Pharmacology and Therapeutics 5:581-610.

35. Bruckner, H.W. and Creasey, W.A. (1974) The Administration of 5-Fluorouracil by Mouth, Cancer 33:14-18.

36. Hahn, R.G., Moertel, C.G., Schutt, A.J., et al (1975) A Double-Blind Comparison of Intensive Course 5-Fluorouracil by Oral Vs. Intravenous Route in the Treatment of Colorectal Carcinoma, Cancer 35:1031-1035.

37. Stolinsky, D.C., Pugh, R.P., and Bateman, J.R. (1975) 5-Fluorouracil Therapy for Pancreatic Carcinoma: Comparison of Oral and Intravenous Routes, Cancer Chemotherapy Reports 59:1031-1033.

38. Ansfield, F., Klotz, J., Nealon, T., et al (1977) A Phase III Study Comparing the Clinical Utility of four Regimens of 5-Fluorouracil. A Preliminary Report, Cancer 39:34-40.

39. Curreri, A.R., Ansfield, F.J., McIver, F.A., et al (1958) Clinical Studies with 5-Fluorouracil, Cancer Research 18:478-484.

40. Jacobs, E.M., Reeves, W.J., Wood, D.A., et al (1971) Treatment of Cancer with Weekly Intravenous 5-Fluorouracil, Cancer 27:1302-1305.

41. Horton, J., Olson, K.B., Sullivan, J., et al (1970) 5-Fluorouracil in Cancer: An Improved Regimen, Annals of Internal Medicine 73:897-900.

42. Lemon, H.M., Modzen, P.J., Mirchandani, R., Farmer, D.A., and Athans, J. (1963) Deceased Intoxication by Fluorouracil when Slowly Administered in Glucose, JAMA 185:1012-1016.

43. Hum, G.J. and Bateman, J.R. (1975) 5-Day IV Infusion with 5-Fluorouracil for Gastroenteric Carinoma After Failure on Weekly 5-FU Therapy, Cancer Chemotherapy Reports 59:1177-1179.

44. Seifert, P., Baker, L.H., Reed, M.L., et al (1975) Comparison of Continuously Infused 5-Fluorouracil with Bolus Injection in Treatment of Patients with Colorectal Adenocarcinoma, Cancer 36:123-128.

45. Tanlon, R.N., Bunnell, I.L., and Cooper, R.G. (1973) The Treatment of Metastatic Carcinoma of the Liver by the Percutaneous Selective Hepatic Artery Infusion of 5-Fluorouracil, Surgery 73:118-121.

46. Ansfield, F.J., Guillermo, R., Shibba, J.L., et al (1971) Intrahepatic Arterial Infusion of 5-Fluorouracil, Cancer 28:1147-1151.

47. Buroker, T., Samson, M., Correa, J., et al (1976) Hepatic Artery Infusion of 5-FUdR After Prior Systemic 5-Fluorouracil, Cancer Treatment Reports 6-:1277-1279.

48. Sullivan, R.D., Young, C.W., Miller, E., et al (1960) The Clinical Effects of the Continuous Administration of Fluorinated Pyrimidines (5-Fluorouracil and 5-Fluoro-2'-Deoxyuridine), Cancer Chemotherapy Reports 8:77-83.

49. Bourke, R.S., West, C.R., Chheda, G., et al (1973) Kinetics of Entry and Distribution of 5-Fluorouracil in Cerebrospinal Fluid and Brain Following Intravenous Injection in a Primate, Cancer Research 33:1735-1746.

50. Chadwich, M. and Rogers, W.I. (1972) The Physiological Disposition of 5-Fluorouracil in Mice Bearing Solid L1210 Lymphocytic Leukemia, Cancer Research 32:1045-1056.

51. Myers, C.E., Young, R.C., and Chabner, B.A. (1975) Biochemical Determinants of 5-Fluorouracil Response *in vivo*, JCI 56:1231-1238.

52. Burchenal, J.H., Holmberg, E.A.D., Fox, J.J., Hemphill, S.C., and Reppert, J.A. (1959) The Effects of 5-Fluorodeoxycytidine, 5-Fluorodeoxyuridine, and Related Compounds on Transplanted Mouse Leukemias, Cancer Research 19:494-500.

53. Martin, D.S. and Stolfi, R.L. (1977) Thymidine Enhancement of Antitumor Activity of 5-Fluorouracil Against Advanced Murine (CD8F1) Breast Carcinoma, Proc. Am. Assoc. Cancer Research 18:126.

54. Santelli, G. (1977) Potentiation of 5-Fluorouracil Cytotoxicity by Thymidine Against Leukemia Cells, Proc. Am. Assoc. Cancer Research 18:148.

55. Jato, J.G., Lake, L.M., Grunden, E.E., and Johnson, B.M. (1975) Effect of Deoxyuridine Coadministration on Toxicity and Antitumor Activity of Fluorouracil and Floxuridine, J. Pharm. Sci. 64:943-946.

56. Vogel, S., Presant, C., Ratkin, G., and Klahr, C. (1978) Phase I Study of Infusion 5-Fluorouracil Plus Thymidine, Proc. Am. Assoc. Cancer Research 19:232.

57. Woodcock, T.M., Martin, D.S., Kemeny, N., and Young, C.W. (1978) Phase I, Evaluation of Thymidine Plus Flourouracil in Patients with Advanced Cancer Proc. Am. Soc. Clin. Oncol. 19:351.

58. Kirkwood, J.M. and Frei III, E. (1978) 5-Fluorouracil with Thymidine: A Phase I Study, Proc. Am. Assoc. Cancer Research 19:159.

59. Martin, D.S., Stolfi, R.L., and Spiegelman, S. (1978) Striking Augmentation of the *in vivo* Anticancer Activity of 5-Fluorouracil by Combination with Pyrimidine Nucleosides: An RNA Effect, Proc. Am. Assoc. Cancer Research 19:221.

60. Heidelberger, C., Griesbach, L., Cruz, O., et al (1958) Fluorinated Pyrimidines. VI. Effects of 5-Fluorouridine and 5-Fluoro-2'-Deoxyuridine on Transplanted Tumors, Proceedings of the Society of Experimental Biology 97:470-475.

61. Reitemeier, R.J., Moertel, C.G., and Hahn, R.G. (1965) Comparison of 5-Fluorouracil and 2'-Deoxy-5-Fluorouridine in the Treatment of Patients with Advanced Adenocarcinoma of Colon or Rectum, Cancer Chemotherapy Reports 44:39-43.

62. Moertel, C.G., Reitemeier, R.J., and Hahn, R.G. (1967) A Controlled Comparison of 5-Fluoro-2'-Deoxyuridine Therapy Administered by Rapid Intravenous Injection and by Continuous Intravenous Infusion, Cancer Research 27:549-552.

63. Birnie, G.D., Kroeger, H., and Heidelberger, C. (1963) Studies of Fluorinated Pyrimidines. XVIII. The Degradation of 5-Fluoro-2'-Deoxyuridine and Related Compounds by Nucleoside Phosphorylase, Biochemistry 2:566-572.

64. Blokhina, N.G., Vozny, E.K., and Garin, A.M. (1972) Results of Treatment of Malignant Tumors with Ftorafur, Cancer 30:390-392.

65. Smart, C.R., Townsend, L.B., Rusho, W.J., et al (1975) Phase I Study of Ftorafur, an Analog of 5-Fluorouracil, Cancer 36:103-106.

66. Cohen, A.M. (1975) The Disposition of Ftorafur in Rats After Intravenous Administration, Drug Metabolism and Disposition 3:303-308.

67. Diasio, R., Bennet, J., and Myers, C.E. (1978) The Mode of Action of 5-Fluorocytosine, Biochemical Pharmacology in press.

Clinical Pharmacology of Anti-Neoplastic Drugs
H. M. Pinedo, editor

CLINICAL PHARMACOLOGY OF CYTOSINE ARABINOSIDE IN ACUTE MYELOID LEUKAEMIA

H.C. VAN PROOIJEN
Division of Hematology, Dept. Int. Med. St. Radboud Hospital, University of Nijmegen, Geert Grooteplein Zuid 16, Nijmegen, The Netherlands.

INTRODUCTION

The compound cytosine arabinoside (Ara-C, 1-β-D-Arabinofuranosylcytosine, Arabinosylcytosine) is an analogue of the naturally occurring nucleoside cytidine (Fig. 1). The drug differs from cytidine in the sterical position of the OH-group at the C_2-atom of the sugar moiety of the molecule.Unlike related derivatives such as thymine arabinoside and uracil arabinoside (1), the drug is not a naturally occurring substance. Several technical procedures have been published for the synthesis of Ara-C (2,3). It is a fairly stable agent that retains 90% of its potency after storage at neutral pH at room temperature for 6 months (4).

Antitumor activity. The first experiments with Ara-C have been reported in 1961; it was demonstrated that the drug inhibits cell growth in a variety of transplantable murine tumors, including Sarcoma 180, Ehrlich ascites carcinoma, Leukaemia L-1210 and Lymphoma L 5178Y (5), resulting in a high incidence of "cures" (6). Later studies reported that the growth inhibiting effect of Ara-C is the result of an inhibition of DNA synthesis (7,8). In man the drug has been used for the treatment of several haematologic malignancies and at present, Ara-C is the drug of choice for treatment of acute myeloid leukaemia.

Related derivatives. 5-Azacytidine, which is an analogue of Ara-C has been first reported on in 1964 (9). The drug is phosphorylated intracellularly to its mono-, di- and triphosphates and is subsequently incorporated into RNA (10). 5-Azacytidine, inhibiting the growth of leukaemic cells in culture and in mice (11), is still under clinical investigation.

Recently a new antitumor agent O2,2'-cyclocytidine (Cyclo-C) has been introduced (12). It is an analogue of cytidine and is slowly hydrolyzed to Ara-C after administration. This results in a long plasma half-life (8 hours (13)) of the active product (Ara-C). This finding is of clinical importance since pharmacologic studies on Ara-C indicate that this drug is rapidly degraded by deaminases, resulting in a plasma half-life of only 12 minutes (14). In some patients the rapid plasma clearance of Ara-C seems to result in drug resistance and in these cases administration of Cyclo-C might be more effective.

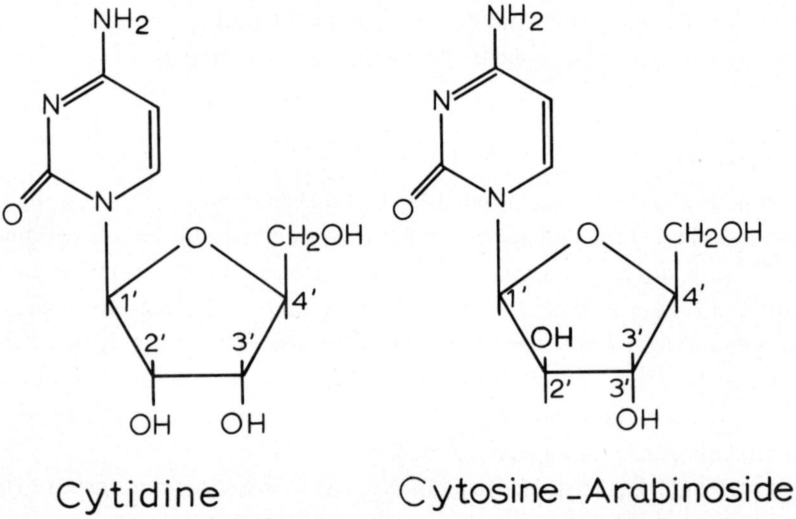

Cytidine

Cytosine-Arabinoside

Fig. 1. Structure of cytidine and cytosine arabinoside.

MECHANISM OF ACTION OF ARA-C

Biochemical studies. The mechanism through which Ara-C inhibits DNA synthesis is not known in detail. Three important biochemical pathways which are influenced by the drug are briefly commented on.

In the first pathway the ribonucleoside diphosphate reductase is involved. This enzyme catalyzes the reduction of ribonucleoside diphosphates to deoxyribonucleoside diphosphates. These enzymatic conversions are essential steps in the synthesis of deoxyribonucleoside 5'-triphosphates which are the DNA nucleotides. The first studies were those of Chu and Fischer (15) and involved murine L-5178Y lymphoblasts in culture. They showed a significant reduction of the intracellular deoxycytidine diphosphate (dCDP) level in the presence of Ara-C, while the level of cytidine diphosphate (CDP) was not affected. They concluded that the mechanism of action of Ara-C might be due to inhibition of CDP reduction by phosphorylated derivates of Ara-C. Moore and Cohen (16) investigated the effect of phosphorylated Ara-C in crude enzyme extracts from Novikoff and Ehrlich ascites tumor cells. They did not find a significant inhibition of the reduction of CDP to dCDP, neither by diphosphates nor by triphosphates of Ara-C. Skoog and Nordenskjöld (17) measured the intracellular pools of deoxyribonucleotide in murine embryo cells in the presence of Ara-C and found a transient decrease in the dCTP pool and an increase in the levels of deoxyribosyladenine triphosphate, deoxyribosylguanine triphosphate and deoxyribosylthymine triphosphate. From these studies it is obvious that the inhibition of CDP-reduction is not the major mechanism which can be held responsible for the inhibition of DNA synthesis by Ara-C.

A second influence mechanism of action is through the incorporation of Ara-C into DNA, which was to be expected since the drug is rapidly phosphorylated to its triphosphate. Indeed, small amounts of radioactivity in the acid insoluble fraction (presumably DNA) have been found during incubation of various cell lines in the presence of tritiated Ara-C (8,18). In some of these studies it was demonstrated by enzymatic degradation of the nucleic acid that the incorporated radioactivity did originate from Ara-C (19,20). Despite the evidence that Ara-C is incorporated into DNA, the problem remains as to how this incorporation relates to the inhibition of DNA synthesis. Graham and Whitmore (21) incubated murine L-cells with labelled Ara-C. After specific enzymatic digestion of DNA they found that more than 70% of the radioactivity was released as 3'-Ara-CMP indicating that the drug is incorporated into DNA.

From these experiments the assumption was made that Ara-C was incorporated into the small DNA fragments (Okazaki pieces). The incorporated Ara-C prevented the assemblage of the small DNA fragments to large DNA molecules. When Ara-C was removed from the medium the assemblage of DNA recovered, probably because of the synthesis of Ara-C-free Okazaki pieces. Despite the consistent finding of small amounts of Ara-C being incorporated into DNA, it has not been clarified how such small amounts do result in cell kill.

The third and probably most important action of Ara-C is the inhibition of DNA polymerase. This enzyme catalyzes the incorporation of the deoxyribonucleoside 5'-triphosphates into the DNA molecule. In crude preparations of DNA polymerase extracted from Ehrlich ascites cells the enzyme was inhibited by Ara-CTP (22). Similar results were found with DNA polymerase extracted from calf thymus (23) and human leukaemic cells (24). Graham and Whitmore (25) reported that in DNA polymerase extracts from murine L-cells, Ara-CTP was a competitive inhibitor of the enzyme. The affinity of this enzyme to dCTP and Ara-CTP was similar and in all these studies the inhibition of DNA polymerase by Ara-CTP could be reversed by dCTP. Experiments with polynucleotide chains in a cell free system confirmed that Ara-CTP competes with dCTP for the active sites on DNA polymerase (26). High concentrations of Ara-CTP in the cell will block the active sites of the enzyme completely and will result in strong inhibition of DNA synthesis. Indeed, experiments with murine leukaemic cells (L1210) demonstrated that the extent of depression of DNA synthesis correlated with the level of Ara-CTP (27). At present the relation between the amount of Ara-CTP and cytotoxicity is still under investigation. Studies indicate that a minimum level of Ara-CTP has to be maintained in the cell for a certain period of time before the Ara-CTP leads to cytotoxicity (28).

Cell kinetic studies. Ara-C is an inhibitor of DNA synthesis exerting its lethal activity on cells in the S-phase. In microfluorimetric experiments on cell suspensions exposed to Ara-C it was found that most of the cells were blocked at their entrance of the S-phase. At low concentrations the blocking effect was only partial and was reversible (29). These data indicate that Ara-CTP is formed probably in the G_1-phase and in the S-phase of the cell cycle and is active only when the cell is in the S-phase. Cell kinetic studies on leukaemic bone marrow from patients with acute myeloid leukaemia reveal that the percentage of proliferating cells is low as compared to that of normal bone marrow cells (30). In clinical studies it has been found that the result of therapy is better when the percentage of proliferating cells in the bone marrow is high (30). Hence, it might be concluded that the cytotoxic effect of Ara-C on the bone marrow cell population depends on the amount of Ara-CTP accumulated in the G_1-phase and/or S-phase as well as on the percentage of proliferating cells.

INTRACELLULAR METABOLISM OF ARA-C

Deamination. The metabolic pathway of Ara-C has been studied in detail. The pharmacodynamic parameters are important as they determine the ultimate effectiveness of this drug. Conversion of Ara-C to uracil arabinoside (Ara-U) *in vivo* was a prominent finding in the first pharmacological studies (31). It appeared that Ara-U had no cytostatic activity. Inactivation of Ara-C is catalyzed by the enzyme cytidine deaminase as was first reported from experiments with *Escherichia Coli* (32). The enzyme occurs naturally and deaminates cytidine and Ara-C to uridine and uracil arabinoside (Ara-U), respectively. Its activity in different tissues in man varies widely. The highest activity has been found in liver and plasma (33).

The biochemical properties of purified preparations of cytidine deaminase obtained from normal granulocytes and from peripheral leukaemic blast cells have been studied by Chabner *et al.* (34). They found that the affinity of the enzyme to its physiologic substrate cytidine was higher than its affinity to Ara-C. They also found that the concentration of the enzyme per mg protein was significantly higher in normal granulocytes than in leukaemic blast cells from AML patients. After separating normal bone marrow into a mature and an immature cell fraction by Ficoll density centrifugation, the enzymatic activities were determined in each fraction. It appeared that the cytidine deaminase activity in lysates of the mature fraction was 3.55 - 14.2 times greater than the activity found in lysates of the immature fractions. The authors suggested that the amount of cytidine deaminase activity is related to the process of granulocyte maturation. The deaminating activity of leukaemic blast cells in the bone marrow seems to be important. From the results of clinical studies Steuart and Burke (35) concluded that the level of cytidine deaminase in the blast cells of AML patients before treatment determines the response to Ara-C in these patients.

Phosphorylation. In 1962 Chu *et al.* (15) reported that phosphorylation of Ara-C is essential to inhibit DNA synthesis and cell growth. In drug resistant cell lines of L1210 and 5178Y it was found that phosphorylation of both deoxycytidine and Ara-C was decreased by over 90% when compared with phosphorylation in drug-sensitive cells (18,36). It was concluded from these studies that phosphorylation of Ara-C was mediated by deoxycytidine kinase and that a low activity of this enzyme could be responsible for resistance to the drug. Deoxycytidine phosphokinase is a naturally occurring enzyme that catalyzes the first phosphorylation step, namely to deoxycytidine 5'-monophosphate and cytosine arabinoside 5'-monophosphate, respectively. The biochemical properties of this enzyme were first studied in crude extracts of calf thymus (37,38). It appears from these studies that the enzyme is rate limiting in the conversion of Ara-C to Ara-CTP. The second phosphorylation step is catalyzed by cytosine monophosphokinase (39.40) and the third one by non-specific nucleoside diphosphokinase (41). In man deoxycytidine kinase has been found in all dividing cells, the highest activity being in the spleen (42).

Coleman *et al.* (43) have determined the biochemical properties of partially purified deoxycytidine phosphokinase from leukaemic blast cells. The enzyme demonstrated a greater affinity to deoxycytidine than to Ara-C. Of particular interest is the relatively weak feed back inhibition upon the phosphorylation of additional Ara-C by Ara-CTP and the strong inhibition of the same reaction by deoxycytidine and deoxycytidine triphosphate. From these data it can be concluded that high intracellular levels of cytosine arabinoside triphosphate have no effect on further drug phosphorylation.

A wide range of phosphorylating activities have been found in crude extracts from AML bone marrow blast cells (42,44). In a recent study intact leukaemic bone marrow cells and peripheral cells were incubated with labelled Ara-C (45,46). About 80% of the total intracellular radioactivity appeared to be Ara-CTP. Large variations in the amount of Ara-CTP in leukaemic bone marrow cells were found between patients suffering from acute lymphocytic leukaemia (ALL), acute myeloblastic leukaemia (AML) and chronic myelocytic leukaemia (CML). The lowest amounts of Ara-CTP were demonstrated in CML and ALL patients.

In AML patients a large variation was found in the quantities of Ara-CTP.

As mentioned before, the relationship between the intracellular concentration of Ara-CTP and the inhibition of DNA synthesis has been studied on murine leukaemia (L1210) by Chou *et al.* (27). The inhibition of DNA synthesis was higher and more pronounced when higher levels of Ara-CTP were found within the cell. Cytotoxicity was demonstrated when DNA synthesis was inhibited to more than 95%. Above this level a direct relationship was found between the amount of Ara-CTP and cytotoxicity. It is assumed that the minimal effective level of Ara-CTP to achieve cytotoxicity, differs for the various cell types.

Dephosphorylation of Ara-CTP. The rate of cytosine arabinoside triphosphate dephosphorylation has not been extensively studied. It is assumed that the nucleoside triphosphatases and diphosphatases have high activities as compared to the monophosphatases. It might thus be supposed that the rate determining dephosphorylation step is the one converting Ara-CMP into Ara-C (40). One might expect that the rate of dephosphorylation of Ara-C nucleotides could be a factor in the response to Ara-C.

However, no differences in the monophosphatase activities have been found between tumor cells which are sensitive to Ara-C and malignant cells which appeared to be insensitive to Ara-C.

INTRACELLULAR RESISTANCE TO ARA-C

The phosphorylation of Ara-C to its triphosphate is a prerequisite for the drug to inhibit DNA synthesis. In both human and murine leukaemic cells the response to Ara-C has been correlated with the ability to accumulate cytosine arabinoside triphosphate (27,48). Resistance to this agent may be the result of a decreased phosphorylating activity and/or an increased deaminating activity (34,35). Thus, the therapeutic effectiveness of Ara-C will be influenced by

-the total amount of drug transported into the target cells and

-the relative proportions of the drug activated by phosphokinases (K) and inactivated by deaminases (D) expressed as a K/D ratio.

A wide variation has been found in the ability of intact peripheral and bone marrow leukaemic blast cells to phosphorylate or deaminate the drug (42). These findings were confirmed in partially purified enzyme extracts of peripheral blast cells from AML-patients (34,43). The wide variations of the deaminating and phosphorylating capacities of AML cells are reflected in the variations in the calculated K/D ratios.

The K/D ratio of peripheral blast cells appeared to be of little value to predict the response of AML patients to Ara-C (43,50). The large variations in *phosphorylating abilities of both peripheral and marrow blast cells* may be due to the large individual differences between patients of the percentage proliferating cells in blood as well as in bone marrow (30).

The deaminating activity of blast cells of bone marrow seems to be important. From the results of clinical studies Steuart and Burke (35) assumed that the level of cytidine deaminase in the blast cells of AML patients before treatment determines their response to Ara-C.

PHARMACOKINETICS OF ARA-C

Ara-C has been used frequently to treat acute myeloid leukaemia (AML). The disease is characterized by an accumulation of immature myeloid cells in bone marrow. Treatment is aimed at the eradication of these cells. The empirical dosage and schedule of administration of Ara-C are based partly on pharmacokinetic animal studies. Knowledge about the distribution and elimination of the drug in man would be helpful to design optimal-treatment schedules. The present knowledge about pharmacokinetic parameters of Ara-C will be discussed briefly.

Plasma half-life. The first studies on distribution and metabolism of Ara-C in man were performed with the tritium-labelled drug. The levels of radioactivity in the body fluids were determined, after which chromatographic separation of Ara-C from its metabolite uracil arabinoside (Ara-U) followed. The plasma disappearance curve after intravenous administration of labelled Ara-C appeared to be biphasic with half-life values of the second phase ranging from 30 to 111 min (49,51). Bioassays, making use of sensitive cell lines or micro-organisms, have been developed for the determination of Ara-C levels in plasma of large numbers of patients. Pitillo and Hunt (52) described a method in which they used an actinobolin resistant strain of *Streptococcus faecalis.* Hanka et al. (53) modified this assay and were able to measure Ara-C levels as low as 0.1 mg/1. These assays, however, are not sensitive enough for clinical studies. Baguley *et al.* (54,55) reported a bio-assay using mouse L-cells or murine tumor cells. Recently van Prooijen *et al.* (56) developed a sensitive bio-assay which is suitable for pharmacokinetic studies in patients. The test is based on the inhibition of the incorporation of tritiated thymidine into DNA of rat bone marrow cells in the presence of Ara-C. Plasma concentrations as low as 0.003 mg/1 can thus be measured. With this assay the plasma disappearance of Ara-C was determined in AML patients after an intravenous bolus of Ara-C in a dose of 100 mg/m^2. The disappearance curve appeared to be biphasic (Fig. 2).

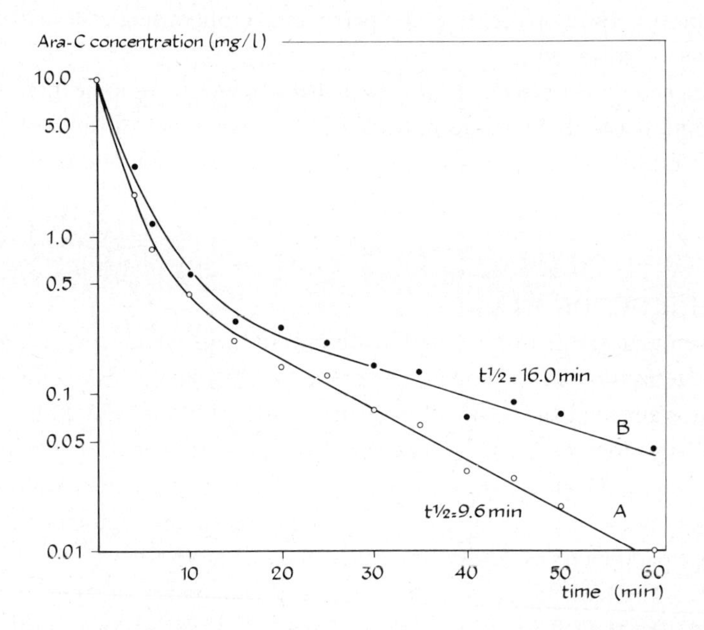

Fig. 2. Biphasic disappearance curves of Ara-C after an intravenous bolus injection (100 mg/m^2) in two AML patients. Half-life values were calculated from the slope of the curves using a two-compartment open model.

The plasma half-life ($T\ ^1/_2$) for the first phase varied from 1.2 to 1.9 min. The $T^1/_2$ of the second phase varied from 8.8 to 18.9 min. The first phase mainly represents the distribution of Ara-C over the total body fluid. The second phase represents the disappearance of Ara-C from the blood (14).

Elimination. The short plasma half-life of Ara-C in the second phase might be due to rapid elimination of Ara-C from the body or to rapid accumulation of the drug in the tissues. Camiener (33) found that the drug was rapidly transformed to Ara-U in the liver by the enzyme cytidine deaminase and presumed a rapid elimination of the drug via this route.

With the use of labelled Ara-C it could be demonstrated that 86 to 96% of the radioactivity recovered in the urine was present as Ara-U (31,49). Similar results were found by Ho *et al.* (51), who recovered 80% of the radioactivity in the urine within 24 hours after administration of labelled Ara-C, 8% being present as Ara-C and 72% as Ara-U.

The possibility of an accumulation of drug in tissues was investigated in whole-body radioautograms in mice (57). Three hours after intravenous administration of a single dose of labelled Ara-C, high amounts of radioactivity were found in the gall bladder, in liver and in the gastrointestinal tract. Those findings indicate the biliary secretion of drug metabolites into the intestine. Enterohepatic recirculation of radioactivity was likely, as 94% of the total administered radioactivity was recovered in the urine within 48 hours and virtually none in the faeces. No specific accumulation of the drug was observed in tissues.

The available data indicate that the drug is rapidly deaminated to Ara-U by cytidine deaminase. A potent inhibitor of cytidine deaminase, tetra-hydrouridine (THU), shows low toxicity in many species including man. Recently, Ara-C blood levels and the elimination curve have been reported for a patient receiving THU and Ara-C simulataneously (58). Oral administration of THU resulted in a twofold increase in Ara-C blood levels without significant changes in the plasma half-life of the second phase. The administration of THU together with Ara-C might be useful in cases where Ara-C is rapidly deaminated.

CLINICAL PHARMACOLOGY OF ARA-C

Ara-C is the drug of choice in the treatment of acute myeloid leukaemia (AML). In most treatment protocols the drug is combined with other cytotoxic agents; complete remission can be achieved in about 60% of the patients (59,60). Despite the improvement in the number of complete remissions in the last few years, failure of therapy still occurs, particularly when patients are treated for relapse. Drug resistance is a fundamental problem in the treatment of leukaemia. Most of the investigations, performed to deal with this problem, concern the intracellular metabolism of the drug. Within the cell the drug is activated by phosphokinases to its triphosphate (Ara-CTP) and inactivated by deaminases to Ara-U. The drug is only active as Ara-CTP as an inhibitor of DNA synthesis. Resistance to the drug at the cellular level is found when the intracellular concentration of Ara-CTP is decreased due to high deaminating and/or low phosphorylating activities.

It is obvious that the intracellular concentration of Ara-CTP depends on the time during which the cells are exposed to an effective drug level in the blood. Pharmacokinetic studies in AML patients demonstrate large variations in the disappearance rate of Ara-C from the blood and ineffective treatment was observed when the plasma half-life of Ara-C was rather short (14). Recently, we studied the relation of the plasma half-life to the intracellular metabolism and also to the therapeutic effect of the drug in AML patients (61). The results of this study are outlined briefly.

TABLE 1
TREATMENT OF AML PATIENTS WITH ARA-C

Patients	Sex	Age Years	Disease stage	Treatment days	
1.	F	30	relapse	14	
2.	F	43	first	10	
3.	M	41	first	14	
4.	M	54	first	10	6*
5.	F	18	first	14	
6.	F	65	first	10	
7.	M	47	first	10	
8.	F	38	first	10	
9.	F	53	first	14	10
10.	F	23	first	14	
11.	M	56	first	10	10
12.	F	19	first	14	
13.	F	28	relapse	14	10*
14.	F	31	relapse	10	14*

*patient received combination therapy
Patients data (sex and age in years)
Stage of disease (first stage, relapse)
Duration of chemotherapy in days (first course:
Ara-C; second course in case of failure:
either Ara-C or, starting Ara-C and day 3, in combination
with adriamycin [day 1] and vincristine [day 2]

TABLE 2
PHARMACOKINETICS OF TREATMENT OF AML PATIENTS

Patients	$T^1/_2$ Ara-C min.	Remission	DNA-inhibition %	$T^1/_2$ nucleated cells h
1.	18.9	++	95	–
2.	15.5	++	90	23
3.	16.6	++	86	33
4.	17.4	++	- -	36
5.	16.0	†	- -	36
6.	13.0	†	83	48
7.	14.7	†	81	- -
8.	13.3	++	81	- -
9.	14.6	++	79	46
10.	14.3	++	78	53
11.	18.0	++	73	- -
12.	11.5	†	69	103
13.	9.5	- -	65	160
14.	8.8	- -	50	82

Plasma half-life of Ara-C ($T^1/_2$ Ara-C in min.), drug effect (complete remission ++, partial remission +, failure - and death † during the aplastic phase after the first treatment course),
inhibition of DNA synthesis (%) in leukaemic bone marrow cells and disappearance of leukaemic (nucleated) cells from blood ($T^1/_2$ nucleated cells in h.; not calculated in cases of leukopenia i.e. nucleated cells $< 3.0 \times 10^9/1$) of 14 AML patients (see Table 1).

Plasma half-life and the inhibition of DNA synthesis. The study was performed in 14 AML patients treated with intravenous bolus injections of Ara-C in a dose of 100 mg/m^2 every 12 hours for 10 or 14 consecutive days. After the first bolus injection blood samples were taken at several time intervals to determine the plasma concentrations of Ara-C with the bio-assay (56). The Ara-C elimination curves appeared to be biphasic (Fig. 2). The plasma half-life for the first phase varied from 1.2 to 1.9 minutes; the plasma half-life values in the second phase were calculated and appeared to range from 8.8 to 18.9 minutes. As a result of rapid elimination, the plasma concentration of Ara-C decreases from 10.0 mg/1 to 0.05 mg/1 in 60 minutes (Fig. 2), during this short time interval the bone marrow cells are exposed to the drug and intracellular metabolism takes place (45). Therefore the result of metabolism was determined in the bone marrow cells one hour after the bolus injection by the *in vitro* incorporation of tritiated thymidine into the leukaemic bone marrow cells. This thymidine uptake was compared with the uptake in marrow cells obtained prior to the Ara-C injections. The of thymidine uptake one hour after Ara-C

A relationship between the plasma half-life and the degree of the inhibition of DNA synthesis in the leukaemic bone marrow cells is quite clearly shown. A strong inhibition of DNA synthesis (> 70%) was observed in 11 patients with relatively long half-life values (> 13.0 min.). All these patients achieved complete remission. (Table 2). Patients with the highest percentage of inhibition achieved complete re-

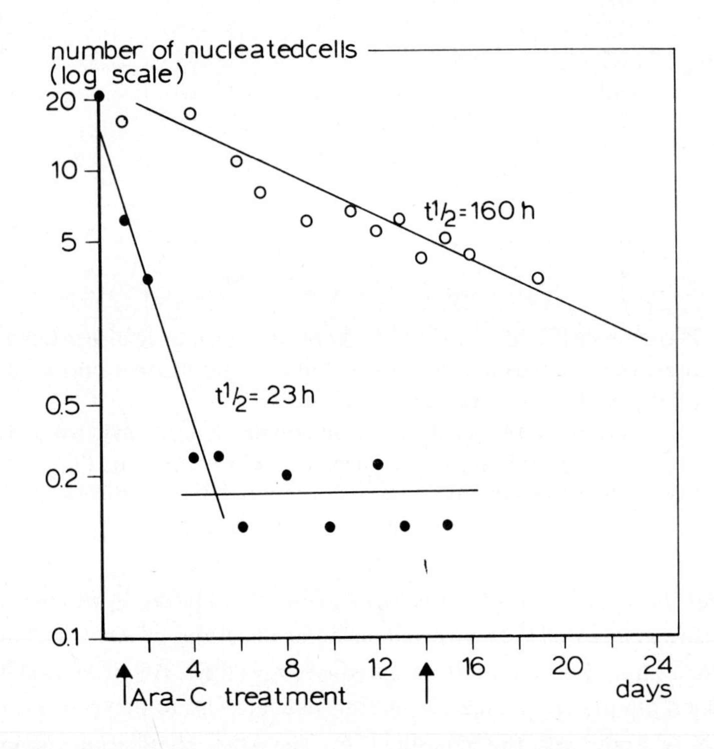

Fig. 3. Plotted are the number of nucleated cells during the first course of treatment in two full blown AML patients (myeloblasts >90%). The leukocyte half-life values were calculated from the slope of the curves.

mission after the first course of treatment. The other patients needed two or more courses of treatment. Three patients with relatively short plasma half-life values showed a weak inhibition of DNA synthesis with values below 70%. Therapy failed in all three patients. Although the number of patients is small, the data indicate that pharmacokinetics and similar metabolic studies render valuable information before treatment of the individual patient.

We observed considerable differences in the disappearance rate of peripheral leukemic blasts, indicated as leukocyte half-life ($T^1/_2$) (Fig. 3). This half-life ranged from 23 to 160 hours. As might be expected, a close relationship was found between the inhibition percentage and the leukocyte half-life values. All patients with high inhibition percentages ($>$ 70%) showed relatively short leukocyte half-life values ($<$ 55 hours). All patients with low inhibition percentages ($<$ 70%) showed higher leukocyte half-life values ($>$ 55 hours). From these data it may be concluded that the disappearance rate of the peripheral cells during the first course of treatment may become a helpful additional parameter in the treatment of leukemic patients.

REFERENCES

1. Bergmann, W., Burke, D.C. (1955) J. Org. Chem. 20, 1501.

2. Kanai, T., Kojima, T., Maruyama, O., Ichino, M. (1970) Chem. Pharm. Bull. (Tokyo) 18, 2569-2570.

3. Darzynkiewics, E., Kusmierek, J.K., Shugar, D. (1972) Biochem. Biophys. Res. commun. 46, 1734-1741.

4. Notari, R.E., Chin, M.L., Wittebort, R. (1972) J. Pharm. Sci. 61, 1189.

5. Evans, J.S., Musser, E.A., Mengel, G.D., Forsblad, K.R., Hunter, J.H. (1964) Cancer Res., 24, 1285.

6. Wodinsky, I., Kensler, C.J. (1965) Cancer Chemother. Rep. 47. 65.

7. Lark, K.G., Lark, C.L. (1964) J. Mol. Biol. 10, 120.

8. Silagi, S. (1965) Cancer Res. 25, 1446.

9. Piscala, A., Sorm, F. (1964) Collection Czech. Chem. Commun. 29, 2060.

10 Jurovcik, M., Raska, K., Sornova, Z., Sorm, F. (1965) Collection Czech. Chem. Commun. 30, 3370.

11. Sorm, F., Vesely, J. (1964) Neoplasma 11, 123.

12. Vendetti, J.M., Baratta, M.C., Greenberg, N.H., Abbott, B.J. (1972) Cancer Chemother. Rep. 56, 483.

13. Ho, D.H.W., Rodriquez, V., Ti Li Loo, Bodey, G.P. and Freireich, E.J. (1975) Clin. Pharmacol. Ther. 17,66.

14. Prooijen van, H.C., Kleyn van der, E., Haanen, C. (1977) Clin. Pharmacol. Ther. 21, 744.

15. Chu, M.Y., Fischer, G.A. (1962) Biochem. Pharmacol. 11, 423.

16. Moore, E.C., Cohen, S.S. (1967) J. Biol. Chem. 242, 2116.

17. Skoog, L., Nordenskjöld, B. (1971) Europ. J. Biochem. 19, 81.

18. Chu, M.Y., Fischer, G.A. (1965) Biochem. Pharmacol. 14, 333.

19. Chu, M.Y., Fischer, G.A. (1968) Biochem. Pharmacol. 17, 753.

20. Momparler, R.L., Lalitan, A., Rossi, M. (1972) Cancer Res. 32, 408.

21. Graham, F.L., Whitmore, G.F. (1970) Cancer Res. 30, 2636.

22. Kimball, A.P., Wilson, M.J. (1968) Proc. Soc. Exptl. Biol. 127, 429.

23. Furth, J.J., Cohen, S.S. (1968) Cancer Res. 28, 2061.

24. Inagaki, A., Nakamera, T., Wakinsoka, G. (1969) Cancer Res. 29, 2169.

25. Graham, F.L., Whitmore, G.T. (1970) Cancer Res. 30, 2627.

26. Momparler, R.L.(1972) Molec. Pharmcol. 8, 362.

27, Chou, T.C., Hutchison, D.J., Schmidt, F.A., Philips, F.S. (1975) Cancer Res. 35, 225.

28. Jones, P.A., Baker, M.S., Benedict, W.F. (1976) Cancer Res. 36, 3789.

29. Yataganas, X., Strife, A., Perez, A., Clarkson, B.D. (1974) Cancer Res. 34, 2795.

30. Hillen, H., Wessels, J., Haanen, C. (1975) The Lancet 15, 609.

31. Papac, R.J., Creasey, W.A., Calabresi, P., Welck, A.D. (1965) Proc.Amer. Ass. Cancer Res. 6, 50.

32. Pizer, L.I., Cohen, S.S. (1960) J. Biol. Chem. 235, 2387.

33. Camiener, G.W. (1967) Biochem. Pharmacol. 16, 1681.

34. Chabner, B.A., Johns, D.C., Coleman, C.N., Drake, J.C., Evans, W.H. (1974) J. Clin. Invest. 53, 922.

35. Steuart, C.D., Burke, P.J. (1971) Nature, 233, 109.

36. Schrecker, A.W., Urshel, M.J. (1968) Cancer Res. 28, 793.

37. Durham, J.P., Ives, D.H. (1968) Molec. Pharmacol. 5, 358.

38. Momparler, R.L., Fischer, G.A. (1968) J. Biol. Chem. 243, 4298.

39. Sigino, Y., Tereoka, H., Shimono, H. (1966) J. Biol. Chem. 241, 961.

40. Schrecker, A.W. (1970) Cancer Res. 30, 632.

41. Nakamura, H., Sugino, Y. (1966) J. Biol. Chem. 241, 4917.

42. Ho, D.H.W. (1973) Cancer Res. 33, 2816.

43. Coleman, C.N., Stoller, R.G., Drake, J.G., Chabner, A. (1975) Blood 46, 791.

44. Tattersall, M.H.N., Ganeshaguru, K., Hoffbrand, A.V. (1974) Brit. J. Haematol. 27, 39-46.

45. Chou, T.C., Arlin, Z., Clarkson, B.D., Philips, F.S. (1977) Cancer Res. 37, 3561-3570.

46. Drenthe, A. (1978) Personal communications.

47. Drakouvsky, D., Kreis, W. (1970) Biochem. Pharmacol. 19, 940.

48. Kessel, D., Hall, T.C., Rosenthal, D. (1969) Cancer Res. 29, 459.

49. Creasy, W.A., Papac, R.J., Markiw, M.E., Calibresi, P., Welch, A.D. (1966) Biochem. Pharmacol. 15, 1417.

50. Smyth, J.F., Robins, A.B., Leese, C.L. (1976) Europ. J. Cancer, 12, 567

51. Ho, D.H.W., Frei, E. (1971) Clin. Pharmacol. Ther. 12, 945.

52. Pitillo, R.F., Hunt, D.E. (1967) Proc. Sic. exp. Biol. 124, 636.

53. Hanka, L.J., Kuentzel, S.L., Neil, G.L. (1970) Cancer Chemoth. Rep. 54, 393.

54. Baguley, B.C., Faulkenhoug, E.M. (1971) Cancer Chemother. Rep, 55, 291.

55. Baguley, B.C., Faulkenhoug, E.M. (1975) Europ. J. Cancer 11, 43.

56. Prooijen van, H.C., Vierwinden, G., Egmond van, J., Wessels, J., Haanen, C. (1976) Europ. J. Cancer 12, 899-905.

57. Liss, R.H., Neil, G.L. (1975) Cancer Chemother. Rep. 59, 501-513.

58. Kreis, W., Woodcock, T.M., Gordon, C.S., Krakoff, I.H. (1977) Cancer treatment Rep. 61, 1347-1353.

59. Clarkson, B.D. (1972) Cancer 30, 1572-1583.

60. Mathé, G., Pouillart, P., De Vasal, F., Delgado, M., Schwarzenberg, L., Misset, J.L., Hayat, M., Jasmin, C., Belpomme, D., Musset, M. (1976) Lancet i, 1130-1131.

61. Prooijen van, H.C. (1977) Thesis, Nijmegen.

62. Talley, R.W., Vaitkevicius, V.K. (1963) Blood 21, 352-362.

63. Benedict, W.R., Karon, M. (1971) Science 171, 680-682.

© 1978 Elsevier/North-Holland Biomedical Press
Clinical Pharmacology of Anti-Neoplastic Drugs
H. M. Pinedo, editor

EXTRACTION PROPERTIES AND LIQUID CHROMATOGRAPHIC SEPARATION OF ADRIAMYCIN AND DAUNORUBICIN AND THEIR HYDROXYL METABOLITES. APPLICATION TO BIOANALYSIS.

STAFFAN EKSBORG
Karolinska Pharmacy, Fack, S-104 01 Stockholm 60, Sweden

ABSTRACT

The extractions of the antraquinone glycosides adriamycin, adriamycinol, daunorubicin and daunorubicinol have been studied using a mixture of chloroform and 1-pentanol as the organic phase. For optimal extraction pH was varied within the range of 8.0-8.6.

Antraquinone glycosides showed a high tendency to form dimers and tetramers in aqueous solutions. The formation constants were found to be in the order of $10^{4.5}$ and 10^{12}, respectively. The degrees of extraction of the compounds were therefore not only dependent upon pH of the aqueous solution, but also upon the solute concentration.

Separation of antraquinone glycosides has successfully been achieved with reversed-phase high performance liquid chromatography using acetonitrile-water as the mobile phase.

The development of analytical methods for the determination of adriamycin-adriamycinol and daunorubicin-daunorubicinol has been based on data obtained by studies of extraction and chromatographic properties. The methods comprise quantitative extraction into an organic solvent, re-extraction into a small acidic aqueous phase and separation by reversed-phase liquid chromatography with photometric (253.7 nm or 500 nm) or fluorimetric (435 nm/550 nm) detection. Quantitation is based on peak area measurement. Determinations in the low ng/ml region with a high accuracy and precision are possible.

INTRODUCTION

Antraquinone glycosides have successfully been used for the treatment of neoplastic diseases (1). Adriamycin (A) and daunorubicin (D) are the most potent drugs within this class of substances (2,3,4). Both drugs are used for the treatment of leukemia, while solid tumors are preferably treated with adriamycin.

Metabolites with cytostatic activity (5,6,7), adriamycinol (AOH) and daunorubicinol (DOH) respectively, are formed by enzymatic reduction of the keto group in the side chains of the drugs. Structure of the drugs and the metabolites are given in Fig. 1.

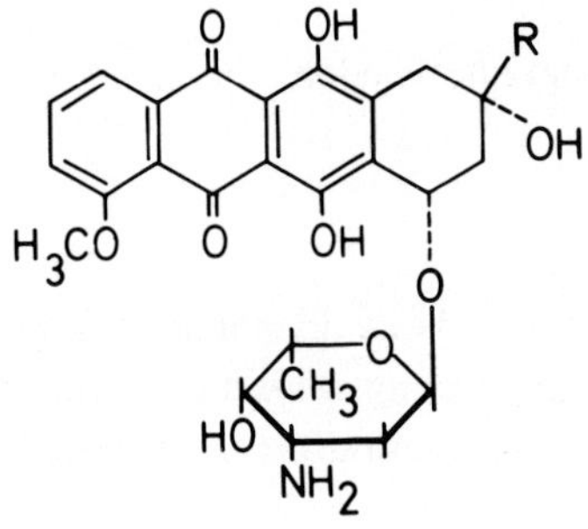

Fig. 1. Structural formulae.
R = $-COCH_2OH$ (adriamycin),
$-CH(OH)CH_2OH$ (adriamycinol),
$-COCH_3$ (daunorubicin),
$-CH(OH)CH_3$ (daunorubicinol).

The cytotoxic effect of antraquinone glycosides has been attributed to complex formation with DNA, resulting in an inhibition of RNA and DNA synthesis (8,9, 10).

Most of the side effects originating from treatment with adriamycin and daunorubicin such as myelotoxicity, stomatitis, nausea, vomiting and alopecia, are reversible, and commonly seen with other neoplastic drugs. Therapy with adriamycin and daunorubicin is restricted due to cardiomyopathy. It is recommended that the cumulative doses of these drugs should not exceed 550 mg/m^2 (11).

Many attempts have been made to overcome the fatal toxicity of high doses of daunorubicin and adriamycin (12,13,14); a promising one is the administration of the drugs as complexes with DNA (15,16).

The aim of our work has been to develop fast and reliable analytical methods for the determination of adriamycin-adriamycinol and daunorubicin-daunorubicinol in biological samples for comparative pharmacokinetic studies. The development of such methods became possible after extensive studies of the extraction properties (17) and of reversed-phase liquid chromatography (18) of antraquinone glycosides.

The pharmacokinetics of adriamycin and daunorubicin have been studied previously with unselective methods such as measurements of total fluorescence (19,20) and radioimmunoassay (RIA) (21). By the use of these methods it is not possible to differentiate between a drug and its hydroxyl metabolite. Other metabolites, e.g. aglycones, may also interfere. Analytical methods including a chromatographic step give a considerable higher selectivity (22-25).

MATERIALS AND METHODS

Chemicals. Adriamycin and adriamycinol were kindly supplied by Farmitalia (Milan, Italy), daunorubicin and daunorubicinol by Pharma Rhodia (Stockholm, Sweden) and desipramine by AB Hässle (Mölndal, Sweden).

Chloroform, analytical grade (E. Merck, Darmstadt, G.F.R.), was equilibrated with water to remove ethanol. All other organic solvents were of analytical grade and used without purification. Carbonate, citrate and phosphate buffers had an ionic strength of 0.1, unless otherwise stated.

Apparatus. This consisted of an Aminco-Bowman 4-8202 B Spectrofluorimeter, a Zeiss PMQ III Spektralphotometer and an Orion Research Model 701/digital pH meter equipped with an Ingold combined electrode type 401.

Glass equipment. All glass equipment, with the exception of pipettes, was silinized by treating with dichlorodimethyl silane (5% by volume) in toluene, followed by washing with dry methanol.

Chromatographic system. The two photometric detectors used were the LDC Spectromonitor I (500 nm) and the Aktex Model 153 (253.7 nm). Both were equipped with a cell of 10 nm path length and a volume of 8 μl. The fluorimetric detector used was the Schoeffel Instrument FS 970 Fluorimetric Detector (435 nm/550 nm) with a cell volume of 5 μl.

The pump was of the LDC 711 Solvent Delivery System type, and the columns were of stainless steel (length 150 mm, ID 4 mm, OD 1/4 in.). The column end fittings were modified Swagelok connectors. A Rheodyne (Model 70-10) injection valve with a sample loop of 300 μl was used.

The LiChrosorb RP-2 and LiChrosorb RP-8 supports (E. Merck) had a mean diameter of 5 μm, and the chromatographic system was thermostated to 25.0± 0.1°C.

Chromatographic technique. The columns were packed by the balanced density slurry technique (26) with tetrachloroethylene as suspending medium. The columns were washed with n-hexane and acetone (100 ml of each) before use.

The mobile phase was passed through the chromatographic system until constant retention of the solutes was obtained. Less than 50 ml was usually required.

Drug administration. The doses adriamycin and daunorubicin were given as intravenous infusions and were within the range of 0.70-1.50 mg per kilogram of mass, either as free drugs or as complexes with DNA (mass ratio of adriamycin or daunorubicin to DNA, 1:12).

Plasma samples. Blood samples (5-7 ml) were collected in 10 ml glass test tubes (Vacutainer) containing 250 IU heparin (freeze dried) immediately prior to and at appropriate times after the start of drug administration. The samples were immediately cooled in an ice bath and centrifuged at 5,000 rpm for 10 min at 0°. The plasma fraction was carefully aspirated and frozen at -20° until assayed.

Analytical methods

Extraction procedure for the determination of adriamycin and adriamycinol. A 1.00 ml sample of plasma or urine is carefully mixed with 0.10 ml phosphate buffer pH 8.6, $\mu = 1.0$, and 1.5 g diatomaceous earth (acid washed Celite 545), and quantitatively transferred onto an extraction column (ID 6 mm). The column is eluated with a mixture of chloroform + 1-heptanol (8:2), the first 7 ml being collected in a centrifuge tube. The organic phase is extracted with 0.300 ml phosphate buffer pH 2.2 containing 10 μg/ml of desipramine for 10 min.

Extraction procedure for the determination of daunorubicin and daunorubicinol. A 2.00 ml sample of plasma or urine is mixed with 0.20 ml phosphate buffer pH 8.1, $\mu = 1.0$, and extracted with 10.0 ml of chloroform + 1-heptanol (9:1) for 10 min. After centrifugation 7.00 ml of the organic phase is extracted with 0.400 ml phosphoric acid 0.1 M containing 5 μg/ml of desipramine for 10 min.

Liquid chromatographic isolation and quantitation. The aqueous (upper) phase obtained from the extraction procedure is transferred into a centrifuge tube with tapered bottom (0.2 ml), containing 2 ml of hexane and is centrifugated. (This step is included to facilitate the transfer of the aqueous phase onto the chromatographic column without contamination with organic phase).

Part of the aqueous (lower) phase (0.050-0.300 ml) is injected onto the chromatographic column (support: LiChrosorb RP-2, 5 μm; mobile phase: acetonitrile - water - 0.1 M phosphoric acid, 20:70:10 by volume for the determination of adriamycin and adriamycinol, 25:65:10 by volume for the determination of daunorubicin and daunorubicinol; mobile phase speed 0.8-1.0 ml/min). The concentration of the solutes in the eluate is measured by photometric (253.7 nm or 500 nm) or fluorimetric (436 nm/550 nm) detection.

Quantitation is based on peak area measurements.

RESULTS AND DISCUSSION

The following symbols not defined in the text are used:

$[\ ], [\ ]_{org}$ = concentrations of molecules and ions in aqueous and organic phases, respectively

C_D = total concentration in aqueous phase

C_{Dorg} = total concentration in organic phase

k_d = $[DOH]_{org} \times [DOH]^{-1}$ = distribution coefficient

a_h = hydrogen ion activity

Protolysis. The protolysis of the antraquinone glycosides studied can be illustrated by the following scheme, in which k'_1, k'_2, k'_{12}, and k'_{21} are equilibrium constants.

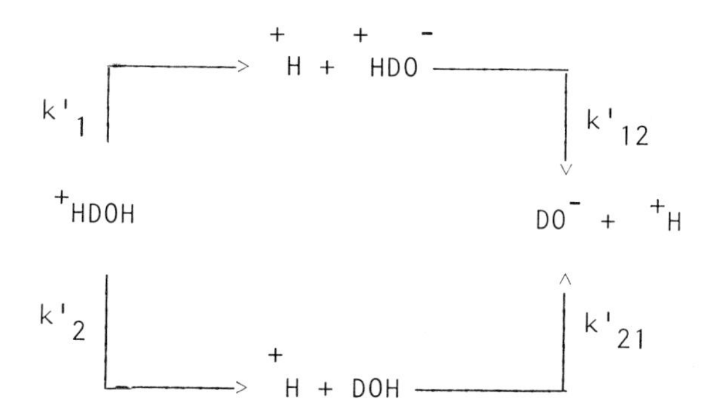

Four forms of the compounds can occur, viz. the ammonium form (^+HDOH), the phenolate form (DO^-), the uncharged form (DOH) and the zwitter ion form ($^+HDO^-$). It was, however, shown (17) that formation of zwitter ions was negligible. By photometric measurements it was possible to determine $pk'_{21} = 9.54$ (a phenolic group) while pk'_2 (an amino group) was determined by partition experiments (Table 1).

TABLE 1
ACID DISSOCIATION CONSTANTS

Substance	pk'_2
Adriamycin	7.20
Adriamycinol	7.69
Daunorubicin	6.4
Daunorubicinol	6.64

Obviously the dissociation constant of the amino group (pk'_2) is strongly dependent on the substitution in the side chain. Studies of molecular models revealed that a hydrogen bond formation between the amino group at the sugar moiety and the keto and/or hydroxyl groups at the side chain is most likely to occur.

Distribution to an organic phase. Partition experiments were performed using chloroform + 1-pentanol as the organic and a buffer solution as the aqueous phase. Antraquinone glycosides are most likely extracted into the organic phase in the uncharged form (17). The distribution ratio, D, is given by (1)

$$D = C_{Dorg} \times C_D^{-1} = k_d \times (a_h/k'_2 + k'_1/k'_2 + k'_{21}/a_h + 1)^{-1} \quad (1)$$

An optimal degree of extraction is obtained when $pH = 1/2\,(pk'_2 + pk'_{21})$

When $pH \leq pk'_{21} - 1$, Eq. (1) can be given the form

$$D^{-1} = k_d^{-1} + a_h(k_d \times k'_2)^{-1} \quad (2)$$

since $k'_1 >> k'_2$ (formation of zwitterion is negligible).

It was possible to evaluate k_d and k'_2 from experimental data by plotting 1/D versus a_h. The influence of pH on the distribution ratio has been calculated from determined constants, and is presented in Fig. 2.

From Fig. 2 it follows that none of the compounds can be quantitatively extracted by a single extractants using equal phase volumes. As described in the Analytical Methods daunorubicin and daunorubicinol were quantitatively extracted by using a ratio organic phase/ aqueous phase of 5. To avoid too large volumes of organic extractions adriamycin and adriamycinol were transferred into an organic phase using column extraction. Aglycones, formed as metabolites, were excluded by re-extraction of the organic phase with an acidic aqueous phase. Addition of desipramine to this aqueous phase eliminated adsorption phenomena.

It was found that the distribution not only is dependent upon pH of the aqueous phase, but also upon the concentration in the aqueous phase. This effect is illustrated in Fig. 3.

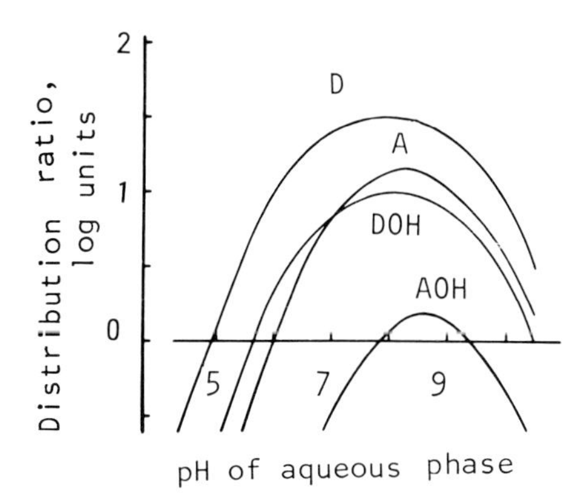

Fig. 2. Distribution ratio and pH of the aqueous phase.
Organic phase: chloroform + 1-pentanol (9 + 1).
Aqueous phase: buffer solution.
A=adriamycin; AOH=adriamycinol; D=daunorubicin; DOH=daunorubicinol.
The curves are calculated from constants given in ref. 17.

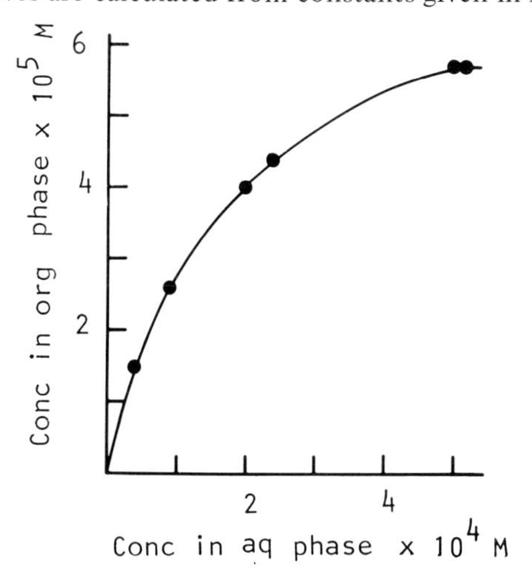

Fig. 3. Distribution equilibrium and concentration of daunorubicin.
Organic phase: chloroform + 1-pentanol (9 + 1)
Aqueous phase: citrate buffer pH 4.9.

The distribution into the organic phase is declined with increasing concentration of the antraquinone glycoside. It was shown that this is due to the formation of dimers and tetramers in the aqueous phase (17), the formation constants being in the order of $10^{4.5}$ and 10^{12}, respectively. The formation constants are of a remarkably high magnitude, and the influence of dimerization and tetramerization often has to be taken into account, e.g. by the evaluation of cytostatic effect of antraquinone glycosides in *in vitro* test systems, evaluation of constants of binding reactions to DNA etc.

Reversed-phase liquid chromatography

Retention and selectivity By the separation of antraquinone glycosides the selectivity and retention were found to be strongly dependent upon the concentration of the organic modifier in the mobile phase (18) (Fig. 4).

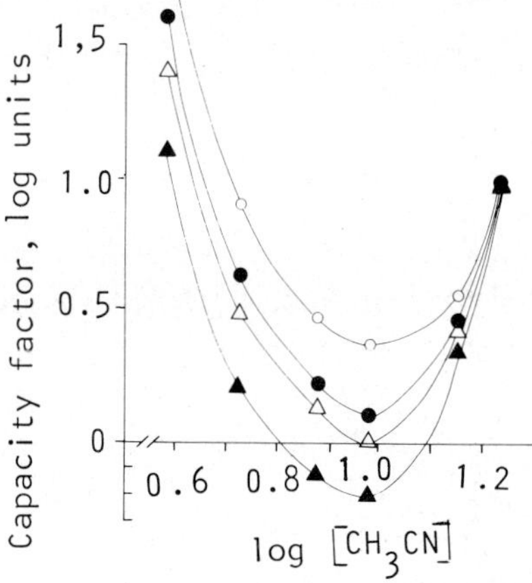

Fig. 4. Retention and concentration of acetonitrile in mobile phase.
Mobile phase: phosphoric acid (10^{-2} M) in acetonitrile + water.
Support: LiChrosorb RP-8 (5 μm).
Solutes: adriamycin (△); adriamycinol (▲); daunorubicin (○); daunorubicinol (●), 2.5 nmole of each in 100 μl of mobile phase.

The minima of the retention within the range $0.9 < \log [CH_3CN] < 1.0$ might be due to solvation of the solutes in the mobile phase as adducts including both water and organic solvent. From Fig. 4 it follows that the selectivity of the chromatographic system increases with decreasing concentration of acetonitrile in the mobile phase. The separation of the four antraquinone glycosides is illustrated in Fig. 5.

Highest performance when separating a drug from the corresponding hydroxyl metabolite was obtained when using LiChrosorb RP-2 (5 μm) as the support. Fig. 6 shows the influence of the concentration of acetonitrile in mobile phase on the retention time of the solutes.

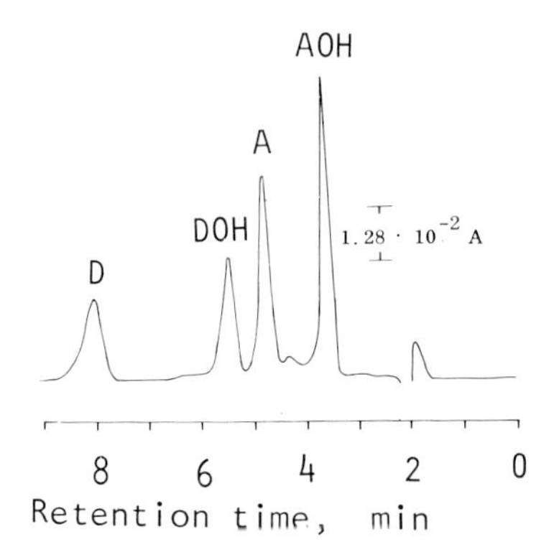

Fig. 5. Liquid chromatographic separation of antraquinone glycosides. Concentration of acetonitrile in mobile phase: 7.6 M.
Solutes: A=adriamycin; AOH=adriamycinol; D=daunorubicin; DOH=daunorubicinol.
Further conditions: see legend Fig. 4.

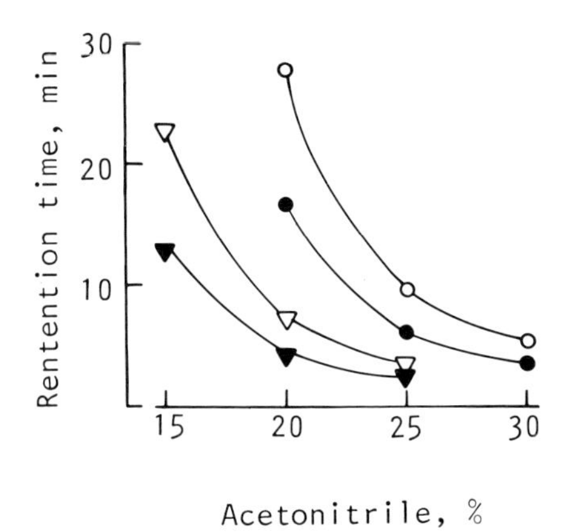

Fig. 6. Retention time and concentration of acetonitrile in mobile phase.
Solutes: adriamycin (▽); adriamycinol (▼); daunorubicin (○); daunorubicinol (●).
Support: LiChrosorb RP-2 (5 μm).
Mobile phase: Phosphoric acid (10^{-2} M) in acetonitrile + water, 1 ml/min.

Detection selectivity and sensitivity. Liquid chromatographic determination of antraquinone glycosides is possible with a very high detection selectivity. A high detector response is obtained by photometric detection at 500 nm as well as by fluorimetric detection at 436 nm/550 nm, i.e. under conditions where almost no endogenous compounds and other drugs may interfere. A considerably lower detection selectivity is obtained when using the commonly used UV detector measuring at 253.7 nm. With such a detector the selectivity in the extraction and chromatographic procedures are sometimes sufficient for quantitative determination in biological samples. Approximately the same sensitivities are obtained with the UV and the fluorimetric detectors.

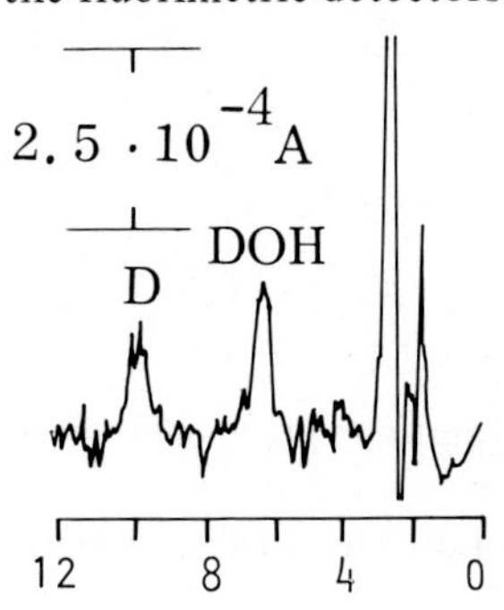

Fig. 7. High sensitivity by chromatography of daunorubicin (D) and daunorubicinol (DOH) with UV detection (253.7 nm).
Amount of sample: 4 x 10^{-3} nM (2.3 ng) of each solute in 100 μl of mobile phase. Chromatographic conditions: according to the Analytical Methods.

A sample containing 2 ng daunorubicin and daunorubicinol of each gives a signal to noise ratio of 3 (Fig. 7). Photometric detection at 500 nm gives an about 3-5 times lower sensitivity. Besides the high detection selectivity and sensitivity, a further advantage of the fluorimetric detector is that, compared to photometric detectors, considerably larger sample volumes can be measured. Only minor disturbances of the base line are caused by the non-retarded solvent peak. Band-broadening of the solute peaks is minimized by using a sample solvent by which the solutes are non-retarded (27).

Quantitative determination

Fluorimetric detection (346 nm/550 nm). Evaluation of the amount of antraquinone glycosides in an unknown sample is based on peak area measurement and the use of a calibration graph, obtained by running known amounts through the chromatographic system. A calibration graph in the low ng range is shown in Fig. 8.

Photometric detection (253.7 nm or 500 nm). Quantitation is based on peak area measurement. The amount of sample in the chromatographic peak can be calculated by means of Eq. (3).

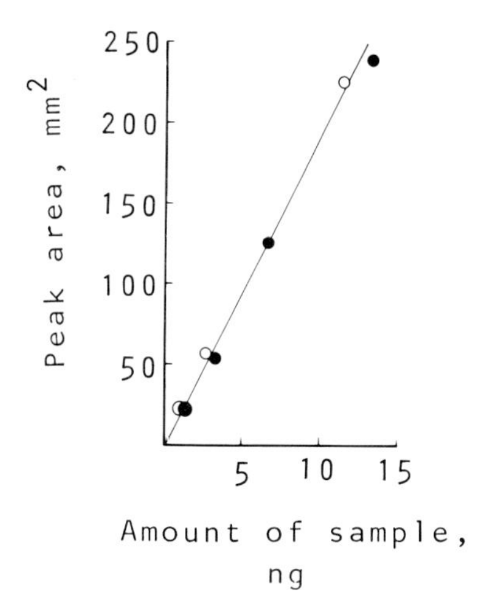

Fig. 8. Calibration graph for quantitation of adriamycin (○) and adriamycinol (●) by fluorimetric detection.
Chromatographic detection at 436 nm/ 550 nm.
Further conditions as given in the Analytical Methods.

$$M = Y \times u \times b \times \epsilon^{-1} \qquad (3)$$

M = amount of sample in mM,
Y = peak area in mm^2,
u = ml/mm chart paper,
b = absorbance/mm chart paper and
ϵ = molar absorptivity of the migrating compound (27).

The molar absorptivities of the four antraquinone glycosides were found to be identical (7.89×10^3 at 500 nm and 1.92×10^4 at 253.7 nm). From Eq. (3) it follows that the peak area is independent of chromatographic parameters such as column efficiency and capacity factors of the solutes, length and diameter of the chromatographic column.

Recovery and precision. The recovery and precision of the Analytical Methods were evaluated by analysing blank plasma samples spiked with 20 - 200 ng of the drugs and corresponding reduced metabolites. Results obtained when testing the Analytical Methods for determination of daunorubicin and daunorubicinol are given in Table 2. It shows that the recovery is very close to 100%. Neither the recovery nor the precision of the Analytical Methods were lowered when daunorubicin and daunorubicinol were added to blank plasma samples as DNA complexes.

TABLE 2

RECOVERY AND PRECISION

Plasma level (ng/ml)	Recovery (%) Daunorubicin	Daunorubicinol	Added as
25	99.3±1.1 [1)]	98.6±2.1	Free drug
100	99.6±1.6	99.7±0.9	-,,-
200	100.0±0.3	103.5±1.8	-,,-
20	99.3±1.7	99.7±1.8	DNA complex
70	99.9±1.5	99.0±1.2	-,,-
200	99.5±1.2	101.0±0.8	-,,-

1) Relative standard deviation (n = 8)
Measuring wave length: 500 nm

Samples from patients. A typical chromatogram of a urine sample from a leukemic patient treated with daunorubicin is shown in Fig. 9. Examples of plasma levels of daunorubicin and daunorubicinol after repeated administration of daunorubicin as free drug to leukemic patients is presented in Fig. 10.

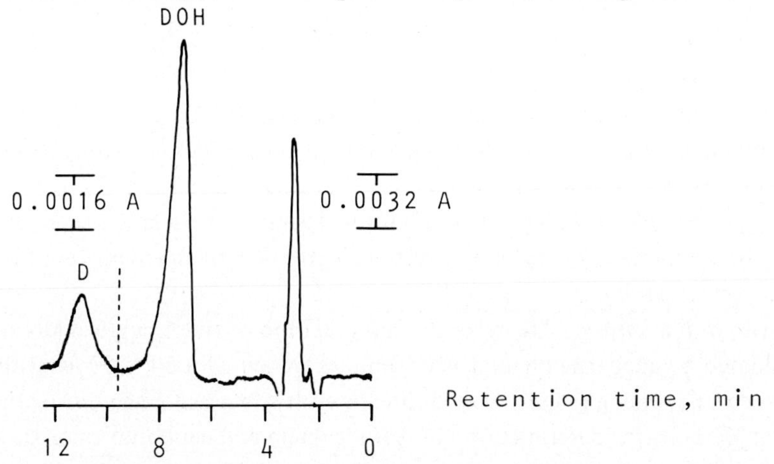

Fig. 9. Chromatogram from a leukemic patient's urine sample containing daunorubicin (D) and daunorubicinol (DOH).
Urine sample treated according to the Analytical Methods.
Measured concentrations: 108 ng/ml daunorubicin and 765 ng/ml daunorubicinol.
Dotted line indicates a change of detector sensitivity setting.

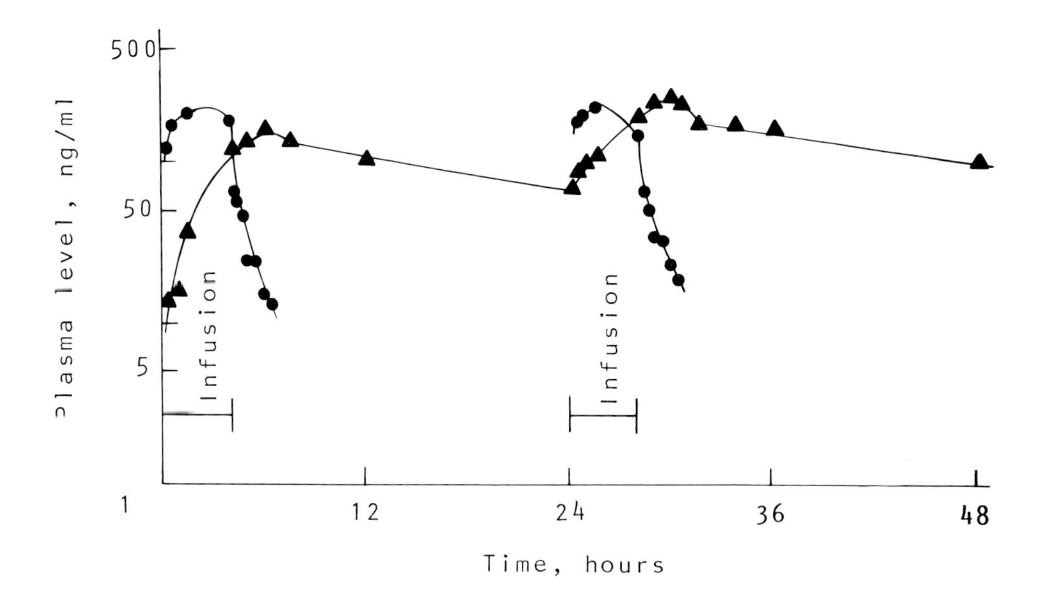

Fig. 10. Plasma levels of daunorubicin (●) and daunorubicinol (▲) after repeated infusion of daunorubicin (1.50 mg/kg)

The plasma concentration of daunorubicin was rather high during the infusion periods. It decreased rapidly when the infusion was terminated, and was below the detection limit about three hours later. The daunorubicinol level rose during the infusion periods to about the same magnitude as the maximum level of daunorubicin, but it declined considerably slower. Plasma levels of daunorubicinol can be measured for more than 24 hours after infusion of daunorubicin.

ACKNOWLEDGMENTS

I express my thanks to Dr. Hans Ehrsson for valuable discussions on the manuscript.

REFERENCES

1. Bachur, N.R. (1976) in Cancer Chemotherapy, Sartorelli, A.C. ed., ACS Symposium Series. Washington, D.C. pp. 58-70.

2. Blum, R.H. and Carter, S.K. (1974) Annals Int. Med., 80, 249-259.

3. Carter, S.K. (1975) J. Nat. Cancer Inst., 55, 1265-1274.

4. Bernard, J., Paul, R., Boiron, M., Jacquillat, C. and Maral, R. (1969) in Rubidomycin. Recent Results in Cancer Research, Springer-Verlag, New York Inc.

5. Bachur, N.R. (1975) Cancer Chemother. Reports Part 3, 6, 153-158.

6. Bachur, N.R. (1974) Biochem. Pharmacol. Suppl. 2, 207-216.

7. Asbell, M.A., Schwartzbach, E., Wodinsky, I. and Yesair, D.W. (1972) Cancer Chemother. Reports Part 1, 56, 315-320.

8. Calendi, E., DiMarco, A., Reggiani, M., Scarpinati, B. and Valentini, L. (1965) Biochem. Biophys. Acta, 103, 25-49.

9. DiMarco, A., Zunino, F., Silvestrini, R., Gambarucci, C. and Gambetta, R.A. (1971) Biochem. Pharmacol., 20, 1323-1328.

10. Pigram, W.J., Fuller, W. and Hamilton, L.D. (1972) Nature (New Biol.), 235, 17-19.

11. Minow, R.A., Benjamin, R.S., Lee, E.T. and Gottlieb, J.A. (1977) Cancer, 39, 1397-1402.

12. Zbinden, G. (1975) Exp., 31, 1058-1060.

13. Kishi, T. and Folkers, K. (1976) Cancer Treat.Rep., 60, 223-224.

14. Myers, C.E., McGuire, W.P., Liss, R.H., Ifrim, I., Grotzinger, K. and Young, R.C. (1977) Science, 197, 165-167.

15. Trouet, A., Deprez-De Campencere, D., Zenebergh, A. and Hulhoven, R. (1975) in Adrimycin Review Part 1, pp. 62-69.

16. Brown, I. and Ward, H.W.C. (1977) Cancer Letters, 2, 227-232.

17. Eksborg, S. (1978) J. Pharm. Sci., in press.

18. Eksborg, S. (1978) J. Chromat., in press.

19. Rosso, R., Ravazzoni, C., Esposito, M., Sala, R. and Santi, L. (1972) Europ. J. Cancer, 8, 455-459.

20. Alberts, D.S., Bachur, N.R. and Holtzman, J.L. (1971) Clin. Pharm. Therapeut., 12, 96-104.

21. Van Vunakis, H., Langone, J.J., Riceberg, L.J. and Levine, L. (1974) Cancer Research, 34, 2546-2552.

22. Chan, K.K. and Harris, P.A. (1973) Res. Com. in Chem. Path. and Pharm., 6, 447-463.

23. Langone, J.J., van Vunakis, H. and Bachur, N.R. (1975) Biochem. Medicine, 12, 283-289.

24. Huffman, D.H., Benjamin, R.S. and Bachur, N.R. (1972) Clin. Pharm. Therapeut., 13, 895-905.

25. Hulhoven, R., Desager, J.P., Sokal, G. and Harvengt, C. (1977) Arch. Int. Pharmacodyn., 226, 344-345.

26. Majors, R.E. (1972) Anal. Chem., 44, 1722-1726.

27. Eksborg, S. and Schill, G. (1973) Anal. Chem., 45, 2092-2100.

Clinical Pharmacology of Anti-Neoplastic Drugs
H. M. Pinedo, editor

CLINICAL PHARMACOLOGY OF ADRIAMYCIN

PETER M. WILKINSON, M.Sc., M.B., M.R.C.P.
Consultant Clinical Pharmacologist, Christie Hospital & Holt Radium Institute, Wilmslow Road, Manchester M20 9BX, England, U.K.

INTRODUCTION

Adriamycin is an antitumour antibiotic consisting of the tetracyclic aglycone, adriamycinone linked to the amino sugar daunosamine. The structure, as determined by Arcomone et al. (1969) (1), is shown in Fig. 1. It is closely related to daunomycin differing from it only by the presence of a hydroxyl group on the acetyl radical of the aglycone moiety. Whilst daunomycin was the first compound to be used clinically, it has little, if any, activity in solid tumours (2) and has been superseded by adriamycin for the treatment of a variety of malignant neoplasms.

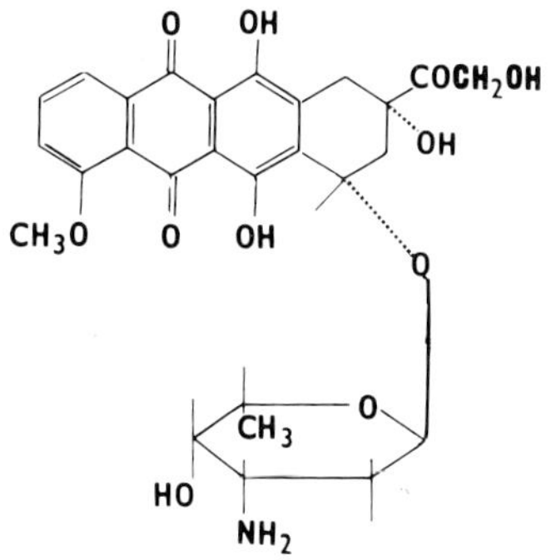

Fig. 1. The structure of adriamycin.

MECHANISM OF ACTION

Both antibiotics bind to DNA thereby inhibiting synthesis (4). Synchronised cells in G1 or G2 are less sensitive to adriamycin than cells in the S phase, and similarly plateau phase cells are less sensitive than cells from log phase cultures (5). If the carboxyl group is masked, the ability to bind to DNA is retained, but antimitotic activity is reduced (6). Masking of the amino group results in reduced binding to DNA and lack of biological activity (6); cleavage of the glycosidic bond produces complete loss of pharmacological activity (7). Adriamycin is more active and less toxic *in vivo* (8,9) and this has been attributed to differences in cellular uptake and intracellular half times of the two drugs (10). This is determined predominantly by the permeability of the cell membrane to the unionised form of the molecule and affinity for intracellular binding sites (11). Attempts have been made to correlate between patient differences in uptake and relate this to response in human leukaemia, but so far, this has not been successful (12).

DETERMINATION OF ADRIAMYCIN AND METABOLITES

Because of the number of unsaturated bonds present within the molecule the compound lends itself well to fluorescent analysis and such assays were first used for the estimation of daunomycin (13,14). Estimation of parent drug and metabolites requires separation by thin layer chromatography with a variety of solvent systems (15), and quantitation is achieved by elution of relevant areas or by use of fluorescent scanner (16). A radioimmunoassay has been developed which is extremely sensitive, but this cannot distinguish between parent compound and the closely related metabolite adriamycinol, and adriamycin aglycone has about a quarter of the reactivity of adriamycin (17). Comparative serum concentrations determined by fluorescent and radioimmunoassay give higher concentrations with the former because aglycones and conjugates are not detected by the latter procedure (18). High pressure liquid chromatography has somewhat overcome the problems associated with more tedious assays (19) and after separation parent compound and metabolites can be quantitated by radioimmunoassay (20). Flow fluorescent detection has further aided quantitation of metabolites directly by HPLC (21).

DOSE

While a variety of schedules have been proposed (3), it is generally administered as a single intravenous push. The reasons for this were based on clinical observations of toxicity and kinetic studies in both man and animals.

In initial Phase 1 and 2 studies it was found that an intermittent dose schedule had fewer toxic effects compared to alternate-day administration (22). A 50% incidence of fatal marrow aplasia was observed when daunomycin was administered daily, but this was reduced by increasing the interval between doses (23). Eventually, Benjamin and co-workers demonstrated the efficacy and safety of a single intravenous dose following information obtained from kinetic studies (24). The intermittent administration of 60 mg/m^2 is well tolerated provided liver function is normal. Dose reductions of 50% are necessary if the serum bilirubin is from 1.2 to 3 mg/% and a dose reduction of 75% is required if the bilirubin is $>$ 3 mg%.

It is unclear whether the total duration of exposure to the drug or the initial peak concentration is the prerequisite for optimal response. The same argument applies to the problem of cardiotoxicity, which limits the total amount of drug that can be administered safely. Prediction from experimental data in animals and *in vitro* studies using a variety of tumours are unhelpful. Compilation of data from several experiments in L1210 and P388 leukaemia show that adriamycin has no definite schedule dependency (25). There is evidence that in sarcoma 180 ascites, daunomycin is schedule dependent, but this does not hold for adriamycin (10). Continuous infusion of adriamycin produces comparable response and toxicity as the same total bolus dose in Wistar Furth myeloid leukaemia. (Wilkinson, P.M., Israel, M., Ensinger, W.D. and Greenberger, J.S., unpublished results).

Studies in man are restricted to reports of fractionated doses. In one study three dose schedules were given for a variety of tumours in either singly, daily x 4, or every 8 hours for six doses. The daily and single schemes were more toxic to platelets; granulocyte toxicity was more severe with the 8 hourly regimen but the within patient toxicity was comparable. A positive response maintained for more than one month was observed in 11 patients, 8 of whom received the daily schedule, one the 8-hourly schedule and two, the single dose schedule (26). Other workers using 30 mg/m^2 daily x 3 observed objective responses and comparable toxicity to that of single intravenous doses (27). Maintenance doses of 0.4 to 0.6 mg/kg every 7 days significantly reduces the incidence of cardiomyopathy and achieves comparable response rates to more intensive schedules (28). Adriamycin has been administered by intra-arterial infusion (29,30) with moderate toxicity, but the overall response rate was no better than that of conventional doses. Continuous hepatic arterial infusion has demonstrated that adriamycin is cleared by the liver parenchyma and that this regimen may avoid myelosuppression (31).

In summary, therefore, the most practical dose for an outpatient setting is 60 mg/m^2

to 75 mg/m^2 (24,32) given at intervals of 3 weeks. Weekly administration with lower doses avoids the problem of cardiotoxicity, but a controlled trial will be necessary to decide which of the two regimes is more efficacious in terms of response.

KINETICS, DISTRIBUTION AND EXCRETION

For clinical pharmacological studies to be of benefit in terms of dose, design and prediction of toxicity, it would be useful to know the precise distribution of any drug in both serum and tissues. Generally, it is not possible to evaluate tissue distribution in man, and therefore theoretical predictions must be made from computer models, or extrapolation made from tissue distribution studies in animals.

Initial distribution studies with daunomycin in mice demonstrated that there was a rapid uptake of drug in liver, spleen, heart and kidneys (13), and high concentrations of drug were observed in the spleen, lymph nodes and bone marrow, particularly during the first 8 hours after administration (33,34). Comparative studies with adriamycin demonstrated that there was a slow decay of drug in the liver, with a gradual increase in concentration in the spleen, lymph nodes and bone marrow (35). A biphasic decay of drug in plasma was observed in the rat (36,37) with preferential accumulation in the liver, lung, spleen and bone marrow and radiographic localisation to the reticuloendothelial system (37).

Determination of tissue distribution in man is quite rightly restricted by ethical considerations. Using [^{3}H]-daunomycin a rapid decay of drug in ascitic fluid was observed and none was detected in the CSF (38). A similar study with [^{3}H]-adriamycin yielded inconclusive results (39). Tissue levels of daunomycin have been determined in man (14), but not for adriamycin.

The plasma concentration/time curve in man decays as a bi- or triphasic function with time (37,40). The decay of total fluorescence is biphasic, but that for adriamycin is triphasic with the half-time of the third phase being 30 hours (40). Complex computer models have been proposed to explain and predict serum and tissue concentrations (41), but for practical purposes, a two compartment model will provide much useful information. Such a model is illustrated in Fig. 2. The volume of the central compartment (19 litres) is slightly in excess of that of the extracellular fluid volume. The large volume of the peripheral compartment (350 litres) is explained by binding of the drug to cellular components. There is a rapid clearance between the two compartments and the elimination clearance (140 ml/min) is greater than that of the creatinine clearance. Such models require experimental confirmation by means of the estimation of drug concentrations in plasma or serum and in the model described a one standard error fit was observed between the predicted concentrations in the central compartment and the observed values (Fig. 3) (37).

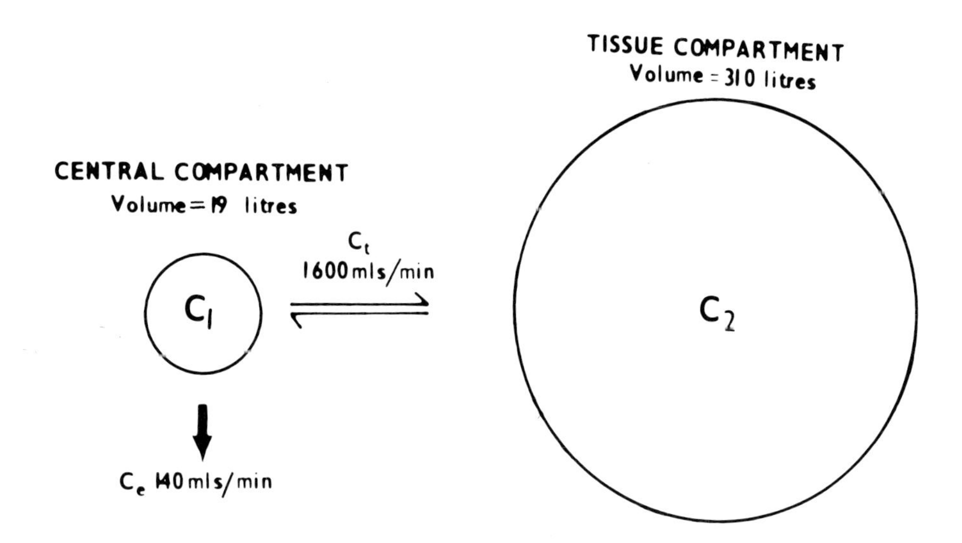

Fig. 2. Two compartment model for adriamycin

The value of such models in predicting, for example, the response is as yet unknown. There is, however, considerable between patient variation in the peripheral compartment volumes reflecting differing degrees of intra-cellular drug concentrations and distribution, which may well be related to the ultimate response and toxicity. Knowledge of the compartmental volumes, transfer and elimination clearances will permit the prediction of drug concentrations in both compartments (Fig. 3). Thus, there is rapid equilibriation of drug between the central and peripheral compartment and 80 minutes after administration the concentration in the latter exceeds that in the former, i.e. plasma or serum. Thereafter there is a gradual exponential decay of drug in both compartments as drug is released from the tissues into the central compartment from which excretion occurs.

The main excretory pathway for adriamycin in animals is via the bile (42,43) and very little is excreted in the urine (44). This is so in man and up to 45% of the total dose may be excreted in the bile as parent drug and fluorescent metabolites (45). In a detailed study in a patient with a biliary fistula, 33% of the administered dose was excreted during the first 72 hours of which 20% was unchanged adriamycin,

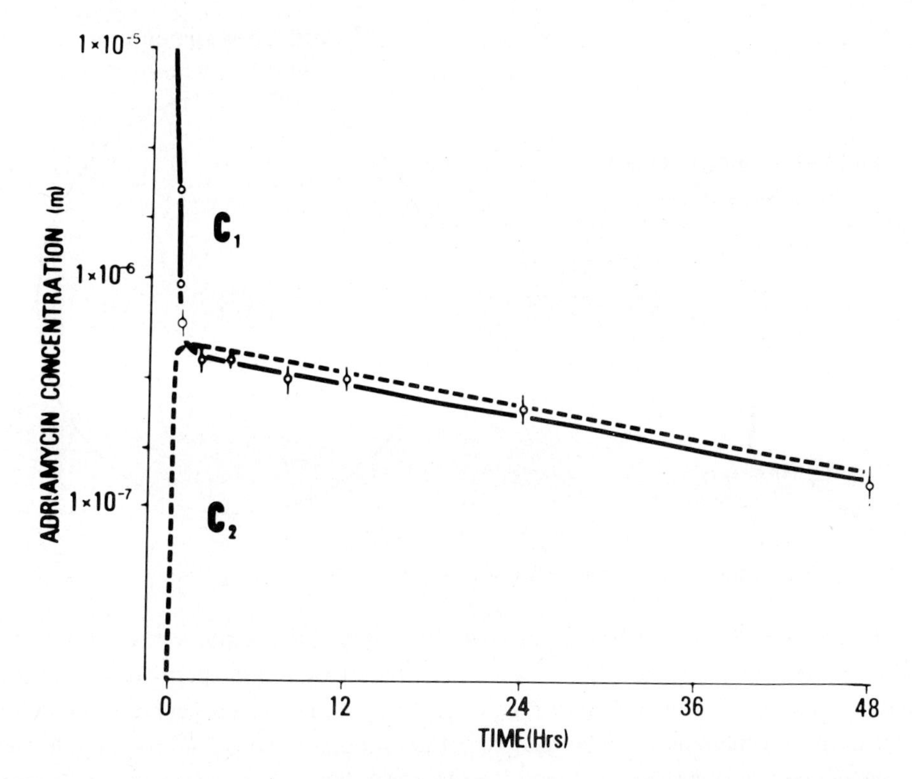

Fig. 3. Predicted concentrations of adriamycin in the central and peripheral compartments. The continuous line represents the concentration predicted by the model (Fig. 2) in the central compartment (C_1) and the interrupted line the concentration in the peripheral compartment (C_2). The points represent the observed values (mean ± S.E.M.).

10% adriamycinol and the remainder polar conjugates (46). Less than 12% of the administered dose is excreted in the urine. The main constituent is adriamycin and adriamycinol with a variable proportion of other fluorescent metabolites (15,46,47).

METABOLISM

The first step in the metabolism of adriamycin is carbonyl reduction at the C14 position to adriamycinol. The small structural change does not prevent adriamycinol from binding to DNA and therefore this metabolite is therapeutically active (48). The enzyme responsible is aldo-keto reductase which has a ubiquitous distribution throughout the body tissues (48). This enzyme has been isolated in a purified form, requires NADPH as a co-factor and has a molecular weight of 39,500 (49). Comparison of the Km values for adriamycin and daunomycin show that the highest activity is always present in the liver and kidney and that the Vmax for daunomycin is greater than that for adriamycin (50). This latter observation may account for the therapeutic superiority of adriamycin *in vivo*.

There is considerable between species variation in the proportion of parent drug metabolised to adriamycinol. The highest rate of activity is seen in the rabbit (51), there is little activity in the rat (43) and man is intermediate between these species (46). Variation in the proportion of adriamycin metabolised to adriamycinol is the most likely explanation for between species variation in response and toxicity.

The further biotransformation of adriamycin and adriamycinol has principally been determined by Bachur (48). Cleavage of both adriamycin and adriamycinol at the glycocydic bond results in formation of the respective aglycones. Both are water insoluble and require conjugation to either a sulphate or with glucuronic acid for excretion. Both these compounds have been identified in rabbit and human bile (45,46,51). Further degradation includes demethylation and a variety of other metabolites have been identified in human urine (15). The above metabolites are therapeutically inactive and probably contribute little to the toxicity of adriamycin.

The proportion of adriamycin converted to metabolites other than adriamycinol varies considerably. Some workers have been unable to identify aglycone products in the urine (46,52), whereas other workers have found substantial metabolites (15). In comparative studies with daunomycin and adriamycin no evidence of adriamycin metabolism was found in rat or mouse tissue extracts, in contrast to a substantial proportion of daunomycin metabolites (35,53). Whilst between or within species variation in metabolism may well explain this divergence, it is possible that an additional factor is the different methodological assays employed. The introduction of high pressure liquid chromatography may help clarify this situation. This has demonstrated that adriamycinol is the major fluorescent metabolite in the urine, and the proportion of other fluorescent metabolites account for only a very small percentage of the total fluorescence (46). Thus variations in the proportion metabolised to adriamycinol may well account for within species variation in response.

As with other drugs in therapeutic use, the concurrent administration of other compounds that increase microsomal enzymes alter the proportion of drug metabolised. In mice bearing L1210 leukaemia, pretreatment with phenobarbitone resulted in a significantly lower survival rate compared to controls (54). It is not known however, whether the concurrent administration of barbiturates in man alters the response or toxicity of adriamycin.

No study to date has succeeded in accounting for 100% of the administered dose; the average recovery figure being 60% when fluorescent assays are employed. Once the ring structure is opened or the bond becomes saturated the chromophore loses its ability to fluoresce and therefore any such metabolites escape detection. The nature of the non-fluorescent species can only be determined by using an appropriate radiolabelled compound and mass spectrographic examination. These techniques carry inherent difficulties and it is likely that it will be some time before the final metabolic pathway is clarified.

TOXICITY

As with other cytotoxic drugs, adriamycin will produce nausea and vomiting, bone marrow depression and epilation. These toxic effects are familiar to all clinicians experienced in the use of cancer drugs and will not be discussed further.

The major toxicity of adriamycin is the damaging effect to the myocardium, seen with repeated doses. Acute cardiac deaths were initially noted with daunomycin but the explanation for this may have been sensitisation of the heart to the action of noradrenaline as daunomycin prevents the uptake of this catecholamine (55). With more widespread clinical use it became clear that a separate effect of the anthracyclines was that of latent cardiomyopathy seen after repetitive courses of treatment. The incidence is 0.25 to 9% with total doses of less than 550 mg/m^2, 10 to 20% with total doses of 550-600 mg/m^2 increasing to 30 to 50% with doses in excess of 600 mg/m^2 (56,57). The incidence is significantly greater in patients who develop a $>$ 30% decrease in limb lead QRS voltage during treatment; concurrent cyclophosphamide and mediastinal radiotherapy lower the accumulative dose of adriamycin necessary for the development of cardiotoxicity. Uncontrolled hypertension is also a risk factor, and congestive cardiac failure is more likely to be fatal if it develops shortly after the last dose (56). A detailed study of daunomycin associated congestive cardiac failure in 5,613 patients revealed an overall incidence of cardiotoxicity of 1.96% and a 1.16% incidence of cardiomyopathy. Age, total dose and length of period of administration were unrelated to the time between the last dose of drug and the onset of congestive cardiac failure, and therefore these parameters did not provide clues to establish a precise time when the patient is at risk (58). Most clinicians accept a limiting dose of

550 mg/m^2, which should be reduced if there is concurrent therapy with cyclophosphamide or following mediastinal irradiation.

Various experimental studies have been carried out to try and explain the aetiology. Cardiolipin, a characteristic component of the inner membrane of mitochondria is abundant in cardiac muscle and effectively concentrates adriamycin (59). This may explain why the anthracycline-DNA complex and acetylated derivatives that do not bind to DNA are not toxic to cardiac muscle (60,61). Co-enzyme Q can prevent cardiotoxicity, as prolonged adriamycin treatment depletes this enzyme (62).

The most interesting development is that of the work of Myers and co-workers (1976) (63). It was noted that cardiac lesions produced by adriamycin were similar to those produced by α-tocopherol deficiency (64,65). Anthracyclines, which possess quinone and hydroxyquinone groups, theoretically, therefore, have the potential to engage in the generation of both free radicals and peroxide *in vivo*, thus promoting tissue damage via mechanisms similar to those of α-tocopheral deficiency. In mice, pretreatment with α-tocopherol produced a significant reduction in drug induced mortality, and greatly diminished but did not abolish the ability of adriamycin to cause cardiac damage. It remains to be seen whether this will have therapeutic relevance in man.

An interesting toxic effect that occurs but rarely, is the nephrotic syndrome. In one patient severe interstitial fibrosis and tubular atrophy developed during treatment. Immuno-fluorescent studies revealed only faint staining with complement, suggesting that this was drug related, and the patient recovered when the drug was discontinued (66). Other antibiotics capable of inducing the nephrotic syndrome are puromycin (67) and daunorubicin directly affects the enzyme systems in isolated glomeruli (68). The low incidence may well be related to the fact that cardiomyopathy supervenes before the onset of the renal damage.

There are few reports of drug interactions with adriamycin. The combination of adriamycin and stretozotocin should be avoided as this produces increased myelosuppression due to altered adriamycin metabolism (69). Patients treated concurrently with 6-mercaptopurine show an increased incidence of cholestasis due to adriamycin potentiating the hepatoxicity of 6-mercaptopurine (70). The possible role of enzyme inducers has been mentioned earlier but little, if anything, is known of interactions with other cytotoxic drugs.

NEW ANALOGUES

There have been various attempts to alter the basic structure of adriamycin with a view to producing an analogue that is therapeutically superior to and less cardiotoxic than adriamycin. Whilst many have been synthesised (71), none to date has satisfied the above criteria with the exception of that synthesised by Israel and co-workers (1975) (72). This compound, N-trifluoracetyl adriamycin-14-valerate (AD32) is a semisynthetic analogue and differs from the natural antibiotic in having a 5-carbon straight chain ester function at the 14-carbonyl position and trifluoracetyl substitution on the glycosidic amino group. It is therapeutically superior to adriamycin and less toxic in animal systems (72,73). It is also less cardiotoxic, using a rabbit model (74); significant cardiotoxicity was noted in adriamycin treated animals, but no severe effects were seen in those animals treated with AD32 (61).

Comparative studies designed to explain the above observations have revealed subtle differences between the two drugs. AD32 is unable to bind to DNA (75) and fluorescence studies have shown that whilst adriamycin appears slowly in living cells and is localised in nuclei and chromosomes, AD32 enters the cell rapidly, is localised to the cytoplasm and does not bind to nuclei or chromosomes (76). However, both drugs produce qualitatively and quantitatively similar effects on the incorporation of [^{3}H]-thymidine into DNA (77). These observations bring into question whether the accepted mechanism for adriamycin's activity, namely DNA binding, is the total explanation.

It is theoretically possible that AD32 could serve as a pro-drug for adriamycin, but to date experimental metabolic studies have failed to reveal that adriamycin is a significant metabolite (43,44, 78). It remains to be seen whether the therapeutic superiority and reduced toxicity observed in animals will be confirmed in man.

ACKNOWLEDGEMENTS

Part of the work described in this article was carried out by the author at the Sidney Farber Cancer Institute, Boston, Massachusetts, U.S.A. The author wishes to express his appreciation to Dr. M. Israel for invaluable help and advice and Dr. W.J. Pegg for skilled technical assistance.

REFERENCES

1. Arcamone, F., Franceschi, G., Penco, S. and Selva, A. (1969) Tetrahedron Letters, 13, 1007-1010.

2. Benjamin, R.S., Wiernik, P.H., Huffman, D.H. and Bachur, N.R. (1973) Clin. Res. 20, 563.

3. Blum, R.H. (1975) Cancer Chemother. Rep. Part 3. 6, 247-251.

4. Zunino, F., Gambetta, R., DiMarco, A. and Zaccara, A. (1972) Biochem. et Biophys. Acta. 277, 489-498.

5. Krishan, A. and Frei, E. III (1976) Cancer Res. 36, 143-150.

6. DiMarco, A., Zunino, F., Silvestrini, R., Gambarucci, C. and Gambetta, R. (1971) Biochem. Pharmacol. 20, 1323-1328.

7. Driscoll, J.S., Hanzard, G.F.Jr., Wood, H.D.Jr. and Goldin, A. (1974) Cancer Chemother. Rep. 4, 7.

8. DiMarco, A., Gaetani, M. and Scarpinato, B. (1969) Cancer Chemother. Rep. 53, 33-37.

9. Sandberg, J.S., Howsden, F.L., DiMarco, A. and Goldin, A. (1970) Cancer Chemother. Rep. 54, 1-7.

10. Silvestrini, R., Lenaz, L., DiFronzo, G. and Sanfilippo, O. (1973) Cancer Res. 33, 2954-2958.

11. Skovsgaard, T. (1977) Biochem. Pharmacol. 26, 215-222.

12. Chervinsky, D.S. and Wang, J.J. (1976) J. Medicine. 7, 63-79.

13. Bachur, N.R., Moore, L.A., Bernstein, J.G. and Liu, A. (1970) Cancer Chemother. Rep. 54, 89-94.

14. Alberts, D.S., Bachur, N.R. and Holtzman, J.L. (1971) Clinic. Pharmacol. Ther. 12, 96-104.

15. Takanashi, S. and Bachur, N.R. (1975). Drug Metabolism and Disposition. 4, 79-87.

16. Watson, E. and Chan, K.K. (1976) Cancer Treat. Rep. 60, 1611-1618.

17. VanVunakis, H., Langone, J.J., Riceberg, L.J. and Levine, L. (1974) Cancer Res. 34, 2546-2552.

18. Bachur, N.R., Riggs, C.E.Jr., Green, M.R., Langone, J.L., VanVunakis, M. and Levine, L. (1977). Clin. Pharmacol. Ther. 21, 70-77.

19. Hulhoven, R. and Desager, J.P. (1976). J. Chromatography. 125, 369-374.

20. Langone, J.J., VanVunakis, H. and Bachur, N.R. (1975) Biochem. Med. 12, 283-289.

21. Israel, M., Pegg, W.J., Wilkinson, P.M. and Garnick, M.B. (1978) in "Biological/Biophysical applications of liquid chromatography". Hank, G.L. Ed. Marcel Dekker Inc. In Press.

22. Bonadonna, G., Monfardini, S., DeLena, M., Fossati-Bellani, F. and Beretta, G. (1970) Cancer Res. 30, 2572-2582.

23. Malpas, J.S. and Scott, R.B. (1969) Lancet 1, 469-470.

24. Benjamin, R.S., Wiernik, P.H. and Bachur, N.R. (1974) Cancer 33, 19-27.

25. Goldin, A. and Johnson, R.K. (1975) Cancer Chemother. Rep. Part 3, 6, 137-145.

26. Creasey, W.A., McIntosh, L.S., Brescia, T., Odujinrin, O., Aspnes, G.T., Murray, E. and Marsh, J.C. (1976). Cancer Res. 36, 216-221.

27. Wang, J.J., Holland, J.F. and Sinks, L.F. (1975) Cancer Chemother. Rep. Part 3, 6, 267-270.

28. Weiss, A.J., Metter, G.E., Fletcher, W.S., Wilson, W.L., Grage, T.B. and Ramirez, G. (1976) Cancer Treat. Rep. 60, 813-822.

29. Haskell, C.M., Silverstein, M.J., Rangel, D.M., Hunt, J.S., Sparks, F.C. and Morton, D.L. (1974) Cancer 33, 1485-1490.

30. Shah, P., Baker, L.H. and Vaitkevicius, V.K. (1977) Cancer Treat. Rep. 61, 1565-1567.

31. Garnick, M.B., Israel, M., Ensminger, W.D. and Glode, L.M. (1978) Proc. Am. Assoc. Cancer Res. 19, 400.

32. O'Bryan, R.M., Luce, J.K., Tolley, R.W., Gottlieb, J.A., Baker, L.H. and Bonadonna, G. (1973) Cancer 32, 1-8.

33. DiFronzo, G. and Gambetta, R. (1971) Rev. Europ. Etudes Clin. et. Biol. 16, 50-55.

34. Rusconi, A., DiFronzo, G. and DiMarco, A. (1968) Cancer Chemother. Rep. 52, 331-335.

35. Yesair, D.W., Schwartzbach, E., Shuck, D., Denine, E.P. and Asbell, M.A. (1972) Cancer Res. 32, 1177-1183.

36. Arena, E., D'Allessandro, N., Dusonchet, L., Gebbia, N., Gerbasi, F., Palazzo-adriano, M., Raineri, A., Ransa, L. and Tubaro, E. Arzneim Forsch. 21, 1258-1263.

37. Wilkinson, P.M. and Mawer, G.E. (1974) Br. J. Clin. Pharmacol. 1, 241-247.

38. DiFronzo, G. and Bonadonna, G. (1970) Europ. J. Clin. Biol. Res. 15, 314-320.

39. DiFronzo, G., Lenaz, L. and Bonadonna, G. (1973) Biomedicine 9, 169-171,

40. Benjamin, R.S., Riggs, C.E.Jr. and Bachur, N.R. (1977) Cancer Res. 37, 1416-1420.

41. Harris, P.A. and Gross, J.F. (1975) Cancer Chemother. Rep. 59, 819-825.

42. Craddock, J.C., Egorin, M.J. and Bachur, N.R. (1973) Arch. Int. Pharmacodyn. Ther. 202, 48-61.

43. Israel, M., Wilkinson, P.M., Pegg, W.J. and Frei, E. III (1978) Cancer Res. 38, 365-370.

44. Israel, M., Pegg, W.J. and Wilkinson, P.M. (1978) J. Pharmacol. Exp. Ther. In press.

45. Riggs, C.E.Jr., Benjamin, R.S., Serpick, A. and Bachur, N.R. (1977) Clin. Phar-macol. Ther. 22, 234-241.

46. Glode, L.M., Israel, M., Pegg, W.J. and Wilkinson, P.M. (1977) Br. J. Clin. Phar-macol. 4, 639.

47. Benjamin, R.S., Riggs, C.E.Jr. and Bachur, N.R. (1973) Clin. Pharmacol. Ther. 14, 592-600.

48. Bachur, N.R. (1975) Cancer Chemother. Rep. Part 3; 6, 153-158.

49. Felsted, R.L., Gee, M. and Bachur, N.R. (1974) J. Biol. Chem. 249, 3672-3679.

50. Loveless, H., Arena, E., Felsted, R.L. and Bachur, N.R. (1978) Cancer Res. 38, 593-598.

51. Bachur, N.R., Hildebrand, R.C. and Jaenke, R.S. (1974) J. Pharmacol. Exp. Ther. 191, 331-340.

52. Rosso, R., Ravazzani, C., Esposito, M., Sala, R. and Santi, L. (1972) Europ. J. Cancer 8, 455-459.

53. DiFronzo, G., Gambetta, R. and Lenaz, L. (1971) Europ. J. Clin. Biol. Res. 16, 572-576.

54. Reich, S.D. and Bachur, N.R. (1976) Cancer Res. 36, 3803-3806.

55. Bernstein, J.G., Bachur, N.R. and Thompson, W.L. (1968) Arch. Int. Pharmacodyn. 176, 11-20.

56. Minow, R.A., Benjamin, R.S., Lee, E.T. and Gottlieb, J.A. (1977) Cancer 39, 1397-1402.

57. LeFrak, E.A., Pitha, J., Rosenheim, S. and Gottlieb, J.A. (1973) Cancer 32, 302-314.

58. VonHoff, D.D., Rozencweig, M., Layard, M., Slavik, M. and Muggia, F.M. (1977) Am. J. Med. 62, 200-208.

59. Duarte-Karim, M., Ruysschaert, J.M. and Hildebrand, J. (1976) Biochem. and Biophys. Res. Comm. 71, 658-663.

60. Rozencweig, M., Kenis, Y., Atassi, G., Staquet, M. and Duarte-Karim, M. (1975) Cancer Chemother. Rep. Part 3; 6, 131-136.

61. Henderson, I.C., Billingham, M., Israel, M., Krishan, A. and Frei, E. III (1978) Proc. Am. Assoc. Cancer Res. 19, 158.

62. Bertazzoli, C. and Ghione, M. (1977) Pharmacol. Res. Comm. 9, 235-250.

63. Myers, C.E., McGuire, W. and Young, R. (1976) Cancer Treat. Rep. 60, 961-962.

64. Van Fleet, J.F., Hall, B.V. and Simon, J. (1968) Am. J. Pathol. 52, 1067-1079.

65. Howes, E.L., Price, M.M. and Blumberg, J.M. (1964) Am. J. Pathol. 45, 599-631.

66. Burke, J.F., Laucius, J.F., Brodovsky, H.S. and Soriano, R.Z. (1977) Arch. Int. Med. 137, 385-388.

67. Frenk, S., Antonowicz, I., Craig, J.M. and Metcoff, J. (1955) Proc. Soc. Exp. Biol. Med. 89, 424-431.

68. Lamberts, B., Buss, H. and Heintz, R. (1973) Clin. Nephrol. 1, 81-85.

69. Chang, P., Riggs, C.E.Jr., Scheerer, M.T., Wiernik, P.H. and Bachur, N.R. (1976) Clin. Pharmacol. Therap. 20, 611-616.

70. Minnow, R.A., Stern, M.H., Casey, J.H., Rodriguez, V. and Luna, M.A. (1976) Cancer 38, 1524-1528.

71. Arcamone, F., Penco, S. and Vigevani, A. (1975) Cancer Chemother. Rep. Part 3; 6, 123-129.

72. Israel, M., Modest, E.J. and Frei, E. III (1975) Cancer Res. 35, 1365-1368.

73. Vecchi, A., Cairo, M., Mantovani, A., Sironi, M. and Spreafico, F. (1978) Cancer Treat. Rep. 62, 111-117.

74. Jaenke, R.S. (1974) Lab. Invest. 30, 292-304.

75. Sengupta, S.K., Seshadri, R., Modest, E.J. and Israel, M. (1976) Proc. Am. Assoc. Cancer Res. 17, 109.

76. Krishan, A., Israel, M., Modest, E.J. and Frei, E. III (1976) Cancer Res. 36, 2114-2116.

77. Parker, L.M., Hirst, M. and Israel, M. (1978) Cancer Treat. Rep. 62, 119-127.

78. Israel, M., Garnick, M.B., Pegg, W.J., Blum, R.H. and Frei, E. III (1978) Proc. Am. Assoc. Cancer Res. 19, 160.

© 1978 Elsevier/North-Holland Biomedical Press
Clinical Pharmacology of Anti-Neoplastic Drugs
H. M. Pinedo, editor

RECENT ADVANCES IN THE STUDY OF CLINICAL PHARMACOLOGY OF BLEOMYCIN

STANLEY T. CROOKE, M.D., Ph.D.[1], ARCHIE W. PRESTAYKO, Ph.D.[2] and JAMES E. STRONG, Ph.D.[3]

1. Associate Director of Research and Development, BRISTOL LABORATORIES and Assistant Professor of Pharmacology, BAYLOR COLLEGE OF MEDICINE and Clinical Assistant Professor, UPSTATE MEDICAL CENTER, Syracuse, New York, U.S.A.

2. Assistant Director of Research and Development, BRISTOL LABORATORIES and Assistant Professor of Pharmacology, BAYLOR COLLEGE OF MEDICINE Syracuse, New York, U.S.A.

3. Instructor, Department of Pharmacology, BAYLOR COLLEGE OF MEDICINE Houston, Texas, U.S.A.

INTRODUCTION

Bleomycin (Blenoxane[R]) is excreted primarily by renal mechanisms. The pharmacokinetics of bleomycin have been reported in patients receiving the drug by a number of routes including intravenous, (Fujita et al. (1), Ohnuma et al. (2), Fujita (3), Crooke et al. (4), Crooke et al. (5), Crooke et al. (6), Broughton et al (7), Broughton et al (8); intramuscular, (Fujita et al. (1), Ohnuma et al. (2); intracavitary, (Alberts et al. (9), Crooke et al. (10); intraarterial, (Fujita et al. (1); subcutaneous, (Hall et al. (11); and intravesical, (Bracken et al. (12).

The early reports (Fujita et al. (1), Ohnuma et al. (2), Fujita (3)) employed a microbiologic assay in a small number of patients using *B. subtilis* ATCC-6633 spore solution which was sensitive to approximately 0.2 milliunit/ml. The elimination of bleomycin from blood was reported to vary, with some patients demonstrating first order kinetics, and others not. The plasma half-life was reported to vary from 14 to 45 minutes after intravenous injection, (Fujita et al. (1)) however, it was unclear whether this time represented $t^1/_2\alpha$ or $t^1/_2\beta$.

Recently two radioimmunoassays were developed which have greater sensitivity and specificity than the microbiologic assay (Broughton and Strong (13); Elson et al. (14)). After the development of these assays, several studies were designed to determine

a) the accuracy of the $[^{125}I]$ radioimmunoassays
b) the comparability of the $[^{57}Co]$ radioimmunoassay to the $[^{125}I]$ radioimmunoassay
c) the comparability of the radioimmunoassays to the microbiologic assay
d) the specificities of the two radioimmunoassays

e) the pharmacokinetics of bleomycin administered to patients as an intravenous bolus, as a prolonged intravenous infusion, intramuscularly and intravesically
f) the effects of varying renal function on the pharmacokinetics and toxicities of bleomycin administered as an intravenous bolus (Table 1).

TABLE 1.

GOALS OF PRESENT STUDIES
Accuracy of the [^{125}I] radioimmunoassay
Comparability of the [^{57}Co] radioimmunoassay to the [^{125}I] radioimmunoassay
Comparability of the radioimmunoassays to the microbiologic assay
Specificities of the two radioimmunoassays
Pharmacokinetics of bleomycin administered to patients as an intravenous bolus, as a prolonged intravenous infusion, intramuscularly and intravesically
Effects of varying renal function on the pharmacokinetics and toxicities of bleomycin administered as an intravenous bolus

In this publication, the results of these studies will be reviewed. In addition, the results of studies on the intracavitary administration of bleomycin performed by Alberts and colleagues (Alberts et al. (9)) will be discussed.

MATERIALS AND METHODS

Assay Procedures

The microbiologic assay was performed employing *B. subtilis* ATCC-6633 spore solution as previously described (Fujita et al. (1)). The radioimmunoassays were performed as previously described (Broughton and Strong (13), Elson et al.(14)). Replicates of each concentration were performed and the results were found to be readily reproducible.

Sample Collection

Blood specimens were obtained in heparinized tubes at specified intervals up to 72 hours after a dose of bleomycin. When serum was to be assayed, blood specimens were collected in non-heparinized tubes. Specimens were refrigerated, centrifuged, and either plasma or serum obtained and stored frozen (-20°C or -70°C) until analyzed. Urine specimens were collected for varying periods of time, stored refrigerated and frozen immediately at termination of the collection period.

Patient Selection

Intravenous Injection

Twenty patients had metastatic testicular tumors and were treated with bleomycin 30 units/week in combination with vinblastine and cis-platinum according to the regimen shown in Table 1 (Einhorn et al. (15)). These patients were chosen for this study for several reasons

1) they were a group of homogeneous and relatively healthy young males
2) they were all treated with the same regimen thereby eliminating possible effects of drugs other than vinblastine and cis-platinum on bleomycin pharmacokinetics
3) most of the patients had normal renal function on entry into the study and since cis-platinum is a nephrotoxic agent, it was possible to determine pharmacokinetics of bleomycin serially in patients with varying creatinine clearance.

Seven other patients had poorly differentiated lymphocytic lymphoma or diffuse histiocytic lymphoma and were treated with 7-10 units bleomycin as a 10-minute intravenous injection.

Intravenous Continuous Infusion

Patients receiving 15-30 units bleomycin per day for 4-5 days as a continuous infusion, had one of the following tumors; squamous cell carcinoma of the tongue, embryonal carcinoma, squamous cell carcinoma of the scrotum, squamous cell carcinoma of the urethra or bronchogenic adenocarcinoma.

Intramuscular Injection

Patients who received 2-30 units bleomycin as an intramuscular injection had various malignancies.

Intravesical Administration

Patients enrolled in this study had stage A or O superficial transitional cell carcinoma of the bladder which was not amenable to local excision, and were treated with intravesical bleomycin at various doses.

RESULTS

Radioimmunoassay Specificity

In Fig. 1, data obtained employing the [^{125}I] radioimmunoassay are compared to the data obtained using the microbiologic assay.

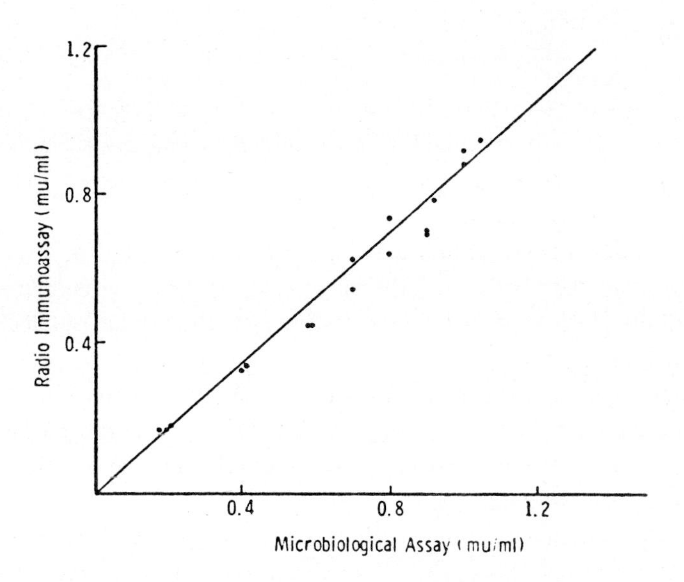

Fig. 1. Correlation of bleomycin determinations by radioimmunoassay and the microbiologic assay.

The coefficient of correlation between the methods within the range of sensitivity of the microbiologic assay was 0.987. Further, these studies demonstrated that both the radioimmunoassay and the microbiologic assays may be employed to assay either plasma or serum.

Fig. 2 shows the general structure of bleomycin, and the terminal amine groups for bleomycin A_2, A_5, and B_2. Bleomycinic acid does not contain a terminal amine structure, and bleomycin B_1 is the amide. Iso-bleomycin A_2 is the product of carba-

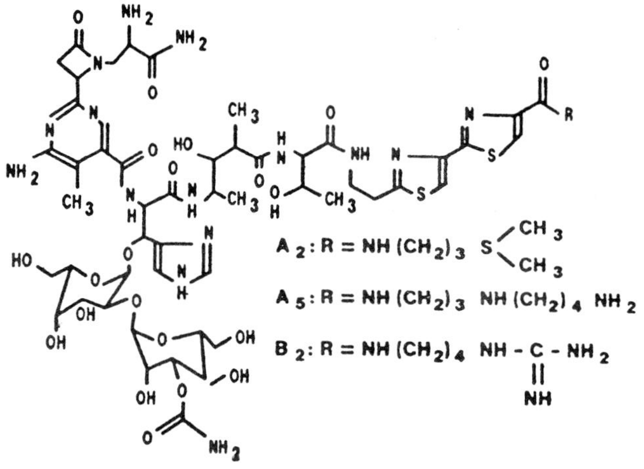

A_2: R = $NH(CH_2)_3\ S(CH_3)_2$

A_5: R = $NH(CH_2)_3\ NH(CH_2)_4\ NH_2$

B_2: R = $NH(CH_2)_4\ NH-C(=NH)-NH_2$

Fig. 2. Structure of bleomycin analogs. (R: Terminal amine)

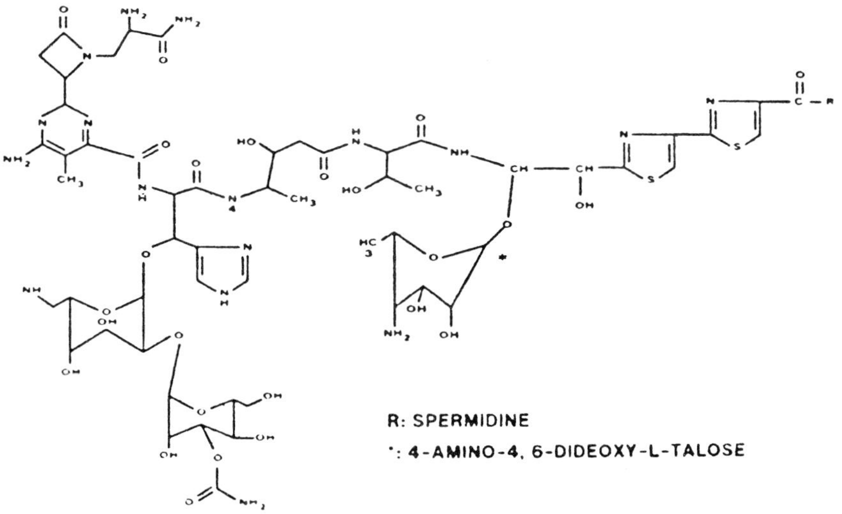

R: SPERMIDINE

*: 4-AMINO-4, 6-DIDEOXY-L-TALOSE

Fig. 3. Structure of Tallysomycin B. (R: Terminal amine)

moyl group migration in which the carbamoyl group is found on the 2-carbon rather than the 3-carbon position of the mannose sugar. Fig. 3 shows the structure of tallysomycin B. The terminal amine, spermidine, is analogous to the terminal amine on bleomycin A_5.

TABLE 2.

CORRELATION FOR COMPARISON OF THREE ASSAY METHODS

Assay Comparison y – x	n	r	Regression equation	Standard Deviation Slope	Standard Deviation Intercept
			Serum Samples		
[^{125}I]RIA – [^{57}Co]RIA	73	.95	y = .75x + .02	± .03	± .01
[^{57}Co]RIA – Microbiologic	42	.91	y = .91x + .10	± .06	± .03
[^{125}I]RIA – Microbiologic	42	.95	y = .75x + .08	± .04	± .02
			Urine Samples		
[^{125}I]RIA – [^{57}Co]RIA	53	.89	y = .76x + 1.47	± .05	± .69
[^{57}Co]RIA – Microbiologic	46	.89	y = 1.33x + .52	± .1	± .97
[^{125}I]RIA – Microbiologic	51	.96	y = 1.26x + .15	± .05	± .52

Table 2 compares the results obtained using the [^{125}I] radioimmunoassay to those obtained employing the [^{57}Co] radioimmunoassay or the microbiologic assay. It demonstrates that the two radioimmunoassays and the microbiologic assay correlate quite well in serum. The correlation of the [^{125}I] radioimmunoassay with the microbiologic assay in urine is also excellent, but the [^{57}C] radioimmunoassay correlated less well with the microbiologic assay in urine.

TABLE 3.

RELATIVE IMMUNOREACTIVITY OF SPECIFIC BLEOMYCIN COMPOUNDS COMPARED TO THE CLINICALLY-USED MIXTURE

	[^{57}Co]RIA	[^{125}I]RIA
Blenoxane$^{(R)}$	100%	100%
Bleomycin A_2	90%	115.4%
Bleomycin B_2	189%	74.5%
Bleomycinic acid	0.6%	$<$ 1%

Table 3 compares the specificity of the [^{125}I] radioimmunoassay to the specificity of the [^{57}Co] radioimmunoassay. Significant differences were observed in the cross-reactivity of the two radioimmunoassays which may account for the differences in the values obtained when urine was assayed. These differences, however, are probably not significant relative to clinical trials since the two assays detect the major components, bleomycin A_2 and B_2, in the clinically employed mixture.

TABLE 4.

PATIENT CHARACTERISTICS

Patient Number	Age	m^2	Performance Status	Initial Creatinine Clearance (ml/min)	Site of Metastases	Tumor Response
1	24	2.0	90	10.7	pulmonary	CR
2	33	1.95	30	21.3	pulmonary, CNS	PR
3	29	2.3	80	62	left inguinal node	CR
4	25	1.8	80	64.6	left cervical node, para aortic	PR
5	27	1.65	90	78	liver	PR
6	46	1.6	80	88	lung	PR
7	21	2.3	80	89	bone, lung, retroperitoneal nodes	PR
8	24	1.9	60	98.6	retroperitoneal mass	PR
9	20	1.9	90	98.7	pelvis, mediastinum, para aortic	PR
10	47	2.1	90	107	pulmonary, mediastinum	PR
11	22	1.5	90	108.5	skull, shoulder, elbow	NE
12	22	2.1	90	109	pulmonary, lymph node	CR
13	25	1.76	90	110	adjuvant therapy	NE
14	26	2.08	90	115	mediastinal mass	PR
15	26	1.68	90	118	pulmonary	CR
16	26	1.88	90	123	lung, retroperitoneal nodes	CR
17	22	2.1	90	128	large retroperitoneal mass, lung	PR
18	18	1.84	90	140	mediastinal mass, pulmonary	CR
19	27	1.7	100	157	lung	PR
20	22	1.98	90	180	pulmonary, liver nodes, para aortic	PR
Median	24	1.9				

CR = complete regression
PR = partiat regression
NE = not evaluable

Intravenous Injection

Table 4 shows the characteristics of twenty patients in whom bleomycin pharmacokinetics were determined. The median age was 24 years. Ages varied from 18 to 47 years. With two exceptions, all initial performance statuses (Karnofsky) were 60 or greater. Initial creatinine clearances varied from 10.7 ml/min to 180 ml/min corrected to 1.73 m^2 body surface area. All evaluable patients achieved either a partial response ($>$ 50% decrease in the cross-sectional area of measurable lesions), or complete response. Two patients were not evaluable for response (NE) because of lack of measurable disease.

Table 5 presents the plasma $t^1/_2\beta$ of bleomycin determined by the microbiologic and radioimmunoassays relative to creatinine clearance. In general, the data shown in Table 5 demonstrate that the plasma $t^1/_2\beta$ of bleomycin determined by both methods was similar, and that the plasma clearance of bleomycin varied with creatinine clearance. The values for areas under curve (AUC) were variable and did not correlate well with the creatinine clearance or $t^1/_2\beta$. This may be explained by slight variations in the timing of the first blood sample relative to the time of bleomycin injection. Since patient 1 received only 15U of bleomycin, AUC data are not presented.

Fig. 4 shows the semi-logarithmic plot of the plasma $t^1/_2\beta$ *vs* the creatinine clearance. These results demonstrate that the inflection point, i.e., the point at which the plasma $t^1/_2\beta$ of bleomycin becomes prolonged, is at a creatinine clearance of approximately 25-35 ml/min. At creatinine clearances in excess of 25-35 ml/min, the mean $t^1/_2\beta$ when determined with the microbiologic assay was 122.7 ± 9.6 minutes and 115.4 ± 8.6 minutes when determined with the radioimmunoassay. Below a creatinine clearance of approximately 25-35 ml/min, the plasma $t^1/_2\beta$ of bleomycin increased exponentially as the creatinine clearances decreased. The mean $t^1/_2\beta$ in patients with creatinine clearances in excess of 70 ml/ min did not differ from the mean of patients with creatinine clearances in excess of 25-35 ml/min (111 or 109 minutes determined by the microbiologic or radioimmunoassays respectively).

Bleomycin pharmacokinetics were evaluated sequentially in eight patients (Table 6). These studies demonstrate that, within a given patient, the plasma half-life of bleomycin varied inversely with the creatinine clearance.

Table 7 shows that the total apparent volume of distribution varied from 14 liters to 35 liters except for two patients who had volumes of distribution of 6.5 liters and 8.3 liters. The mean volume of distribution of bleomycin was 22.7 ± 6.02 liter and 19.8 ± 1.46 liters in patients with creatinine clearances greater or less than 35 ml/min respectively (Table 8).

TABLE 5.

PLASMA $t\frac{1}{2}\beta$ BLEOMYCIN *vs* CREATININE CLEARANCE

Patient's Number	Creatinine Clearance (ml/min)	MICRO		RIA	
		$t\frac{1}{2}$ (min)	AUC	$t\frac{1}{2}$ (min)	AUC
1	10.7	1260	–	1260	–
1	15.2	660	–	660	–
2	21	375	255	341	452
11	35	276	670	178	480
7	48	119	172	–	–
3	62	157	378	114	309
4	65	171	532	177	256
7	89	158	210	117	142
15	98	129	160	150	318
8	99	92	159	68	141
9	99	114	168	133	350
12	105	123	173	103	249
10	107	100	71	106	146
11	108	41	74	25	145
12	109	121	72	86	146
13	110	85	217	74	292
14	115	94	73	117	155
15	118	173	149	129	257
7	120	63	137	79	188
20	122	134	209	209	270
16	123	114	155	103	184
14	127	115	139	98	191
18	140	112	183	98	189
18	146	121	218	98	270
20	149	114	137	124	218
20	180	95	89	140	185

TABLE 6.

CHANGES IN RENAL STATUS AND PLASMA $t\frac{1}{2}\beta$ BLEOMYCIN

Patient's Number	Week of Therapy	Creatinine Clearance (ml/min)	$t\frac{1}{2}$ (min)
15	0	118	129
15	5	98	150
14	0	115	117
14	6	127	98
18	0	140	98
18	6	146	98
12	0	109	86
12	5	105	103
20	0	180	95
20	6	149	114
20	9	122	134
11	0	108	41
11	9	35	276
7	0	89	158
7	3	120	63
7	6	48	119
1	0	10.7	1260
1	1	15.2	660

TABLE 8.

VOLUME OF DISTRIBUTION *vs* CREATININE CLEARANCE

Creatinine Clearance	Mean Volume of Distribution
$\leq$ 35 ml/min	22.7 ± 6.02
> 35 ml/min	19.8 ± 1.46

TABLE 7.

CREATININE CLEARANCE *vs* VOLUME OF DISTRIBUTION

Patient	Creatinine Clearance (ml/min)	Volume Distribution (1)
1	15	34.8
2	21	16.3
11	35	17.2
7	48	33.1
3	62	13.9
4	65	6.5
7	89	29.4
15	98	18.8
9	99	14.5
8	99	19.1
12	105	15.8
10	107	23.6
11	108	16.3
12	109	22.9
13	110	8.3
14	115	30.1
15	118	19.8
7	120	18.1
20	122	26.7
16	123	29.4
14	127	19.7
18	140	18.8
18	146	13.6
20	149	23.4
20	180	28.6

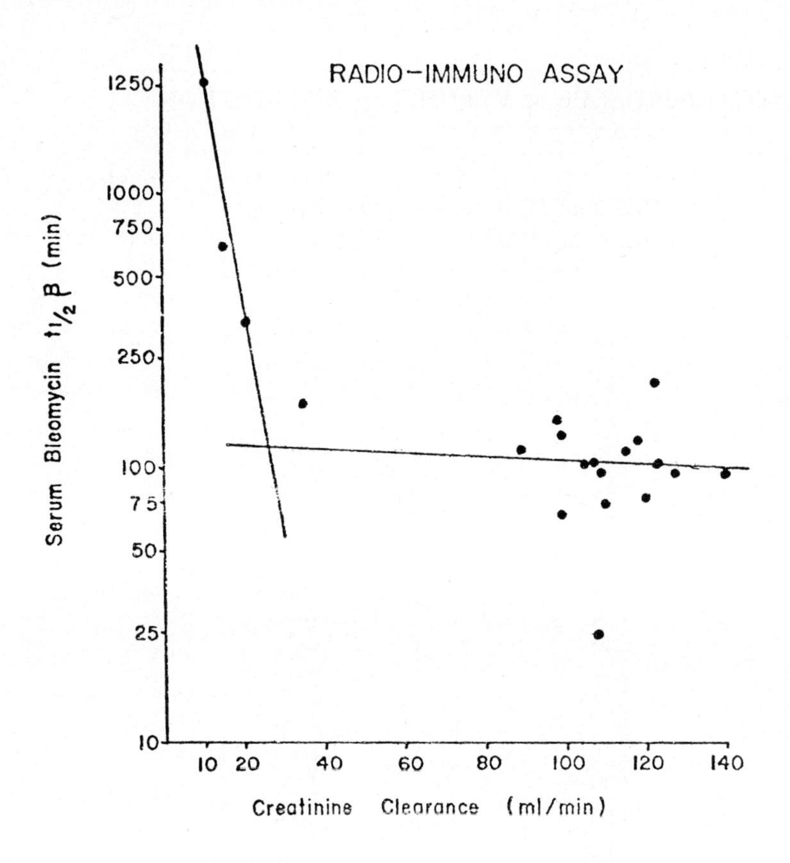

Fig. 4. Semi-logarithmic plot of plasma and serum $t^1/_2\beta$ of bleomycin *vs.* creatinine clearance from values determined using the radioimmunoassay.

Table 9 shows the urinary excretion of bleomycin relative to creatinine clearance. In patients with creatinine clearances approximately 50 ml/min or greater, approximately 50% (mean) of the total dose was excreted during the first four hours post-dose. Within 24 hours post-dose, approximately 70% of the total dose was excreted in the urine.

In another study (Broughton et al. (7)) using a 10-minute infusion in patients with non-Hodgkin's lymphoma, the mean $t^1/_2\beta$ for bleomycin was approximately 122 minutes and approximately 60% of the administered dose was recovered in urine in 24 hours after injection. Six of the seven patients had a creatinine clearance >60 ml/min. Fig. 5 shows the semi-logarithmic plot of the serum bleomycin con-

treated with intravesical bleomycin at various doses.

TABLE 9.

BLEOMYCIN EXCRETION *vs* CREATININE CLEARANCE

Patient	Creatinine Clearance (ml/min)	$t\frac{1}{2}\beta$ (min)	Cumulative % bleomycin excreted in urine 0 – 4 h	0 – 8 h	0 – 12 h	0 – 24 h
7	48	119	50	58.3	59.9	60.6
3	62	157	29	40.6	46.2	53.8
4	65	171	35.3	46.9	52.9	58.2
7	89	158	53	69.0	71.3	75.6
15	98	150	54	70.0	75.0	77.6
12	105	103	57.3	63.3	67.9	69.5
14	115	117	62.6	76.6	80.6	82.1
20	122	134	50	62.0	70.3	70.3
18	140	98	47.6	63.6	66.4	67.9
Mean	93.7 ± 10.1	134 ± 8.7	48.7 ± 3.5	61.1 ± 3.7	65.6 ± 3.6	68.4 ± 3.1

centration in microunits per ml vs time for these patients. The $t^1/_2\beta$ and 24 hour bleomycin excretion after a 10 minute infusion agree well with that determined by Crooke et al. (4) using an i.v. bolus bleomycin dose.

Continuous Infusion

Fig. 6 shows the semi-logarithmic plot of serum bleomycin concentration *vs* time for 4 patients receiving a 4-5 day continuous infusion of bleomycin. Steady state con centration was approached approximately 12 hours after initiation of infusion and ranged from 0.132 to 0.312 mu/ml. The half-life of bleomycin in the post-infusion decay period was approximately 180 minutes when values less than 10 μU/ml were excluded. These results compare reasonably closely to the $t^1/_2\beta$ for a single injection. However, when all values measured were used in the determination of $t^1/_2\beta$, the half-life of bleomycin post infusion, was approximately 10-14 h. Approximately 63% of the dose of bleomycin administered by continuous infusion, was recovered in the urine and was similar to that observed after a single injection.

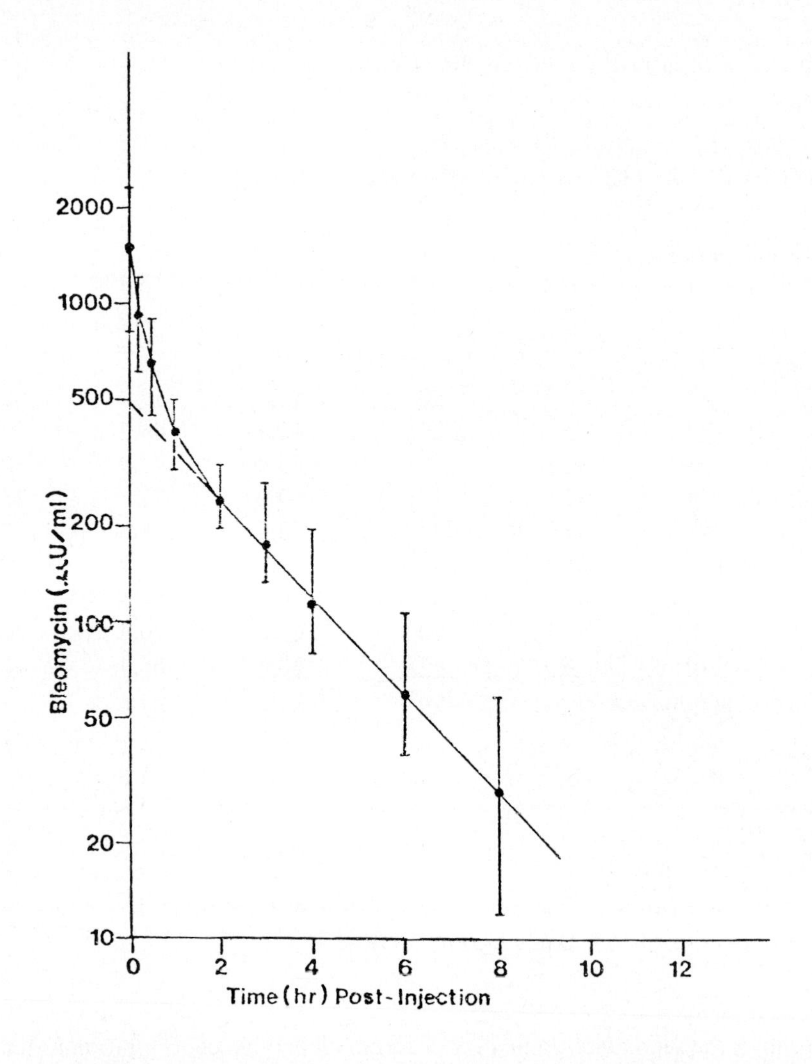

Fig. 5. Semi-logarithmic plot of serum bleomycin *vs* time. Each point represents the average of bleomycin determinations for six patients administered 7-10 units intravenously by 10 minute infusion. The standard deviation for each time point is indicated by vertical bars (from Broughton et al. 1977) (7).

Intramuscular Injection

Bleomycin pharmacokinetic studies were carried out in patients receiving bleomycin by intramuscular injection. Serum concentrations of bleomycin were determined by both [^{57}Co] and [^{125}I] radioimmunoassays (Broughton and Strong (13), Elson et al. (14)) and by the microbiologic assay when blood levels of drug were

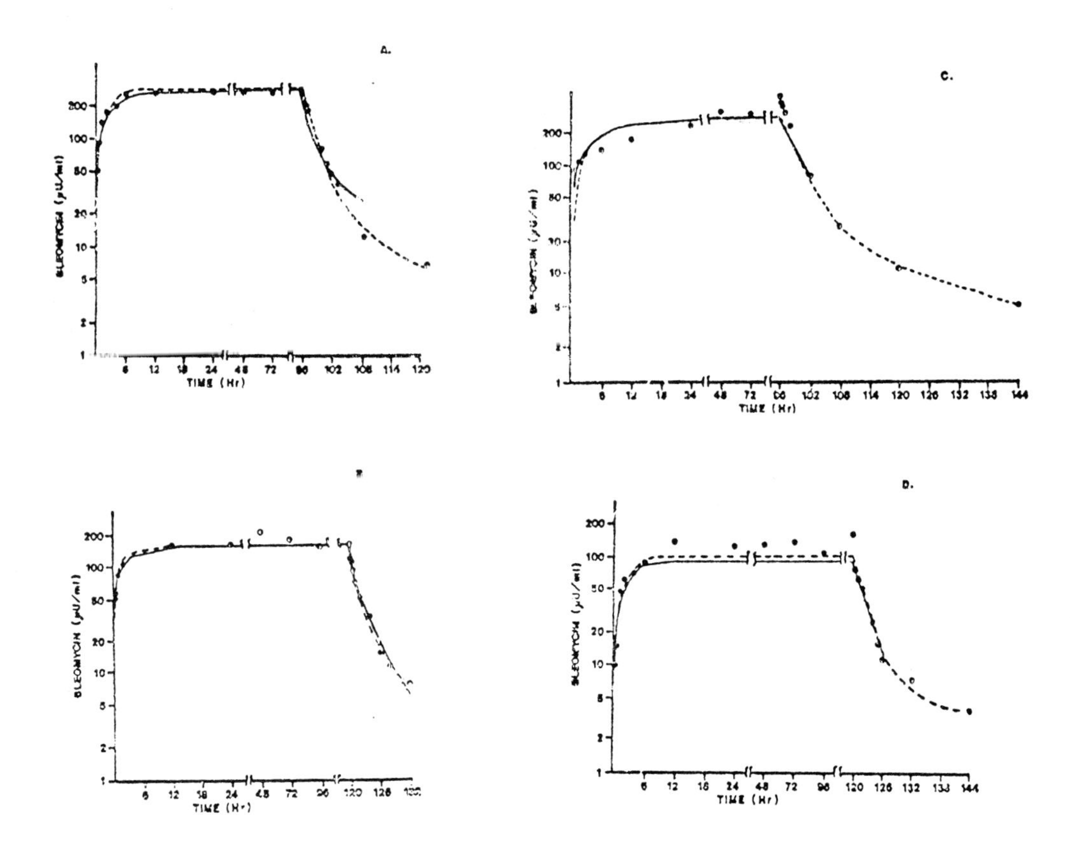

Fig. 6. Semi-logarithmic plots of serum bleomycin concentration *vs* time for four patients receiving 15-30 units per day bleomycin as a continuous 4-5 day intravenous infusion. The experimental data are shown as (o), the curve predicted by the analysis of all the data as (- - - - -) and that predicted by excluding data less than 10 μU/ml as (——). A through D represents patients 1-4 respectively (from Broughton et al. 1977 (7); Broughton et al. 1977a) (8).

high enough for detection. Doses ranged from 2-30 units. Maximum serum levels of bleomycin ranged from 0.13 to 0.35 mu/ml at one hour after injection and no bleomycin could be detected in serum at 24 hours after injection.

Table 10 compares the $t^1/_2\beta$ of IM bleomycin determined by three methods in 6 patients. In only one patient was the creatinine clearance below normal ($<$ 70 ml/min). The microbiologic assay was capable of detecting serum bleomycin only in patients who

TABLE 10.

COMPARISON $T\frac{1}{2}\beta$ BLEOMYCIN FOR MICROBIOLOGIC AND RADIOIMMUNOASSAYS

Patient	Total Dose Units Bleomycin	Creatinine Clearance (ml/min)	RIA(^{125}I) $t\frac{1}{2}$ min	RIA(^{57}Co) $t\frac{1}{2}$ min	Microbiologic $t\frac{1}{2}$ min
1	20	133	160	145	190
2	10	111	145	110	–
3	4	109	180	165	–
4	2	99	135	150	–
5	17	89	170	150	160
6	15	57	310	255	320
Creatinine Clearance > 70 ml/min		Mean	158 ± 8.2	144 ± 9.1	

received ≥ 15 unit dose. In patients with a creatinine clearance of ≥ 70 ml/min, the mean $t^1/_2\beta$ was 158 ± 8.2 and 144 ± 9.1 as determined by the [^{125}I] and [^{57}Co] RIA respectively and was independent of the dose.

Table 11 shows that bleomycin elimination was predominantly via urinary excretion. Urinary bleomycin recovery was 32.2 ± 5.0% (mean) in 0-4 h and 57.8 ± 5.9% (mean) in 0-24 hours of the administered dose. The amount of bleomycin excreted in urine did not appear to correlate with the creatinine clearance.

Table 12 summarizes the $t^1/_2\beta$ for bleomycin administered by i.v. injection, i.v. prolonged infusion, or intramuscular injection and shows that the radioimmunoassays and microbiologic assay gave equivalent results.

Pharmacokinetics after Intracavitary Administration

Alberts and colleagues (Alberts et al. (9)) have studied the pharmacokinetics of bleomycin after intraperitoneal and intrapleural administration in a small number of patients. In patients who received 60 U/m^{2}bleomycin intraperitoneally, the peak plasma concentrationed varied from 0.6 to 3.2 mμ/ml, and the mean terminal half-

TABLE 11.

BLEOMYCIN EXCRETION

Patient	Total Dose Units Bleomycin	Creatinine Clearance (ml/min)	Cumulative % Urine Bleomycin 0 – 4 h	0 – 24 h
1	20	133	48	69
2	10	111	46	72
3	4	109	27	58
4	2	99	32	65
5	17	89	22	33
6	15	57	19	50
	Mean	99 ± 10.4	32.3 ± 5.0	57.8 ± 5.9

TABLE 12.

COMPARISON OF $t_{\frac{1}{2}}\beta$ BLEOMYCIN WITH ROUTE OF ADMINISTRATION*

Route	$t_{\frac{1}{2}}\beta$ RIA [^{125}I] (min)	$t_{\frac{1}{2}}\beta$ RIA [^{57}Co] (min)	$t_{\frac{1}{2}}\beta$ Microbiologic (min)
i.v. Rapid Injection	109	–	111
i.v. 10 min Injection	122	–	–
i.v. Continuous Infusion	9.53	–	–
	234 min (< 10 μU/ml values excluded)		
i.m. Injection	158	144	175

* These values are for patients with creatinine clearance ≥ 60 ml/min

life was 6.3 ± 2.2 hours. In patients who received $60 U/m^2$ intrapleurally, the peak plasma concentrations were approximately equal to those observed after intraperitoneal administration, and the mean terminal half-life in the patients with normal renal function was 3.6 ± 0.8 hours. In one patient with a creatinine clearance of 46 ml/min, the terminal half-life was 9.3 hours.

The terminal half-life of bleomycin when administered intrapleurally was found to be comparable to the elimination half-life after an intravenous bolus. However, after intraperitoneal administration, the terminal half-life was significantly longer. Nonetheless, the bioavailability of bleomycin when administered either intrapleurally or intraperitoneally was shown to be approximately 50%.

Pharmacokinetics after Intravesical Administration

Bleomycin was administered to patients with superficial transitional cell carcinoma of the bladder at doses of 15 U to 120 U weekly for 8 weeks. Following the first dose, the serum and urine concentrations of bleomycin were monitored, using the microbiologic assay. In three patients of the more than 30 studied, bleomycin at a concentration of 0.2 mU/ml was detected in the plasma, an insignificant concentration. Thus, very little of an intravesical dose of bleomycin is absorbed.

DISCUSSION

The conclusions which may be derived from the pharmacokinetic study after i.v. bolus injection of bleomycin are

1) bleomycin is cleared principally by renal mechanisms;
2) at creatinine clearances > 25-35 ml/min, the $t^1/_2\beta$ of bleomycin is approximately 115 minutes;
3) at creatinine clearances < 25-35 ml/min, the $t^1/_2\beta$ increases exponentially as the creatinine clearance decreases;
4) even in frank failure, no bleomycin was detectable in the blood 48-72 hours after a bolus injection;
5) in patients with creatinine clearances ≥ 50 ml/min, approximately 50% of a total dose of bleomycin is excreted in the urine in 4 hours, and > 70% in 24 hours;
6) the mean total volume of distribution is approximately 20 liters, and does not vary with creatinine clearances;
7) bleomycin is probably not dialyzable;
8) pharmacokinetic model describing bleomycin pharmacokinetics does not vary with varying renal function, i.e., a two compartment model best ex-

plains the data in all patients;

9) both the microbiologic and radioimmunoassays give comparable results in plasma or serum.

After continuous infusion of bleomycin, the half-life was approximately 10-14 hours when all detectable levels of bleomycin were used in the determinations. When values $< 10\ \mu U/ml$ were excluded, the bleomycin half-life was approximately 3 hours which approximates that for rapid i.v. injection of bleomycin. Possible explanations for the 10-14 h half-life determination include interference in the radioimmunoassay by an unknown metabolite and/or strong binding of drug to tissues with release at a rate much less than the apparent half-life.

The results from the pharmacokinetic studies after intramuscular injection of bleomycin indicate that the $t^1/_2\beta$ determined by either radioimmunoassay or microbiologic assay is similar to that after an i.v. injection, i.e., approximately 2 hours. Also approximately 60-70% of bleomycin administered by this route is excreted in the urine in 24 hours.

Studies are in progress to determine whether patients who have impaired renal functions and who experience prolonged elevated blood levels of bleomycin, also experience greater pulmonary toxicity. Results of these studies should provide a basis on which to make specific recommendations for dose reduction of bleomycin in patients with compromised renal function.

REFERENCES

1. Fujita, H., Kimura, K. (1970) Blood levels, tissue distribution, excretion and inactivation of bleomycin in progress in antimicrobial and anticancer chemotherapy. *Proc. 6th Internat. Cong. of Chemother. 12*: 309-314, Baltimore University Park Press.

2. Ohnuma, T., Holland, J.F., Masuda, H., Waligunda, J.A. and Goldberg, G.A. (1974) Microbiologic assay of bleomycin: Inactivation, tissue distribution and clearance. *Cancer 33*: 1230-1238.

3. Fujita, H. (1971) Comparative studies on the blood level, tissue distribution, excretion and inactivation of anticancer drugs. *Jap. J. Clin. Oncol. 12*: 151-162.

4. Crooke, S.T., Comis, R.L., Einhorn, L.H., Strong, J.E., Broughton, A. and Prestayko, A.W. (1977) The effects of variations in renal function of the clini-

cal pharmacology of bleomycin administered as an intravenous bolus, *Cancer Treatment Reports 61*: 1631-1636.

5. Crooke, S.T., Comis, R.L., Einhorn, L.H., Strong, J.E., Broughton, A. and Prestayko, A.W. (1977a) Studies on the clinical pharmacology of bleomycin, Carter, S.K., Umezawa, H. (eds.), Proceedings of the U.S.-Japan Conference May 12-13, 1977. Springer-Verlag, New York, in press.

6. Crooke, S.T., Luft, F.T., Broughton, A.W., Strong, J.L., Casson, K. and Einhorn, L. (1977b) Bleomycin serum concentrations in a patient with varying renal function. *Cancer 39*: 1430-1434.

7. Broughton, A., Strong, J.E., Holoye, P., Hall, S., Feldman, S. and Kramer, W. (1977) Pharmacokinetics of bleomycin following long and short term infusion. Manuscript submitted for publication.

8. Broughton, A., Strong, J.E., Holoye, P. and Bedrossian, C. (1977a) Clinical pharmacology of bleomycin following intravenous infusion as determined by radioimmunoassay. *Cancer*: in press.

9. Alberts, D., Chen, H.S., Liu, R., Himmelstein, K., Gross, J., Broughton, A. and Salmon, S. (1978) Bleomycin pharmacokinetics in man, in bleomycin current status and new developments. S.K. Carter, H. Umezawa, S.T. Crooke (eds.). *Academic Press,* N.Y.

10. Crooke, S.T. and Bradner, W.T. (1976) Bleomycin, A Review, *J. of Medicine 7*: No. 5, 333-428.

11. Hall, S., Broughton, A., Strong, J. and Benjamin, R. (1977) Clinical pharmacology of bleomycin by radioimmunoassay, *Clin. Res. 25*: 407A.

12. Bracken, R., Johnson, D., Rodriquez, L., Samuels, M. and Ayala, A. (1977) Treatment of multiple superficial tumors of bladder with intravesical bleomycin, *Urology 9*: No. 2, 161-163.

13. Broughton, A. and Strong, J. (1976) Radioimmunoassay of bleomycin, *Cancer Research 35*: 1418-1421.

14. Elson, M., Oken, M. and Shafer, R. (1977) A radioimmunoassay for bleomycin, *Journal of Nuclear Medicine 18*: 296-299.

15. Einhorn, L., Furnas, B. and Powell, N. (1976) Combination chemotherapy of disseminated testicular carcinoma with Cis-platinum diamminedichloride (CPPD) vinblastine (VLB) and bleomycin (Bleo), *Amer. Assoc. Clin. Oncol. 17*: 240.

Clinical Pharmacology of Anti-Neoplastic Drugs
H. M. Pinedo, editor

A REVIEW OF THE PHARMACOLOGY AND CLINICAL USE OF CYCLOPHOSPHAMIDE

MICHAEL COLVIN
Pharmacology Laboratory, The Johns Hopkins Oncology Center, 601 North Broadway, Baltimore, Maryland 21205 U.S.A.

INTRODUCTION

Cyclophosphamide was developed by Arnold and coworkers at the Astra company in Germany and reported in 1958 (1). The rationale for the synthesis of this compound was a hypothesis first advanced by Seligman and Friedman in 1954 (2). This hypothesis suggested that a phosphate substituted nitrogen mustard might be tumor specific by virtue of selective activation by phosphamidase enzymes thought to be elevated in certain types of tumors. Cyclophosphamide was found to have a high therapeutic index in several animal tumor models (3), and the drug was moved rapidly into clinical trials (4).

Cyclophosphamide has proven to be clinically effective against a variety of tumors and is widely used both as a single agent and in combination chemotherapy. In particular it is used in the treatment of lymphomas (5), carcinoma of the breast (6), multiple myeloma (7), carcinoma of the lung (8), and sarcomas (9,10). In addition, because of its immunosuppressive properties, the drug has been used for organ transplantation (11) and in the treatment of diseases thought to be of autoimmune origin (12,13).

Cyclophosphamide contains the bis-chloroethylamino group of the nitrogen mustards, demonstrates strong activity against tumors which are traditionally sensitive to alkylating agents and demonstrates a significant degree of cross resistance to other alkylating agents. Thus it seems likely that this agent is functioning as an alkylating agent.

STRUCTURE AND METABOLISM

The structure of cyclophosphamide is shown in Fig. 1. The nitrogen mustard moiety (bis-chloroethylamino) group of the molecule is attached to a six membered oxoazaphosphorine ring. It is the structure of this unusual heterocyclic ring which is responsible for the complex metabolic transformations which this drug undergoes. The parent molecule exhibits no alkylating activity and is not cytotoxic *in vitro*, but is activated *in vivo* to alkylating and cytotoxic metabolites (14,15).

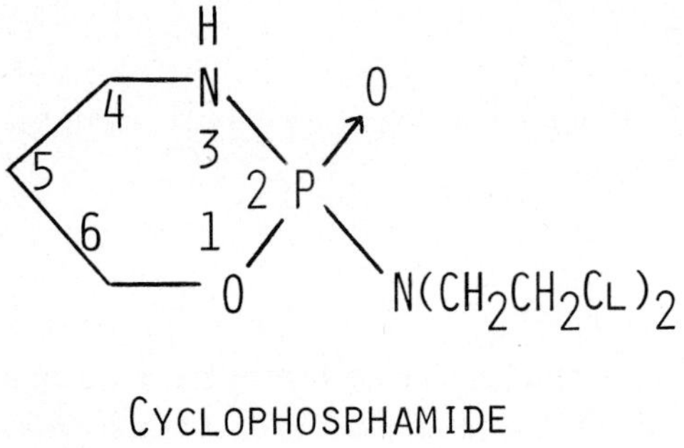

CYCLOPHOSPHAMIDE

Fig. 1. Structure of Cyclophosphamide.

However, this activation occurs not in tumor cells, as originally postulated, but is initiated by the mixed function oxidase enzymes of the liver microsomes (15,16). The complex metabolic scheme which cyclophosphamide undergoes is shown in Fig. 2.

The initial metabolic alteration of cyclophosphamide is the hydroxylation of the 4-carbon, which is adjacent to the nitrogen of the heterocyclic ring. This hydroxylation produces a hemiaminal structure, 4-hydroxycyclophosphamide (IIa) (17-19), which is in spontaneous equilibrium with the open ring aldophosphamide (IIb) (20,21). The majority of the 4-hydroxycyclophosphamide-aldophosphamide equilibrium mixture is oxidized enzymatically to 4-ketocyclophosphamide (VI) and carboxyphosphamide (VII) (22,23). These latter two compounds are not significantly cytotoxic (22) but are quantitatively important in that well over 50% of a dose of cyclophosphamide is excreted in the urine as carboxycyclophosphamide (the major metabolite) and 4-ketocyclophosphamide (a minor metabolite) in several animal species (22,23). The enzymes which carry out the oxidation of the initial activation products are located in the cytosol of the cell (24) and have been found to be highest in the rat in the liver, kidney, and the intestinal epithelium, with low levels in bone marrow and tumor tissue (25). This finding has led to the hypothesis that normal tissues may be protected from the drug by these inactivating enzymes.

The aldophosphamide which has escaped enzymatic oxidation spontaneously eliminates acrolein (IV) (26) to form phosphoramide mustard (III) (27). This compound is an active alkylating agent which is likely the metabolite which alkylates biological molecules, since the primary metabolites, 4-hydroxy-cyclophosphamide and aldophosphamide, have low alkylating activity (28,29). To what extent the activated cyclophosphamide enters cells as the primary metabolites (IIa or IIb) or as phosphoramide mustard remains uncertain.

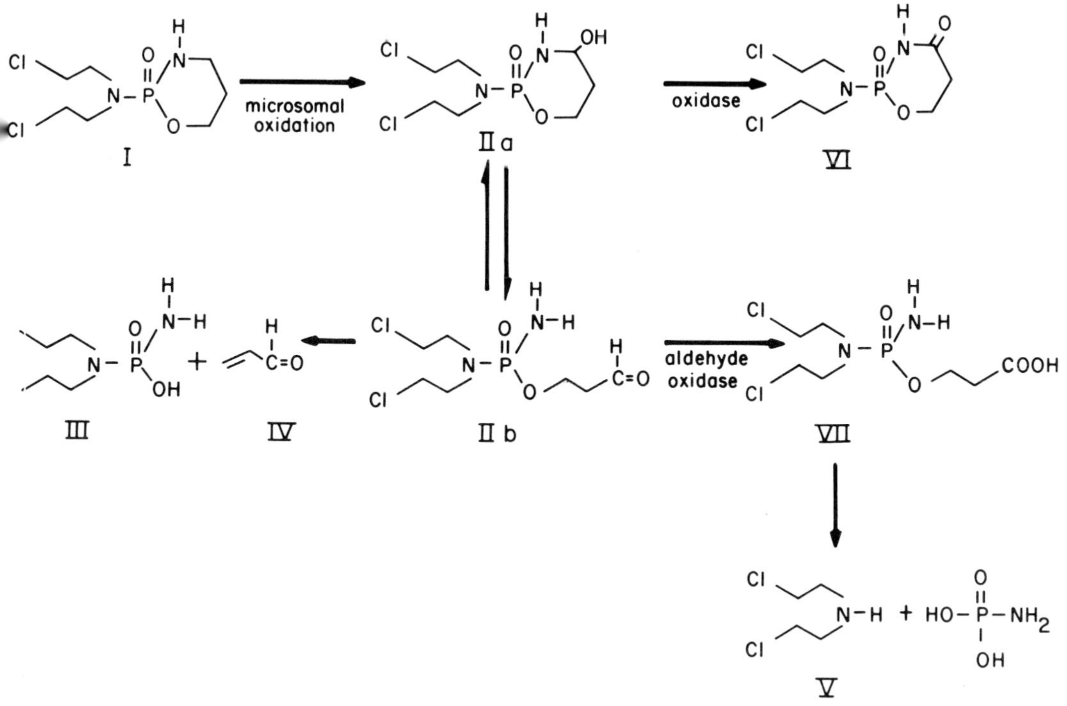

Fig. 2. Metabolic Scheme of Cyclophosphamide.

The fact that the primary metabolites are up to 20 times more cytotoxic to cells *in vitro* than phosphoramide mustard, on a molar basis (18,30), supports the hypothesis that the primary metabolites enter target cells more facilely than phosphoramide mustard and thus serve as "transport forms" of the drug. Furthermore, in animal studies and its limited clinical trials, phosphoramide mustard lacks certain characteristic properties of the parent compound. Perhaps the most important difference is that phosphoramide mustard appears to have a lower therapeutic index in both animals and man than the parent compounds (28,31). In addition, phosphoramide mustard possesses little immunosuppressive activity (32) and does not produce alopecia (31,33), both characteristic effects of the parent compound. These observations are consistent with the postulate that a metabolite prior to phosphoramide mustard is responsible for some of the specific actions of the parent compound.

MECHANISM OF ACTION

Studies on the molecular mechanism of action of cyclophosphamide utilizing metabolites are limited. Several studies have shown that the metabolites bind to nucleic acid after *in vivo* administration of cyclophosphamide (34,35). Nucleic acid synthesis is rapidly inhibited in sensitive cells exposed to cyclophosphamide metabolites *in vitro* (36), and our studies show that the inhibition of DNA synthesis occurs prior to the inhibition of RNA and protein synthesis. The decline in viability of the cells coincides with the inhibition of DNA synthesis. These observations are consistent with the hypothesis that the cytotoxic effects of cyclophosphamide are mediated through the alkylation of DNA by a reactive metabolite (or metabolites), most likely phosphoramide mustard, which has been shown to alkylate the 7-nitrogen of guanylic acid (37). However, considerably more evidence will be required to demonstrate convincingly that such is the case.

CLINICAL DOSES AND SCHEDULES

Cyclophosphamide is administered in a wide variety of doses and schedules. The drug is as active by mouth as by parenteral administration and is assumed to be completely absorbed from the gastrointestinal tract, although no bio-availability studies have been carried out in man. A common dosage by the oral route is 100 to 200 mg per day given either continuously or for two-week periods. Animal studies and limited clinical experience indicate that intermittent high doses of cyclophosphamide may be given by mouth as effectively as parenterally, but the drug has seldom been used in this fashion.

A wide range of parenteral doses and schedules has also been used. A single dose of up to 25 mg/kg is usually well tolerated without serious hematologic depression, and single doses of up to 75 mg/kg may be given if severe leucopenia and thrombocytopenia can be tolerated. In our experience doses above this level have often produced severe hemorrhagic cystitis and at least one instance of fatal myocardial damage occurred with a single dose of 100 mg/kg. If doses greater than 75 mg/kg are desired, the dose should be divided over several days to diminish the acute toxicity (38,39). This author recommends a maximum single dose of 60 mg/kg, which produces severe leucopenia, but not usually marked thrombocytopenia or serious non-hematologic toxicity. Such doses can be repeated every 3-4 weeks, and we have not seen cumulative hematologic toxicity. It is important that such high doses of cyclophosphamide be given on the basis of ideal body weight (or the corresponding body surface dose), since we have seen severe toxicity in markedly obese patients dosed on actual body weight.

Although intermittent schedules of cyclophosphamide are superior to daily administration regimens in virtually all animal studies (40,41), no convincing evidence of schedule dependency has been demonstrated in man. In some instances daily oral cyclophosphamide has been claimed to be superior to intermittent cyclophosphamide, but these studies have not compared equivalent doses of intermittent drug with oral cyclophosphamide.

CLINICAL PHARMACOLOGY

Studies of the clinical pharmacology of cyclophosphamide have been limited, since the key metabolites and techniques for quantitating them have not been available. Investigations utilizing radioactive cyclophosphamide have demonstrated that the plasma half-life of the parent compound in man varies from 2 hours to 10 hours (42,43), and these values have now been confirmed by direct measurement of cyclophosphamide levels by mass spectrometric techniques (44,45). Only recently have measurements of individual metabolites been reported (44). Shown in Fig. 3 are the levels of cyclophosphamide, phosphoramide mustard, and nornitrogen mustard in the plasma of a patient who received 75 mg/kg of cyclophosphamide. These measurements were made by gas chromatography selective ion monitoring. The plasma half-life of cyclophosphamide in this patient was 3.5 hours, and in the other patients studied varied up to 7 hours, which is in agreement with the results published using less direct measurements of the cyclophosphamide.

As can be seen in Fig. 3 most of the patients we studied showed high initial levels of nornitrogen mustard, which then declined rapidly. However, there was a marked variation in the nornitrogen mustard levels between patients. Also, significant decomposition of other metabolites, especially carboxyphosphamide, to nornitrogen mustard occurs during storage and extraction from plasma and urine.

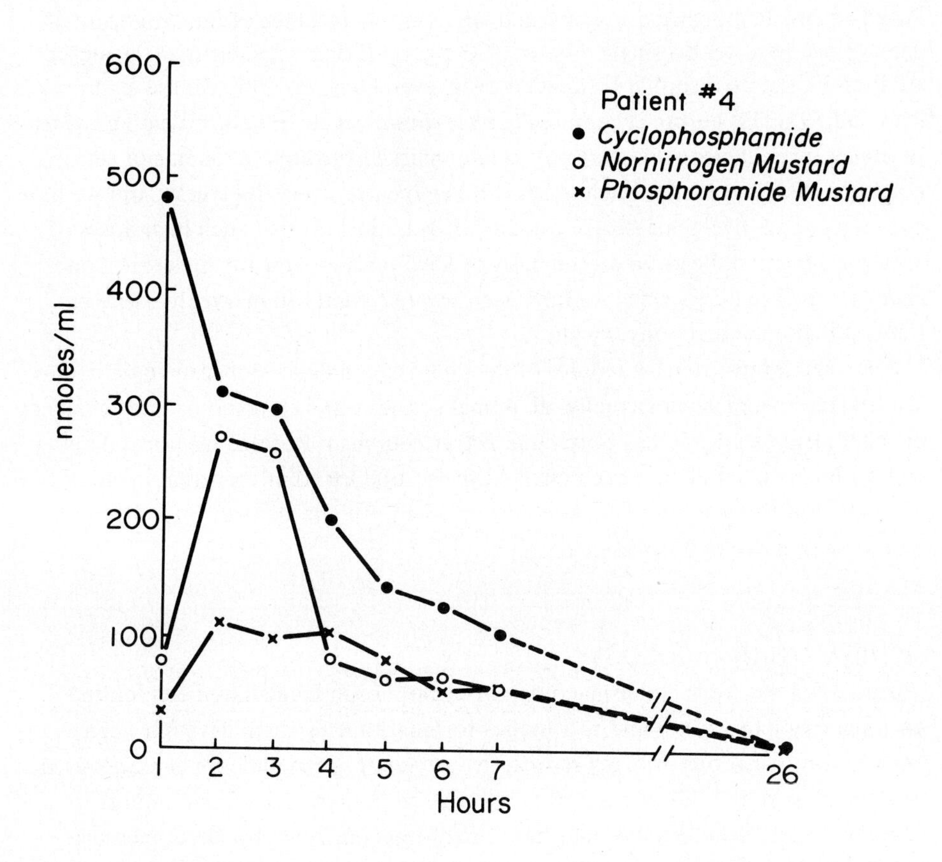

Fig. 3. Plasma Levels of Cyclophosphamide and Metabolites.

These findings suggest that the levels of nornitrogen mustard which have been seen in our studies and animal studies (46) may be artefactually elevated by *in vitro* decomposition of other metabolites. However, significant levels of nornitrogen mustard are probably present *in vivo* and may play a role in the toxic and therapeutic effects of cyclophosphamide. Since nornitrogen mustard is a potent alkylating agent at acid pH, but not at physiological pH (46,47), it is especially likely to contribute to renal and bladder damage.

Significant levels of phosphoramide mustard are present in the plasma after cyclophosphamide administration and remain elevated for several hours. We are confident that the levels measured represent the actual level of phosphoramide mustard present in the plasma *in vivo* since none of the other metabolites (except aldophosphamide) decompose to phosphoramide mustard *in vitro* to a significant degree.

TABLE 1
24-HOUR URINARY EXCRETION OF CYCLOPHOSPHAMIDE AND METABOLITES

	Excretion (mmoles)		
	Patient 2	Patient 3	Patient 4
Cyclophosphamide	2.8 (19.5)[a]	5.4 (25.1)	2.0 (16.3)
Phosphoramide mustard	0.4 (2.8)	0.3 (1.2)	0.2 (1.8)
Nornitrogen mustard	1.4 (10.4)	2.4 (11.0)	1.8 (14.5)
Total	4.6 (32.7)	8.1 (37.3)	4.0 (32.6)

[a] Numbers in parentheses, percentage of dose.

As can be seen in Table 1, about 20% of the administered dose of cyclophosphamide is excreted in the urine in the first 24 hours. During this time approximately 2% of the dose is excreted as phosphoramide mustard and about 12% as nornitrogen mustard. The time course of urinary excretion of the compounds which were measured in this study are shown in Fig. 4. After 24 hours only negligible amounts of these compounds are excreted. Of interest is the fact that there is a delayed peak of nornitrogen mustard excretion, occurring at a time when the plasma levels have fallen to low levels.

The plasma levels of phosphoramide mustard found in these studies are within the levels which have been found to be cytotoxic to cells *in vitro* (48). Therefore it is probable that circulating phosphoramide mustard plays some role in the therapeutic and toxic effects of cyclophosphamide. However, because of the properties of the primary metabolites it will be important to quantitate the levels of 4-hydroxycyclophosphamide and aldophosphamide in plasma after cyclophosphamide administration. Recently techniques for detecting and quantitating the primary metabolites either as the mercaptan derivative of 4-hydroxycyclophosphamide (49) or as the cyanohydrin derivative of aldophosphamide (21) have been described. Since the two primary metabolites are in equilibrium, the measurement of either derivative should measure the total of the two metabolites. The application of these techniques to measure the primary metabolites should further clarify the clinical pharmacology of cyclophosphamide.

Since cyclophosphamide is activated by the microsomal enzymes it is not surprising that drugs which stimulate or inhibit these enzymes can alter the pharmacokine-

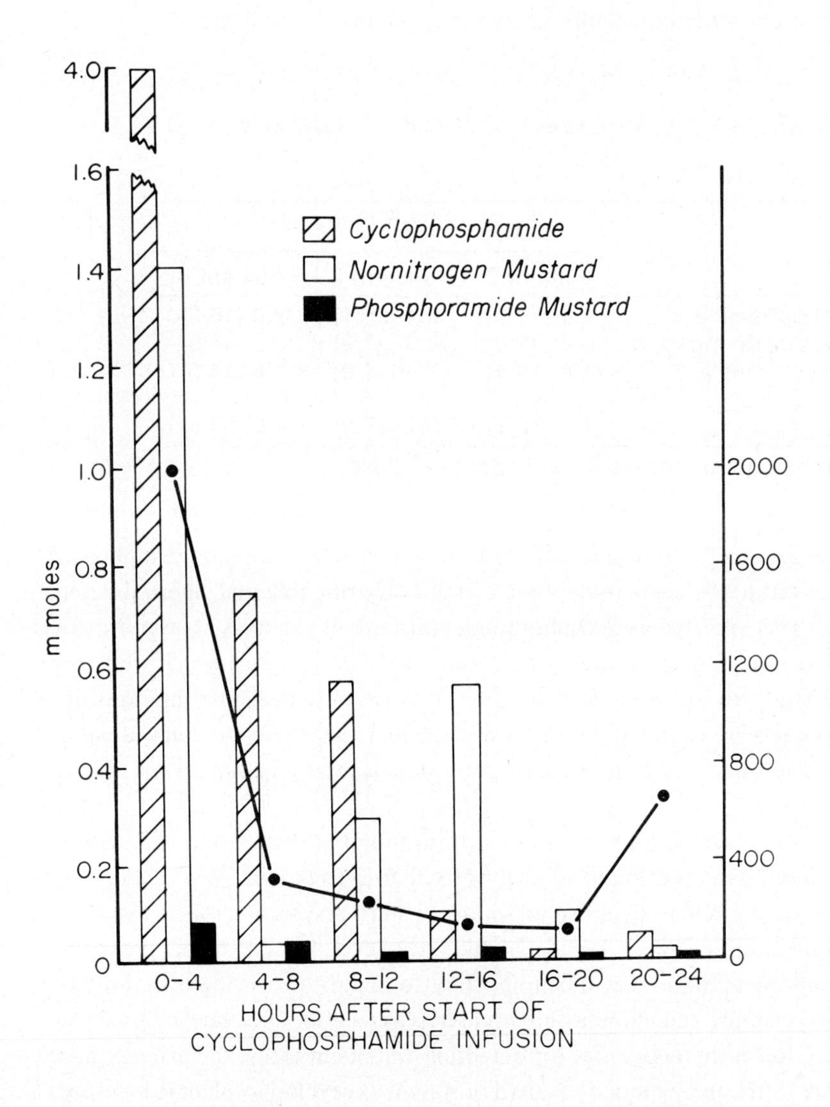

Fig. 4. Time Course of Urinary Excretion of Cyclophosphamide and Metabolites.

tics of the drug. The effects of these alterations in pharmacokinetics on the therapeutic and toxic effects of the drug are complex, and conflicting reports have appeared in animals (50-53). It has been demonstrated that the pharmacokinetics of the parent compound are altered in man by other drugs which affect the microsomes (42), and it is likely that the variations in plasma half-life of cyclophosphamide which have been reported are due to this phenomenon (43). However, there has been no definitive evidence that the therapeutic index or toxicities of cyclophosphamide are altered in man as the result of the concomitant administration of other drugs.

At least two authors have reported that plasma levels of the cyclophosphamide metabolites are elevated and prolonged in the presence of renal failure (43,54), and on this basis a reduction in dose has been recommended for such patients. However, it has not been established that these elevated metabolite levels are associated with increased toxicity, and in The Johns Hopkins Oncology Center we have given full doses of cyclophosphamide to patients with severe renal impairment without an increase in the hematologic and other toxicities of the drug (55).

TOXICITIES

The major toxicities of cyclophosphamide are listed in Table 2. The most consistent toxicity of the agent is depression of the hematopoietic system. After a single dose of cyclophosphamide the nadir of the leucocyte count is at 10-12 days and recovery is usually complete by 21 days (Fig. 5). As the dose of the drug is increased the nadir of the leucocyte depression is decreased, but the time to recovery of the leucocyte count is not significantly prolonged. In contrast to most cytotoxic agents, the drug is relatively platelet sparing, and significant depression of the platelet count is usually not seen unless single doses of 50 mg/kg or higher are employed.

TABLE 2
TOXICITIES OF CYCLOPHOSPHAMIDE

1. Hematopoietic Depression
2. Nausea and Vomiting
3. Alopecia
4. Hemorrhagic Cystitis
5. Water Retention
6. Cardiac Damage
7. Gonadal Atrophy
8. Carcinogenicity

Cumulative or irreparable damage to the bone marrow does not appear to occur in that most patients can receive multiple courses of cyclophosphamide without showing decreasing tolerance of the hematopoietic system to the drug.

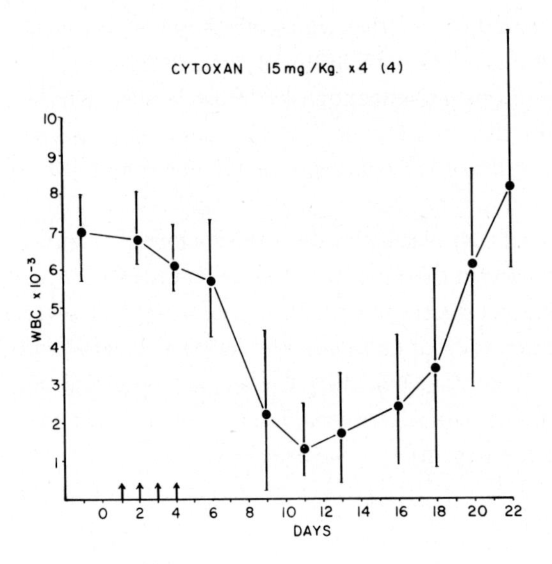

Fig. 5. Leucocyte Count After Cyclophosphamide Therapy.

While nausea and vomiting are not life-threatening toxicities, they are a significant source of discomfort to patients. The degree of this side effect is quite variable from patient to patient, with some patients tolerating very large intravenous doses of drug with little or no discomfort, while other patients become severely nauseated with very small doses. The onset of the nausea and vomiting is usually delayed for 6-8 hours following administration of the drug, but rarely lasts more than 48 hours. Therefore, patients who continue to be nauseated with repeated daily doses of the drug may find an intermittent, higher dose schedule more tolerable.

Another toxicity which is not life-threatening, but is distressing to patients, is alopecia. A degree of hair fragility and loss occurs at even low doses and at high doses significant to complete alopecia will occur. However, this effect is invariably reversible, although the rate of hair regrowth will vary among patients. The structural requirements for depilation have been studied in sheep (33) and at least two chloroethyl groups and the intact ring structure are required. Phosphoramide mustard is not depilating in sheep (33) or man (31), suggesting that this toxic effect is due to entry of the more lipophilic metabolites into the hair follicles.

A unique toxicity which occurs in 10-20% of patients is sterile cystitis. Within a few hours after a dose of cyclophosphamide, the patient may experience dysuria, which may proceed to frank hematuria. The hematuria may be quite severe, and in some instances has either been fatal or required cystectomy to prevent fatal bleeding. While a variety of approaches to the treatment of this hemorrhagic cystitis have been used, we have found that a conservative approach, with irrigation of the bladder to prevent clot formation and transfusions to keep up with blood loss, has been the most successful. Prevention of the hemorrhagic cystitis is most satisfactory, and we have found that adequate hydration and frequent emptying of the bladder will minimize the incidence of hemorrhagic cystitis, even with doses of 60 and 75 mg/kg. The bladder toxicity appears to be due to the presence of alkylating metabolites in the urine (56,57), but the damage may be potentiated by an effect of blood-borne metabolites on the submucosa (58). Phosphoramide mustard also produces hemorrhagic cystitis (31), indicating that this compound and its degradation products, such as nornitrogen mustard, are responsible for the bladder damage. In experimental animals, bladder damage from cyclophosphamide and isophosphamide can be prevented by irrigation with N-acetylcysteine, and this maneuver has been used clinically to avoid cystitis. In mice, systemic administration of N-acetylcysteine in conjunction with cyclophosphamide will prevent bladder damage but does not diminish the antitumor activity (59).

A toxicity which is probably mediated through an effect on the kidney is that of acute water retention. Patients who receive an acute dose of 50 mg/kg or greater may show a syndrome of decreased urinary output, weight gain, increase in urine osmolality, and decrease in plasma osmolality (60). In extreme cases the patient may develop serious effusions. The onset of this syndrome coincides with the peak excretion of alkylating metabolites in the urine, suggesting that this effect is due to a direct action of the metabolites on the renal tubules. The syndrome is self-limited, and by 12-16 hours after the dose of drug the fluid retention spontaneously reverses. Attempts to reverse the fluid retention immediately by vigorous diuretic therapy may lead to electrolyte imbalance.

The dose limiting toxicity for acute cyclophosphamide administration is cardiac damage (61,62). This syndrome is manifested in its most fulminant form by the rapid onset of intractable heart failure, leading to death in 10-14 days. High dose patients who do not show the complete syndrome may have decreased electrocardiographic voltage and a transient increase in heart size. Cardiac damage has been seen only in patients receiving doses of over 100 mg/kg during a 48-hour period, and has been seen mainly in bone marrow transplant patients receiving more than 200 mg/kg (over 4 days) in preparation for bone marrow transplantation. There is no evidence for cumulative damage to the heart following repeated doses of cyclophosphamide. The histologic appearance of the heart after cyclophosphamide damage is different from that of anthracycline damage, and there is no evidence for an additive effect of these two agents on the heart.

Cyclophosphamide, like other alkylating agents, produces severe effects on the gonads (63,64). Aspermia and amenorrhea are seen in men and women after prolonged therapy, and the clinical effects are correlated with atrophy of the Sertoli cells in males and ovarian atrophy in females. These lesions are often reversible, and both men and women have become the parents of normal children after documented gonadal atrophy from cyclophosphamide (63,65,66). The drug is teratogenic in animals (67) and one case of a malformed child born to a woman treated with cyclophosphamide in early pregnancy has been reported (68). However, there have been several instances in which a normal pregnancy and child occurred despite cyclophosphamide therapy in the first trimester (69).

Cyclophosphamide is carcinogenic in animals (70), and the increasing number of reports of new tumors in patients treated with the agent make it almost certain that this complication occurs in man. While most of the new tumors have been acute leukemias and reticulum cell sarcomas, a variety of new tumors have now been described. The occurrence of this complication makes it imperative to attempt to define the minimum effective therapy for responsive malignancies.

ANALOGUES

Although many analogues of cyclophosphamide have been synthesized and tested, only two are currently in clinical use, isophosphamide and trophosphamide (Fig. 6). Trophosphamide is similar to cyclophosphamide in its effects but has been reported to be better tolerated orally (71). Isophosphamide has been the more extensively tested of the two, and has been reported to be more effective against solid tumors than cyclophosphamide (72). However, the compound has not been compared directly with cyclophosphamide at equally toxic doses. The metabolism of isophosphamide has been studied (24,71,73), and is analogous to the metabolism of cyclophosphamide. However, the oxidation of a chloroethyl side chain, which is a very minor pathway in cyclophosphamide metabolism is quantitatively important in the metabolism of isophosphamide (73). While the hematopoietic toxicity of isophosphamide appears to be lower than that of cyclophosphamide renal toxicity is increased and is the dose limiting toxicity (74).

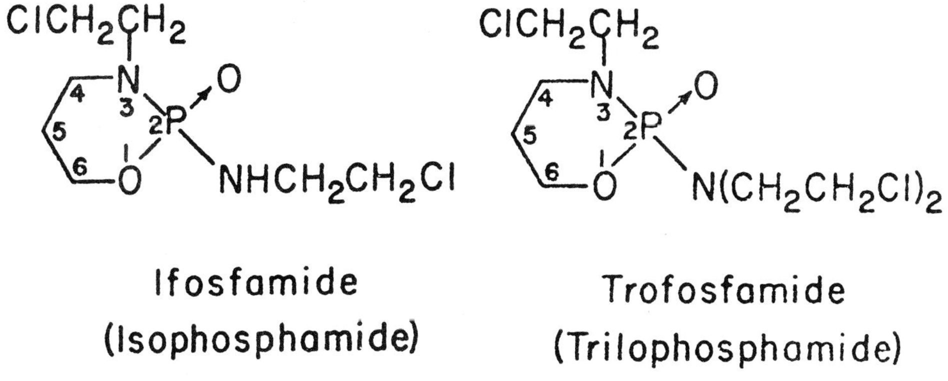

$ClCH_2CH_2$ — N — P(→O) — $NHCH_2CH_2Cl$

Ifosfamide
(Isophosphamide)

$ClCH_2CH_2$ — N — P(→O) — $N(CH_2CH_2Cl)_2$

Trofosfamide
(Trilophosphamide)

Fig. 6. Structures of Isophosphamide and Trophosphamide.

REFERENCES

1. Arnold, H. and Bourseaux, F. (1958) Angew. Chem., 70, 539.

2. Friedman, O.M. and Seligman, A.M. (1954) J. Am. Chem. Soc., 76, 655.

3. Arnold, H., Bourseaux, F. and Brock, N. (1958) Naturwissenschaften, 45, 64.

4. Brock, N. and Wilmanns, H. (1958) Dtsch. Med. Wochenschr., 83, 453.

5. Lenhard, R.E.Jr., Prentice, R.L., Owens, A.H.Jr., Bakemeier, R., Horton, J.H., Shnider, B.I., Stolbach, L., Berard, C.W. and Carbone, P.P. (1976) Cancer, 38, 1052.

6. Carter, S.K. (1972) Cancer, 30, 1543.

7. Humphrey, R.L., Kvols, L.K., Braine, H.G. and Abeloff, M.D. (1973) Proc. Am. Assoc. Cancer Res., 14, 54.

8. Livingston, R.B. and Carter, S.K. (1970) in Single Agents in Cancer Chemotherapy, Plenum Press, Inc., New York, p. 28.

9. Heyn, R.M., Hollan, R., Newton, W.A.Jr., Tefft, M., Breslow, N. and Hartmann, J.R. (1974) Cancer, 34, 2128.

10. Fernandez, C.H., Lindberg, R.D., Sutow, W.W. and Samuels, M.L. (1974) Cancer, 34, 143.

11. Santos, G.W., Sensenbrenner, L.L., Anderson, P.N., Burke, P.J., Klein, D.L., Slavin, R.E., Schacter, B. and Borgaonkar, D.S. (1976) Transpl. Proc., 8, 607.

12. Cooperating Clinics Committee of the American Rheumatism Association (1970) N. Engl. J. Med., 283, 883.

13. Laros, R.K.Jr. and Penner, J.A. (1971) J. Am. Med. Assoc., 215, 445.

14. Foley, G.E., Friedman, O.M. and Drolet, B.P. (1960) Proc. Am. Assoc. Cancer Res., 3, 111.

15. Brock, N. and Hohorst, H.-J. (1963) Arzneim.-Forsch., 13, 1021.

16. Cohen, J.L. and Jao, J.Y. (197) J. Pharmacol. Exp. Ther., 174, 206.

17. Connors, T.A., Cox, P.J., Farmer, P.B., Foster, A.B. and Jarman, M. (1974) Biochem. Pharmacol. 23, 115.

18. Takamizawa, A., Matsumoto, S., Iwata, T., Katagiri, K., Tochino, Y. and Yamaguchi, K. (1973) J. Am. Chem. Soc., 95, 985.

19. Brock, N. (1976) Cancer Treatment Rep., 60, 301.

20. Sladek, N.E. (1973) Cancer Res., 33, 1150.

21. Fenselau, C., Kan, M.-N.N., Subba Rao, S., Myles, A., Friedman, O.M. and Colvin, M. (1977) Cancer Res., 37, 2538.

22. Struck, R.F., Kirk, M.C., Mellett, L.B., El Dareer, S. and Hill, D.L. (1971) Mol. Pharmacol., 7, 519.

23. Bakke, J.E., Feil, V.J. and Zaylskie, R.G. (1971) J. Agr. Food Chem., 19, 788.

24. Hill, D.L., Laster, W.R.Jr., Kirk, M.C., El Dareer, S. and Struck, R.F. (1973) Cancer Res., 33, 1016.

25. Cox, P.J., Phillips, B.J. and Thomas, P. (1975) 35, 3755.

26. Alarcon, R.A. and Meienhofer, J. (1971) Nature (New Biol.), 233, 250.

27. Colvin, M., Padgett, C.A. and Fenselau, C. (1973) Cancer Res., 33, 915.

28. Hohorst, H.-J., Draeger,U., Peter, G. and Voelcker, G. (1976) Cancer Treatment Rep., 60, 309.

29. Struck, R.F., Kirk, M.C., Witt, M.H. and Laster, W.R.Jr. (1975) Biomed. Mass Spectrometry, 2, 46.

30. Colvin, M. Unpublished results.

31. Nathanson, L., Hall, T.C., Rutenberg, A. and Shadduck, R.K. (1967) Cancer Chemotherapy Rep., 51, 35.

32. Sensenbrenner, L.L., Marini, J.J. and Colvin, M. Unpublished results.

33. Feil, V.J. and Lamoureux, C.J.H. (1974) Cancer Res., 34, 2596.

34. Wheeler, G.P. and Alexander, J.A. (1964) Cancer Res., 24, 1331.

35. Murthy, V.V., Becker, B.A. and Steele, W.J. (1973) Cancer Res., 33, 664.

36. Padgett, C.A. and Colvin, M. (1972) Fed. Proc., 31, 554.

37. Colvin, M. (1974) Proc. Am. Assoc. Cancer Res., 15, 70.

38. Mullins, G.M. and Colvin, M. (1975) Cancer Chemotherapy Rep., Pt. 1, 59, 411.

39. Santos, G.W. and Mullins, G.M. (1975) Cancer, 36, 1950.

40. Lane, M. (1959) Cancer Chemotherapy Rep., 3, 1.

41. Venditti, J.M., Humphreys, S.R. and Goldin, A. (1959) Cancer Chemotherapy Rep., 3, 6.

42. Cohen, J.L., Jao, J.Y. and Jusko, W.J. (1971) Br. J. Pharmacol., 43, 677.

43. Bagley, C.M.Jr., Bostick, F.W. and DeVita, V.T.Jr. (1973) Cancer Res., 33, 226.

44. Jardine, I., Fenselau, C., Appler, M., Kan, M.-N., Brundrett, R.B. and Colvin, M. (1978) Cancer Res., 38, 408.

45. Jarman, M., Gilby, E.D., Foster, A.B. and Bondy, P.K. (1975) Clin. Chim. Acta, 58, 61.

46. Struck, R.F., Kirk, M.C., Witt, M.H. and Laster, W.R.Jr. (1975) Biomed. Mass Spectrometry, 2, 46.

47. Colvin, M., Brundrett, R.B., Kan, M.-N.N., Jardine, I. and Fenselau, C. (1976) Cancer Res., 36, 1121.

48. Maddock, C.L., Handler, A.H., Friedman, O.M., Foley, G.E. and Farber, S. (1966) Cancer Chemotherapy Rep., 50, 629.

49. Wagner, T., Peter, G., Voelcker, G. and Hohorst, H.-J. (1977) Cancer Res., 37, 2592.

50. Hart, L.G. and Adamson, R.H. (1969) Arch. Int. Pharmacodyn., 180, 391.

51. Field, R.B., Gang, M., Klein, I., Venditti, J.M. and Waravdekar, V.S. (1972) J. Pharmacol. Exp. Ther., 180, 475.

52. Sladek, N.E. (1972) Cancer Res., 32, 535.

53. Alberts, D.S. and Van Daalen Wetters, T. (1976) Cancer Res., 36, 2785.

54. Mouridsen, H.T. and Jacobsen, E. (1975) Acta Pharmacol. et Toxicol., 36, 409.

55. Humphrey, R.L. and Kvols, L.K. (1974) Proc. Am. Assoc. Cancer Res., 15, 84.

56. Philips, F.S., Sternberg, S.S., Cronin, A.P. and Vidal, P.M. (1961) Cancer Res., 21, 1577.

57. Bellin, H.J., Cherry, J.M. and Koss, L.G. (1974) Lab. Invest., 30, 43.

58. Slavin, R.E., Millan, J.C. and Mullins, G.M. (1975) Human Pathology, 6, 693.

59. Botta, J.A.Jr., Nelson, L.W. and Weikel, J.H.Jr. (1973) J. Natl. Can. Inst., 51, 1051.

60. DeFronzo, R.A., Braine, H.G., Colvin, M. and Davis, P.J. (1973) Ann. Int. Med., 78, 861.

61. Colvin, M. and Santos, G. (1970) Proc. Am. Assoc. Cancer Res., 11, 17.

62. Buckner, C.D., Rudolph, R.H., Fefer, A., Clift, R.A., Epstein, R.B., Funk, D.D., Neiman, P.E., Slichter, S.J., Storb, R. and Thomas, E.D. (1972) Cancer, 29, 357.

63. Fairley, K.F., Barrie, J.U. and Johnson, W. (1972) Lancet, 1, 568.

64. Kumar, R., Biggart, J.D., McEvoy, J. and McGeown, M.G. (1972) Lancet 1, 1212.

65. Hinkes, E. and Plotkin, D. (1973) J. Am. Med. Assoc., 223, 1490.

66. Blake, D.A., Heller, R.H., Hsu, S.H. and Schacter, B.Z. (1976) Johns Hopkins Med. J., 139, 20.

67. Mohn, G.R. and Ellenberger, J. (1976) Mutation Res., 32, 331.

68. Greenberg, L.H. and Tanaka, K.R. (1964) JAMA, 188, 423.

69. Lergier, J.E., Jimenez, E., Maldonado, N. and Veray, F. (1974) Cancer, 34, 1018.

70. Brock, N. and Schneider, B. (1971) Arzneim.-Forsch., 21, 435.

71. Drings, P., Allner, R., Brock, N., Burkert, H., Fischer, M., Fölsch, E., Gerhartz, H., Götzky, P., Hoppe, I., Kanzler, G., Klein, H.O., Mainzer, K., Martin, H., Obrecht, P., Palme, G., Paulisch, H., Riegg, H., Schubert, J.C.F., Treske, U., Weise, W., Willems, D., Wilmanns, H., Witte, S. and Wohlenberg, H. (1970) Dtsch. Med. Wochenschr., 95, 491.

72. Schnitker, J., Brock, N., Burkert, H. and Fichtner, E. (1976) Arzneim.-Forsch., 26, 1783.

73. Norpoth, K. (1976) Cancer Treatment Rep., 60, 437.

74. Van Dyk, J.J., Falkson, H.C., Van der Merse, A.M. and Falkson, G. (1972) Cancer Res., 32, 921.

Clinical Pharmacology of Anti-Neoplastic Drugs
H. M. Pinedo, editor

PHARMACOLOGY OF NITROSOUREA ANTITUMOR AGENTS

JOANNA M. HEAL, B. ROBERT FRANZA AND PHILIP S. SCHEIN
Division of Medical Oncology, Vincent T. Lombardi Cancer Research Center, Georgetown University School of Medicine, Washington, D.C. 20007 U.S.A.

INTRODUCTION

In 1959, 1-methyl-1-nitroso-3-nitrosoguanidine (MNNG) was reported to have limited but reproducible antitumor activity against murine L1210 leukemia (1). Although it was recognized that the therapeutic potential of this compound was insufficient to warrant extensive clinical trial, the observation formed the basis of the intensive evaluation of the N-nitroso containing compounds as antitumor agents that has since occurred. During the subsequent 19 years there has been a series of advances and structure-activity analyses that has resulted in the development of a class of drugs which represent some of the most clinically useful therapeutic agents. Major contributions were made by Dr. Baker and co-workers at Stanford Research Institute. In a sequence of structure-activity studies they demonstrated that the nitroso group of the MNNG molecule was an essential requirement for antitumor activity, and that substitution of a chloroethyl for the methyl group considerably enhanced this cytotoxicity. These findings led to the synthesis of 1-(2-chloroethyl)-1-nitrosourea, CNU, a drug that possesses curative activity for mice bearing the L1210 leukemia (2). Concurrently, Dr. John Montgomery and his colleagues at the Southern Research Institute undertook a study of compounds with structural similarities to MNNG that would have the potential of releasing diazomethane. 1-methyl-1-nitrosourea, MNU, was found to produce greater antitumor activity against the intraperitoneally implanted L1210 leukemia than MNNG (3). In addition, MNU penetrated the blood-brain barrier and increased the life-span of mice bearing intracranially implanted L1210 cells. This property was subsequently correlated with the lipid solubility of MNU. At the time this was an important finding since the majority of clinically available anticancer drugs did not achieve cytotoxic concentration in the central nervous system. It had become recognized that the central nervous system was a pharmacologic sanctuary for leukemic cells, and that meningeal leukemia was the cause of relapse from complete remission in one-half of cases with acute lymphocytic leukemia. Montgomery and Johnston proceeded to synthesize over 200 congeners of the original MNU molecule. This work led to the development and clinical use of a series of chloroethyl derivatives including 1,3-bis(2-chloroethyl)-1-nitrosourea, BCNU (4), a compound with curative activity in mice implanted either intraperitoneally or intracranially with L1210 leukemia cells (5); substitution of a cyclohexyl group resulted in the synthesis of CCNU and eventually methyl-CCNU.

The original methylnitrosourea, MNU, has now undergone extensive clinical testing in the U.S.S.R. and has been demonstrated to have useful activity for the treatment of lymphomas and small cell carcinoma of the lung (6). Streptozotocin, MNU attached to the C-2 position of glucose, was found to occur naturally as a product of the fermentation of Streptomyces achromogenes; this compound is a potent toxin for the pancreatic islet beta cell of rodents and higher animal species (7). We have demonstrated that the diabetogenic activity of streptozotocin is mediated by a rapid reduction in pyridine nucleotides and that one can prevent the beta cell destruction and the associated reduction in NAD by the use of pharmacological doses of nicotinamide (8). Recent work has suggested that the reduction in NAD can be correlated with a significant increase in the activity of poly-ADP ribose polymerase, a chromatin-associated enzyme that uses NAD as a substrate (9). Streptozotocin is now used effectively in the treatment of islet cell carcinoma (10).

The major clinical emphasis has been directed towards the more active chloroethyl nitrosourea derivatives. They have established clinical antitumor activity for a broad range of human malignancies including acute lymphocytic leukemia, lymphomas, myeloma, melanoma, gliomas and gastrointestinal neoplasms (11). Unfortunately, these same agents produce delayed and cumulative bone marrow toxicity which seriously limits their clinical application. This review will describe current research that is being directed towards the identification of the mechanism of nitrosourea antitumor activity and toxicity, and the progress that is being made towards the development of new analogs that may have reduced toxicity for the normal bone marrow.

DECOMPOSITION AND METABOLISM

Under physiological conditions the nitrosoureas decompose spontaneously (12, 13). The chemical half-life of the individual compounds, in phosphate buffered saline (pH 7.4), varies from 5 minutes to as long as 2 hours. In the process of degradation a series of alkylating moieties are formed of which an alkyldiazohydroxide precursor and the chloroethyl carbonium ion are considered the most important. Organic isocyanates are also generated which carbamoyle intracellular proteins (14, 15). Thus there are two chemical activities, alkylation and carbamoylation. In addition to their spontaneous chemical dissociation, the nitrosoureas are now known to be metabolized by the liver microsomal mixed function oxidase system to more polar hydroxylated products that retain both the cyclohexyl ring structure and the cytotoxic nitrosoureido moiety (16,17). May et al. have identified five metabolites in *in vivo* experiments in rats and in *in vitro* studies with rat liver microsomes; these included the cis- and trans-pairs of the 3- and 4- isomers and the cis 2-isomer (18). Hilton and Walker, utilizing a similar system, identified the 3- and 4- isomers and the trans-2-isomer as products of *in vitro* incubation and also in the plasma of rats (19). The cis-4 hydroxy form is the major metabolite and accounts for approximately 50 percent of administered CCNU, and over 60 percent after phenobarbital pretreatment. Studies of metabolism in man have been conducted using CCNU, administered by slow intravenous infusion. Hilton and Walker found that approximately 75% of the plasma drug concentration, after one hour of infusion was in the form of hydroxylated products and that hydroxylation proceeded faster than the drug infusion rate (20). Two-thirds appeared as trans-4-hydroxy CCNU and one-third appeared as the cis-4-isomer. Current data indicate that the rate of metabolic hydroxylation of CCNU exceeds the rate of chemical dissociation, and that as a result it is probable that hydroxylated metabolites are the immediate precursors of the therapeutic and toxic moieties. Metabolism of CCNU produces compounds in which the chemical properties of the parent compound are significantly modified. Wheeler et al. have shown that all of the hydroxylated derivatives of CCNU are more water soluble, have higher alkylating activities and lower carbamoylating activities than CCNU (21). In addition to the hydroxylation of nitrosourea ring structures Hill et al. have presented evidence that both BCNU and MNU are denitrosated by liver microsomal enzymes (22). We have used the TA 100 strain of S. typhimurium in the Ames assay to evaluate the effect of microsomal activation on one aspect of toxicity, mutagenicity (23). All the nitrosoureas in clinical use, except ACNU, demonstrated greater mutagenic activity (12-40%) after incubation with S9, a liver microsomal fraction, than before. Both the trans-2 and trans-4 hydroxy isomers of CCNU had higher initial mutagenicity than the parent compound. Since these two metabolites of CCNU also have greater alkylating activity than CCNU, alkylation probably plays a role in the induction of mutations. However, there was no direct linear relationship between the *in vitro* alkylating activity and the mutagenic potential of the nitrosourea studied before microsomal activation. The alkylating activity of chlorozotocin is 40% higher than ACNU but chlorozotocin has only 47% of the mutagenic potential. This data also suggests that all the clinically available nitrosoureas, except ACNU, are metabolized by S9 and that the metabolic products have mutagenic activity equivalent to metabolized 3-methylcholanthrene (23). This may have relevance in regard to potential carcinogenic activity in man.

ALKYLATION

The relative alkylating activities of the nitrosoureas have been estimated in reactions with 4- (p-nitrobenzyl) pyridine (NBP) (24). Of the large number of compounds we have tested by this assay, CNU (1), RPCNU, chlorozotocin or 2-(3-(2-chloroethyl) -3-nitrosoureido)-D-glucopyranose, GANU, and the trans-2-hydroxy isomer of CCNU have demonstrated the highest alkylating activity. There is an inverse linear relationship between the relative alkylating activity of each analogue and its respective chemical half-life (25, 42). In addition, we have found an inverse linear correlation between the molar LD10 dose in mice and alkylating activity. However, there is no statistical relationship with the degree of bone marrow toxicity and relative alkylating activity in this species (25).

While alkylation is widely accepted as the principal mechanism of nitrosourea antitumor activity, our structure-activity analysis failed to demonstrate a linear correlation between the NBP alkylating activity of chloroethyl nitrosoureas and antitumor activity for the murine L1210 leukemia (25,26). Recent studies with water-soluble analogues have suggested a parabolic relationship with the optimal relative alkylating activity estimated to be approximately 60 percent of that produced by chlorozotocin (26). Nevertheless there are several sets of evidence to support a primary role of alkylation for cytotoxicity. Cheng et al. have shown that the chloroethyl group of CCNU binds to nucleic acid and proteins, whereas the cyclohexyl group was extensively and almost exclusively bound to protein (27,28). We have recently confirmed these data in studies in which L1210 cells were incubated with radiolabelled CCNU and chlorozotocin; the degree of covalent binding of the respective chloroethyl groups to DNA was in rough proportion to their relative NBP alkylating activities (29).

Ludlum et al. have reacted BCNU with the polynucleotides poly C, poly G, poly A and poly U and were able to isolate several derivative nucleotides including 3-(B-hydroxyethyl) CMP, 3,N^4-ethano-CMP and 7-(B-hydroxyethyl) CMP (30). Hilton et al. have shown that CCNU produces a concentration and time-dependent damage to L1210 DNA that is expressed as single-strand breaks on exposure to alkali (31). These studies have also suggested that the rate and extent of repair after CCNU alkylation is slow and incomplete when compared to the rapid repair following X-irradiation damage. Recently, Kohn has proposed that the single alkylating function of the chloroethyl nitrosoureas can cross-link DNA as determined by inhibition of alkali-induced strand separation (32). The reaction occurs in two steps, the initial chloroethylation of a nucleophilic site on the first strand, followed by the gradual displacement of Cl^- by a nucleophilic site on the opposite strand, resulting in an ethyl bridge.

CARBAMOYLATION

A number of investigators have suggested an important biological role for the carbamoylating activity of isocyanates generated on decomposition of a nitrosourea. The contribution of carbamoylation to antitumor activity or toxicity has been largely inferred from *in vitro* studies. Among such reports the clinically active nitrosoureas BCNU, CCNU and methyl-CCNU and their respective isocyanates have been shown to inhibit rat liver (33) and human leukemia (34) DNA polymerase II. A reduction of nucleolar RNA processing by organic isocyanates has been reported by Kann and co-workers (35) and cyclohexyl isocyanates generated by CCNU were shown to bind to the lysine rich H-1 histone fraction of L1210 cells (36). The demonstration that isocyanates can inhibit the repair of X-irradiation damage to DNA (37) is particularly important since inhibition of repair processes could enhance the therapeutic effect of drugs causing alkylation damage but may also increase their carcinogenic potential and toxicity to normal tissues. We have investigated the effect of carbamoylating activity on the repair of DNA alkylation damage produced by the nitrosoureas themselves (38). Two methylnitrosoureas were studied, streptozotocin, in which the cytotoxic moiety is attached to the C-2 position of a glucose carrier and GANU, a C-1 substituted analog. Streptozotocin has similar alkylating activity (100%) to GANU (92%), a comparable half-life, but widely differing carbamoylating activity (3% versus 24% for GANU). There was no statistical difference in the frequency of single strand breaks produced in L1210 cells after a 2-hour exposure to 0.5 mM concentration of either drug. After incubation with streptozotocin, full repair of these lesions was documented 8 hours after drug removal. In contrast, the repair of GANU induced damage was not complete for 12 hours. The cytotoxicity of the two drugs for L1210 cells both *in vitro* using a colony cloning assay and *in vivo* in mice was not statistically different. Thus, although the carbamoylating activity of GANU can be correlated *in vitro* with a delay in repair of single strand breaks, the antitumor activity of this drug both *in vitro* and *in vivo* is not significantly increased by either the carbamoylating activity or the delay in repair of alkylated lesions. Other reports have also questioned whether the *in vitro* effects of carbamoylation contribute significantly to nitrosourea cytotoxicity *in vivo*. Wheeler and Bowden found that incubation of BCNU with intact L1210 cells reduced the total DNA polymerase activity in cell free extracts of these cells. However, administration of BCNU to mice bearing either L1210 in the ascitic or solid tumor form did not alter the total DNA polymerase activity measured in tumor extracts (39). A prolongation of S phase in L1210 cells by cyclohexyl isocyanates has been demonstrated but this was not associated with any antitumor activity in mice bearing

L1210 cells (40). Similarly, in an analysis of the biological effects of 17 nitrosourea in mice, Wheeler found no correlation of carbamoylating activity with antitumor activity but suggested that carbamoylating activity might play a role in toxicity *in vivo* (41).

We have conducted a series of structure-activity analyses of methyl and chloroethyl nitrosoureas in an attempt to define a biological correlate for carbamoylation activity. Linear regression analyses of carbamoylating activity with lethal toxicity, granulocyte suppression, and antitumor activity failed to demonstrate a significant correlation (25,38,42). The excellent antitumor activity of chlorozotocin, despite its negligible carbamoylating activity, suggests that this chemical reaction is not a major factor in antitumor activity, in contrast to the conclusions reached in other studies (41).

NEWER NITROSOUREA ANTICANCER AGENTS

Chlorozotocin. Structure-activity studies with the nonmyelosuppressive methylnitrosourea, streptozotocin, and its cytotoxic group MNU, suggested that bone marrow toxicity could be reduced by attachment of the nitrosourea cytotoxic group to the carbon-2 position of glucose (43). To further evaluate the influence of the glucose carrier for the more active chloroethyl nitrosourea class, a new water soluble compound, chlorozotocin, was synthesized for our studies by Johnston et al. (44). Chlorozotocin has NBP alkylating activity that is two-fold greater than that produced by an equimolar concentration of BCNU, but has negligible carbamoylating activity (25), probably the result of intramolecular carbamoylation. Using the L1210 leukemia model, chlorozotocin was demonstrated to have curative antitumor activity comparable to BCNU and CCNU at 50 percent of the molar dose. In addition, chlorozotocin was nonmyelosuppressive at the LD10 dose; this was confirmed by measurement of absolute peripheral neutrophil counts, bone marrow histology and DNA synthesis, and measurement of the marrow stem cells committed to granulocyte-macrophage differentiation (CFU-C) (45,46). We have subsequently compared the *in vitro* sensitivity of human bone marrow to chlorozotocin and BCNU over a range of plasma concentrations similar to those obtained after intravenous administration to patients (46). The threshhold concentration of chlorozotocin for toxicity to the CFU-C was 1×10^{-4} M which resulted in a 25% reduction in marrow colonies. In contrast, 5×10^{-5} M BCNU decreased human CFU-C to 47 percent of control, and 1×10^{-4} M eliminated all colony formation (46). Twenty-four hours after *in vitro* exposure to a 1×10^{-4} M concentration of chlorozotocin there was no reduction in human bone marrow DNA synthesis in contrast to a 42 percent reduction with 1×10^{-4} M BCNU.

This relative bone marrow sparing property of chlorozotocin has now been confirmed clinically. During the Phase I clinical trial of chlorozotocin, a dose of 120 mg/m^2 was demonstrated to be therapeutically active, but did not produce myelosuppressive toxicity in previously untreated cases or in patients who had less than six months of prior chemotherapy (47). Thrombocytopenia did occur at higher doses. In pharmacology studies, rapid intravenous administration of a 120 mg/m^2 dose of chlorozotocin produced a peak concentration in excess of 1×10^{-4} M, comparable to a 150 mg/m^2 dose of BCNU. After an initial distribution phase, the half-life of the prolonged phase of N-nitroso intact chlorozotocin was 7 minutes compared to 9 minutes for BCNU. Both drugs remained at a concentration in excess of 1×10^{-5} M for a minimum of 10 minutes (46). It should be emphasized that at equimolar plasma concentrations, chlorozotocin has the potential of exposing the normal bone marrow, and the tumor, to twice the alkylating activity of BCNU. Nevertheless, chlorozotocin has been demonstrated to be significantly less myelosuppressive.

Seventy-one evaluable patients with advanced measurable malignancies have now been treated in an ongoing Phase II trial utilizing 120 mg/m^2 i.v. every 6 weeks (48). A total of 12 objective partial responses have been recorded. These include 4/20 with malignant melanoma, 4/24 with colon cancer, and a single patient each with breast cancer, adenocarcinoma of the lung, nodular poorly differentiated lymphoma and acute lymphatic leukemia. As in the Phase I study patients with no prior therapy did not develop significant white blood cell or platelet depression, and no cumulative toxicity has occurred with up to one year of treatment.

Recently completed studies in our laboratory have served to clarify the mechanism for chlorozotocin's reduced bone marrow toxicity (29). The quantitative alkylation and carbamoylation of bone marrow and L1210 leukemia DNA, cytoplasmic RNA and protein was studied *in vitro*, and correlated with antitumor and myelosuppressive activities. The covalent binding of the ethyl-[^{14}C] group to L1210 DNA and RNA was 2.3 fold greater for chlorozotocin than that of CCNU at equimolar concentrations. This greater alkylation of L1210 DNA by chlorozotocin correlated with its four-fold increased *in vitro* cytotoxicity for L1210 cells in cloning assays, and the lower molar dose required for optimal *in vivo* L1210 antitumor activity; the optimal antitumor dose of chlorozotocin (48-64 $\mu M/kg$) is one-third to one-half that of CCNU (128 $\mu M/kg$). In contrast to the results with L1210 cells, the *in vitro* alkylation of murine bone marrow DNA was found to be equivalent for the two drugs at equimolar concentrations. The ratio of alkylation of L1210 DNA to bone marrow DNA was 1.3 for chlorozotocin compared to 0.6 for CCNU.

The result is a reduction in the alkylation of bone marrow DNA by chlorozotocin compared to CCNU at drug doses that produce comparable alkylation of L1210 DNA and antitumor activity.

Studies are now being conducted to determine whether specific differences in subchromatin binding exist between L1210 and bone marrow cells. Enzymatic limit digest experiments are carried out using: micrococcal nuclease, which preferentially cleaves at the nucleosomal-bridge region of chromatin, or DNase 1, which cleaves within the nucleosome core particle. Initial results demonstrate that in L1210 cells, chlorozotocin alkylation sites were primarily within the nucleosome core particles. In contrast, the murine bone marrow alkylation sites were predominantly located on the more exposed DNA of the internucleosome bridges (49).

GANU. GANU is a water soluble sugar analogue which differs from chlorozotocin by the placement of the cytotoxic group on the carbon-1 position of glucose. It has NBP alkylating activity equivalent to chlorozotocin, but with an eight-fold increased carbamoylating activity when compared to the latter carbon-2 substituted glucose derivative (50). Like chlorozotocin, GANU demonstrated essentially no myelosuppressive activity at the LD10 dose. In addition, GANU has significant *in vitro* antitumor activity for the L1210 leukemia. However, on a molar basis, the LD10 dose of GANU in our studies was found to be one-half that of chlorozotocin, thus limiting the μM of alkylating agent that can be administered *in vivo* to the tumor (50). It is possible that the significant carbamoylating activity of GANU may contribute in part to its increased lethal toxicity.

ACNU. ACNU, 1-(4-amino-2-methyl pyrimidin-5-y) methyl-3-(2-chloroethyl)-3-nitrosourea, is a water soluble nitrosourea which has produced delayed hematologic toxicity in man during its recently completed Phase I clinical trials (51). ACNU has *in vitro* alkylating activity 40 percent less than that of chlorozotocin but shares the latter compound's properties of water solubility and negligible carbamoylating activity (52). The latter property appears to result from a nonenzymatic intramolecular carbamoylation, as demonstrated by Tanaka and co-workers (53). ACNU has excellent activity for the L1210 leukemia (54). However, the maximum therapeutic dose produced an 85 percent reduction in circulating neutrophils in normal mice (52). While ACNU, a pyrimidine analogue, possesses many of the chemical properties of chlorozotocin, including water solubility and low carbamoylating activity, it does not share the latter compound's reduced myelotoxicity at therapeutic doses. The glucose carrier of the chlorozotocin molecule appears to impair the selective sparing of the normal bone marrow.

2-Hydroxy Metabolites of CCNU. Wheeler et al. have studied six water soluble hydroxylated isomers of CCNU and found all, on a molar basis, to be more active against the L1210 leukemia than CCNU. In addition, all the hydroxylated derivatives have better therapeutic indices (ED_{50}/LD_{10}) than either CCNU or chlorozotocin (21). The trans-2 isomer appeared to be the most promising, with alkylating activity and carbamoylating activity similar to chlorozotocin, but with a higher index and therapeutic activity for the intracranially implanted leukemia. We have recently completed an analysis of the lethal and bone marrow toxicity, and antitumor activity of the cis-2 and trans-2 hydroxy metabolites. We have confirmed Wheeler's findings of reduced carbamoylating activity and increased alkylating and antitumor activity when compared to an equimolar dose of the parent compound, CCNU. However, despite the low carbamoylating activity and increased water solubility, like chlorozotocin, neither 2-hydroxy isomer demonstrated the bone marrow sparing property of the latter drug, either in the murine model or in the human CFU-C assay (55).

RFCNU. RFCNU is a relatively new lipid soluble ribofuranosyl analogue which has demonstrated both therapeutic activity and typical delayed myelotoxicity during Phase I clinical trial in France. In studies by Imbach et al. this analogue was found to have a high therapeutic index and, unlike other nitrosoureas, was not immunosuppressive in mice (56).

FUTURE DRUG DEVELOPMENT

As previously mentioned, the chloroethylnitrosoureas currently available for clinical use produce treatment-limiting myelosuppression. The decreased myelotoxicity of chlorozotocin and GANU may be largely mediated by the glucose carrier for the chloroethylnitrosourea cytotoxic group. Recommendations for future synthetic work for nitrosourea antitumor agents will have to await completion of the current Phase I and II trials of chlorozotocin, GANU, and RFCNU. If the initial results with chlorozotocin demonstrating antitumor activity without myelosuppression, are confirmed additional analogues should be examined. Placement of the cytotoxic group on positions other than the C-1 or C-2 of the glucose carrier may enhance antitumor activity. In addition, the substitution of other sugars will determine whether glucose is the optimal sugar carrier for the phenomenon of antitumor activity with reduced myelotoxicity.

ACKNOWLEDGEMENTS

NIH Grant #N01 - 17583 and Amer. Cancer Soc. #CH - 13.

ABBREVIATIONS

ACNU, 1-(4-amino-2-methylpyrimidin-5-5yl) methyl-3-(2-chloroethyl)-3-nitrosourea;
BCNU, 1,3-bis(2-chloroethyl-1-nitrosourea;
CCNU, 1-(2-chloroethyl)-3-cyclohexyl-1-nitrosourea;
CNU, 1-(2-chloroethyl)-1-nitrosourea;
GANU, 1-(2-chloroethyl)-3-(B-D-glucopyranosyl)-1-nitrosourea;
MNNG, 1-methyl-1-nitroso-3-nitrosoguanidine;
MNU, 1-methyl-1-nitrosourea;
RFCNU, (chloro-2-ethyl) 1-ribofuranosyl-isopropylidene-2'-3'paranitrobenzoate-5')-3-nitrosourea;
RPCNU, (chloroethyl-2-ethyl)-1 (ribopyranosyl triacetate -2',3'4')-3 nitrosourea.

REFERENCES

1. Greene, M.O. and Greenberg, J. (1960) Cancer Research, 20, 1166-1173.
2. Hyde, K.A., Acton, E., Skinner, W.A., Goodman, L., Greenberg, J. and Baker, B.R. (1962) Med. Pharmaceut. Chem., 5, 1-14.
3. Skipper, H.E., Schabel, F.M.Jr., Trader, M.W., et al. (1961) Cancer Research, 21, 1154-1164.
4. Johnston, T.P., McCaleb, G.S. and Montgomery, J.A. (1963) J. Med.Chem. 6, 669-681.
5. Schabel, F.M.Jr., Johnston, T.P., McCaleb, G.S., Montgomery, J.A., Laster, W.R. and Skipper, H.E. (1963) Cancer Research, 23, 725-733.
6. Emmanuel, N.M., Vermel, E.M., Ostrovoskaga, L.A. and Korman, N.P. (1974) Cancer Chemotherapy Report, 58, 135-148.
7. Rakieten, N., Rakieten, M., and Nadkarni, M. (1963) Cancer Chemotherapy Report, 29, 91-98.
8. Schein, P.S., Cooney, D.A. and Vernon, M.L. (1967) Cancer Research, 27, 2324-2332.
9. Smulson, M.E., Stark, P., Gazzoli, M. and Roberts, J. (1975) Exper. Cell Res. 90, 175-182.
10. Schein, P.S., O'Connell, M.J. and Blom, J. (1974) Cancer 34, 993-1000.

11. Wasserman, T.H., Slavik, M. and Carter, S.K. (1975) Cancer, 36, 1258-1268.

12. Colvin, M., Brundhett, R.B., Cowens, W., Jardin, I. and Ludlum, D.B. (1976) Biochem. Pharmacol. 25, 695-699.

13. Montgomery, J.A., James, R., McCaleb, G.S., Kirk, M.C. and Johnston, T.P. (1975) J. Med. Chem. 18, 568-571.

14. Schmall, B., Cheng, C.J., Fujimura, S., Gersten, N., Grunberger, D. and Weinstein, I.B. (1973) Cancer Research, 33, 1921-1924.

15. Wheeler, G.P., Bowdon, B.J. and Struck, R.F. (1975) Cancer Research, 35, 2974-2984.

16. May, H.E., Boose, R. and Reed, D.J. (1974) Biochem. Biophys. Res. Commun. 57, 426-433.

17. Reed, D.J. and May, H.E. (1975) Life Sci. 16, 1263-1270.

18. May, H.E., Boose, R. and Reed, D.J. (1975) Biochemistry, 14, 4723-4730.

19. Hilton, J. and Walker, M.D. (1975) Biochem. Pharmacol. 24, 2153-2158.

20. Walker, M.D. and Hilton, J. (1976) Cancer Treatment Rept. 60, 725-728.

21. Wheeler, G.P., Johnston, T.P., Bowdon, B.J., McCaleb, G.S., Hill, D.L. and Montgomery, J.A. (1977) Biochem. Pharm. 26, 2331-2336.

22. Hill, D.L., Kirk, M.C. and Strucj, R.F. (1975) Cancer Research, 35, 296-301.

23. Franza, B., Schein, P., Saslaw, L. and Oeschger, M. (1978) Proc. Am. Soc. Clin. Oncol. 19, 234, abstract 934.

24. Wheeler, G.P., Bowdon, B.J., Grimsley, J. and Lloyd, H.H. (1974) Cancer Research, 34, 194-200.

25. Panasci, L.C., Green, D.C., Nagourney, R., Fox, P. and Schein, P.S. (1977) Cancer Research, 37, 2615-2618.

26. Heal, J.M., Fox, P.A. and Schein, P.S. Biochemical Pharm. (In Press).

27. Cheng, C.J., Fujimura, S., Granberger, D. and Weinstein, I.B. (1972) Cancer Research, 32, 22-27.

28. Schmall, B., Cheng, C.J., Fukimara, S., Gersten, N., Grunberger, D. and Weinstein, I.B. (1973) Cancer Research, 33, 1921-1924.

29. Panasci, L.C., Green, D., Fox, P. and Schein, P.S. (1977) Submitted to Jour. Clin. Inv.

30. Ludlum, D.B., Kramer, B.S., Wang, J. and Fenselau, C. (1975) Biochem. 14, 5480-5485.

31. Hilton, J., Bowie, D.L., Gutin, P.H., Zito, D.M. and Walker, M.D. (1977) Cancer Research, 37, 2262-2266.

32. Kohn, K.W. (1977) Cancer Research, 37, 1450-1454.

33. Baril, B.E., Baril, E.F., Laszlo, J. and Wheeler, G.P. (1975) Cancer Research, 35, 1-5.

34. Chuang, R.Y., Laszlo, J. and Keller, P. (1976) Biochim. Biophys. Acta, 425, 463-468.

35. Kann, H.E., Kohn, K.W., Widerlite, L. and Gullion, A. (1974) Cancer Res, 34, 1982-1988.

36. Woolley, P.V., Dion, R.L., Kohn, K.W. and Bono, V.H. (1976) Cancer Research, 36, 1470-1474.

37. Kann, H.E., Kohn, K.W. and Lyles, J.M. (1974) Cancer Research, 34, 398-402.

38. Heal, J.M., Fox, P., Sinks, L.F. and Schein, P. Proc. Am. Soc. Clin. Oncol. (1978) 19, 234, abstract 934.

39. Wheeler, G.P. and Bowdon, B.J. (1968) Cancer Research, 28, 52-59.

40. Bray, D.F., DeVita, V.T., Adamson, R.H. and Oliverio, V.T. (1971) Cancer Chemotherapy Report, 55, 215-220.

41. Wheeler, G.P., Bowdon, B.J., Grimsley, J. and Lloyd, H.H. (1974) Cancer Research, 34, 194-200.

42. Panasci, L.C., Fox, P.A. and Schein, P.S. (1977) Cancer Research, 37, 3321-3328.

43. Schein, P.S. (1969) Cancer Research, 29, 1226-1232.

44. Johnston, T.P., McCaleb, G.S. and Montgomery, J.A. (1975) J. Med. Chem. 18, 104-106.

45. Anderson, T., McMenamin, M. and Schein, P.S. (1975) Cancer Research, 35,

761-765.

46. Schein, P.S., Bull, J.M., Doukas, D. and Hoth, D. (1978) Cancer Research, 38, 257-260.

47. Hoth, D., Woolley, P., Green, D., MacDonald, J. and Schein, P.S. Clinical Pharmacology and Therapeutics (In Press).

48. Hoth, D., Butler, T., Winokur, S., Kales, A., Woolley, P. and Schein, P. (1978) Proc. Am. Soc. Clin. Oncol. 19, 381, abstract C-297.

49. Tew, K., Green, D. and Schein, P.S. (1978) Proc. Am. Soc. Clin. Oncol. 19, 115, abstract 458.

50. Fox, P.A., Panasci, L.C. and Schein, P.S. (1977) Cancer Research, 37, 783-787.

51. Cooperative Study Group of Phase I Study on ACNU (1976) Jap. J. Clin. Oncol. 6(2), 55-62.

52. Nagourney, R.A., Fox, P. and Schein, P.S. (1978) Cancer Research, 38, 65-68.

53. Tanaka, M., Kakajima, T., Nishigaki, T., Shigehara, E. and Nakao, H. (1977) Proc. 10th Intern. Cong. Chemotherap. Abst. $570, Sept. 18.

54. Arakawa, M., Shimizo, F. (1975) Gann, 66, 149-154.

55. Heal, J.M., Fox, P.A., Doukas, D. and Schein, P.S. (1978) Cancer Research, 38, 1070-1074.

56. Imbach, J.L., Montero, J.L., Moruzzi, A., Serrou, B., Chenu, E., Hayat, M. and Mathe, G. (1975) Biomedicine, 23, 410-413.

© 1978 Elsevier/North-Holland Biomedical Press
Clinical Pharmacology of Anti-Neoplastic Drugs
H. M. Pinedo, editor

THE CLINICAL PHARMACOLOGY OF THE VINCA ALKALOIDS, EPIPODOPHYLLOTOXINS, AND MAYTANSINE

DON V. JACKSON, Jr. AND RICHARD A. BENDER
Medicine Branch, National Cancer Institute, Bethesda, Maryland 20014.

VINCA ALKALOIDS

The early uses in herbal medicine of the periwinkle plant, *Vinca rosea* Linn, have been described by Johnson et al., and include remedies for controlling hemorrhage, scurvy, toothaches, diabetes, and the cleaning of chronic wounds (1). Investigation of extracts from this plant for possible hypoglycemic activity led to the isolation of the cytotoxic agents, vinblastine and vincristine (1,2), which were subsequently entered into clinical trials (3,4). Recently, a new synthetic derivative of vinblastine, vindesine (desacetyl vinblastine carboxyamide), has been entered into clinical trials (5-7). The vinca alkaloids are large, dimeric structures composed of an indole nucleus (catharanthine) linked to a dihydroindole nucleus (vindoline) and are illustrated in Fig. 1.

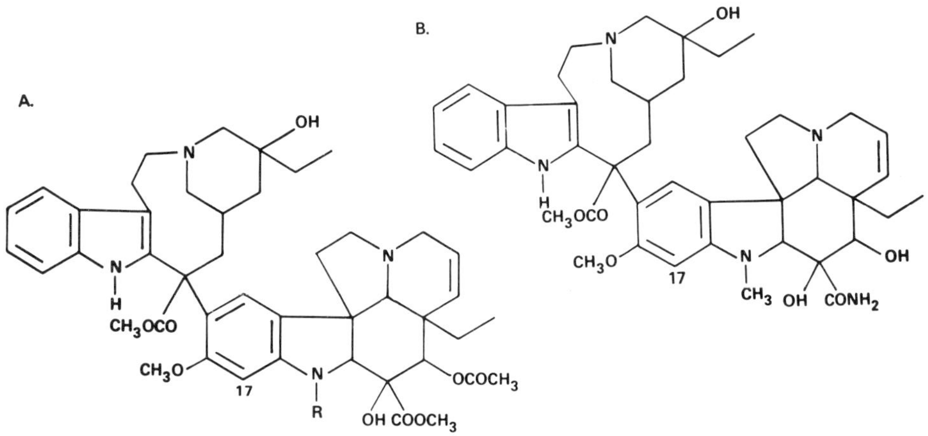

Fig. 1. A. Chemical structure of vinblastine (R=CH_3) and vincristine (R=CHO); B. Vindesine.

Although vincristine and vinblastine differ structurally only at the substitution on the nitrogen atom in the vindoline molecule (a formyl for a methyl group, respectively), these agents differ in their clinical spectrum and toxicity. Vinblastine has been most widely empoyed in the treatment of Hodgkin's disease and testicular neoplasms, whereas vincristine has exhibited substantial activity in the non-Hodgkin's as well as Hodgkin's lymphomas, acute lymphoblastic leukemia, breast carcinoma, Wilms' tumor, neuroblastoma, and embryonal rhabdomyosarcoma (8,9).

The antitumor effects of the vinca alkaloids appear to be several. The major effect, however, appears to be related to the high affinity binding of these agents to the basic protein subunit of microtubules, tubulin, which results in disruption of the mitotic spindle apparatus and arrest of cells in metaphase (10-12). The binding constants (K_a) for tubulin by vincristine and vinblastine have been reported as 8.0×10^6 and 6.0×10^6 M^{-1}, respectively, with maximal binding occurring within less than five minutes (10). Inhibition of tubulin polymerization into microtubular structures *in vitro* has been shown to be affected by vincristine, vinblastine, and vindesine to a similar degree. However, considerably higher concentrations of the separate catharanthine and vindoline portions of the dimeric molecule were required to inhibit tubulin polymerization, consistent with the lack of cytotoxicity of these individual moieties (11).

Several investigators have noted a lack of reversibility of the mitotic arrest of cells exposed to the vinca alkaloids (12,13). Induction of mitotic arrest by these agents, however, may not be translated into loss of cell viability. Tucker et al., demonstrated spindle dissolution in 50% of Chinese hamster fibroblasts after a brief exposure to vinblastine without subsequent cell death as determined by colony formation (14). These results are consistent with earlier reports of the reversibility of vinca alkaloid-induced mitotic arrest following resuspension of cells in fresh media (15) although recovery may not be complete (16). Cell death has generally been thought to occur following metaphase arrest, but these agents may also be cytolytic in interphase (14,17-19). Activity in this phase of the cell cycle may be related to inhibition of microtubular functions other than those associated with cell division or the reported inhibitory effects on DNA, RNA, and protein biosynthesis which have recently been reviewed by Creasey (20). However, many of the latter studies have employed pharmacologic doses of drug (i.e. 10μM) and also used labeled precursors whose incorporation into macromolecules may be adversely affected by inhibition of cellular uptake by the vinca alkaloids (21,22). Inhibition of the entry of glutamic acid into Ehrlich ascites carcinoma cells (23) and thymidine and uridine into P-815 murine mastocytoma cells (22) by vinblastine and vincristine, respectively, suggests that inhibition of the transport of precursor molecules may be an additional mechanism of cytotoxicity. Bleyer et al. have provided evidence for carrier-mediated transport of vinca alkaloids in L1210 and P388 murine leukemia cell lines (24). Furthermore, these investigators noted reduced uptake and binding of vincristine in vincristine-resistant P388 murine leukemia cells *in vitro* and suggested these phenomena may be possible mechanisms of drug resistance (24). Recent work by Bender and Nichols on human lymphoblasts *in vitro* further confirms a carrier-mediated mechanism for vincristine transport in neoplastic cells (25). Further characterization of vinca alkaloid cellular transport in resistant and non-resistant tumors remains an important area of investigation.

Cytotoxic concentrations of vinca alkaloids have been investigated in L1210 murine leukemia cells using soft agar cloning techniques (26,27). These have demonstrated that vincristine concentrations of $\sim 4 \times 10^{-8}$ M are 100% lethal and that concentrations of $\sim 1 \times 10^{-8}$ M produced a 50% cell kill (27). Wilkoff et al., have calculated the minimum effective concentration of vincristine in this cell line to be between 1.2×10^{-8} and 1.2×10^{-9} M by the use of a bioassay in mice (28). Constant *in vitro* exposure of a human lymphoblastic leukemia cell line, CEM, to vincristine revealed a maximally effective concentration of $\sim 10^{-8}$ M which may be clinically achieved (27). A differential *in vitro* cytocidal level has been noted between normal lymphocytes and those of chronic lymphocytic leukemia as determined by morphologic changes. A 90% cell kill was found following a 7 day exposure to 1.2×10^{-5} M and 9.7×10^{-7} M, respectively (19).

Investigation of the human pharmacology of the vinca alkaloids has been greatly assisted by the use of tritiated radiochemicals and, more recently, a radioimmunoassay (29). Two and a half minutes following an intravenous dose of 2 mg of tritiated vincristine in patients with non-Hodgkin's lymphoma, Bender et al. noted an instantaneous peak blood level of 3.6×10^{-7} M (30). Decay of blood radioactivity was triphasic with half-lives of 0.85, 7.4, and 164 minutes, respectively (Fig. 2). Extensive binding of vincristine to formed blood elements was noted with greater than 50% of the radiolabel bound 20 minutes after injection. Over a 72 hour period of study, 12% of radiolabel was excreted in the urine of which one-half was metabolites and ~69% was excreted in the feces with about 40% as metabolites (30). The high percentage of radioactivity in the feces of these patients and previous reports of substantial biliary excretion in animals (31-33) suggested the biliary route to be the principal source of elimination of vincristine in man. This was documented by Jackson et al. employing intravenously administered tritiated vincristine in a patient with a choledochal T-tube (34). Vincristine and its metabolic and/or decomposition products were rapidly concentrated within the bile. Following a total dose of 0.5 mg, the highest concentration attained in the bile (6×10^{-7} M) occurred 2-4 hours after injection and was more than 100 times higher than the concentration recorded in a simultaneous plasma sample (Fig. 3).

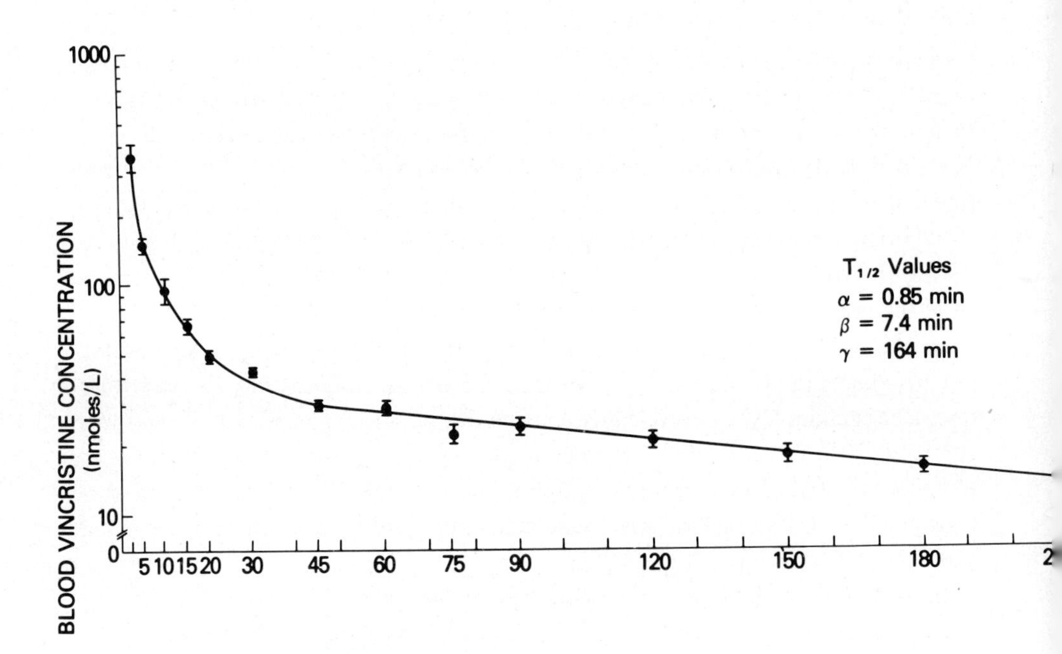

Fig. 2. The blood disappearance curve of [^{3}H]-vincristine in man. The $T^1/_2$ values are derived by linear regression analysis. Correction for metabolism and/or decomposition is not included in concentration measurements. (From Bender et al. Clin. Pharmacol. Ther. 22:430, 1977).

The first 24 hour bile sample contained 21.7% of the total administered dose and 76.4% of the cumulative biliary excretion. During a three day period of observation, 4.2, 45.6, and 49.6% of the excreted radiolabel was present in the feces, urine, and bile, respectively. Products of vincristine metabolism and/or decomposition rapidly appeared in the bile and only 46.5% of the drug was in the parent form in the 2 hour collection following injection. Although hepatic metabolism of vincristine appeared to be implicated, the origin of the species appearing in the bile was unclear since the labeled drug was found to decompose when incubated in a physiologic buffer at 37° (34).

Owellen et al. have similarly noted a triphasic blood decay of vinblastine and its closely related congener, vindesine, although the terminal half-lives (~20 hours) were more prolonged than reported for vincristine which may reflect, in part, differences in technique as a radioimmunoassay was used (29,35). Peak blood concentrations following intravenous administration of these agents were similar to those reported for vincristine and extensive binding to formed blood elements was also noted. Excretion of radioactivity in the urine and feces over a 72 hour period accounted for 13.6 and 9.7% of the administered tritiated vinblastine, respectively. These investigators also identified a major metabolite of vinblastine in the urine and feces, deacetyl vinblastine, which was shown to be a more potent cytotoxic agent than the parent drug in experimental tumors (35).

Following administration of tritiated vincristine and vinblastine, avid tissue binding has been apparent with excretion of only 57-88% (30,34) and 24% (35) of the total administered dose, respectively. Extensive protein (36) and tissue binding and probable enterohepatic recirculation may account for the prolonged blood levels in man (29,34,35). Disruption of microtubules (neurotubules) in isolated nerve fibers of cats and anterior horn cells of rabbits has been observed as a result of exposure to the mitotic inhibitors (37,38) and may affect growth of developing nerve fibers (neurites) (39) and axoplasmic transport of neural proteins (40,41). Therefore the vinca alkaloids, particularly with repeated dosage, may slowly accumulate within microtubule-rich neural tissue and produce neurotoxicity. Furthermore, patients with preexisting liver disease have been found to develop unusually severe neuropathies while receiving relatively small doses of the vinca alkaloids (42) which may relate to delay of biliary excretion causing prolonged exposure to neural tissue.

Despite such close structural similarities and association constants for tubulin (10), vincristine and vinblastine exhibit remarkably different toxicities. Neuropathy has been most frequently observed following vincristine administration (42-46) although it was not uncommon in the early clinical trials of vinblastine with relatively large doses (47). Myelosuppression, especially leukopenia, has been the dose-limiting toxicity of vinblastine with a nadir leukocyte count occurring 4-7 days after administration (48). Alopecia has been observed with both agents in

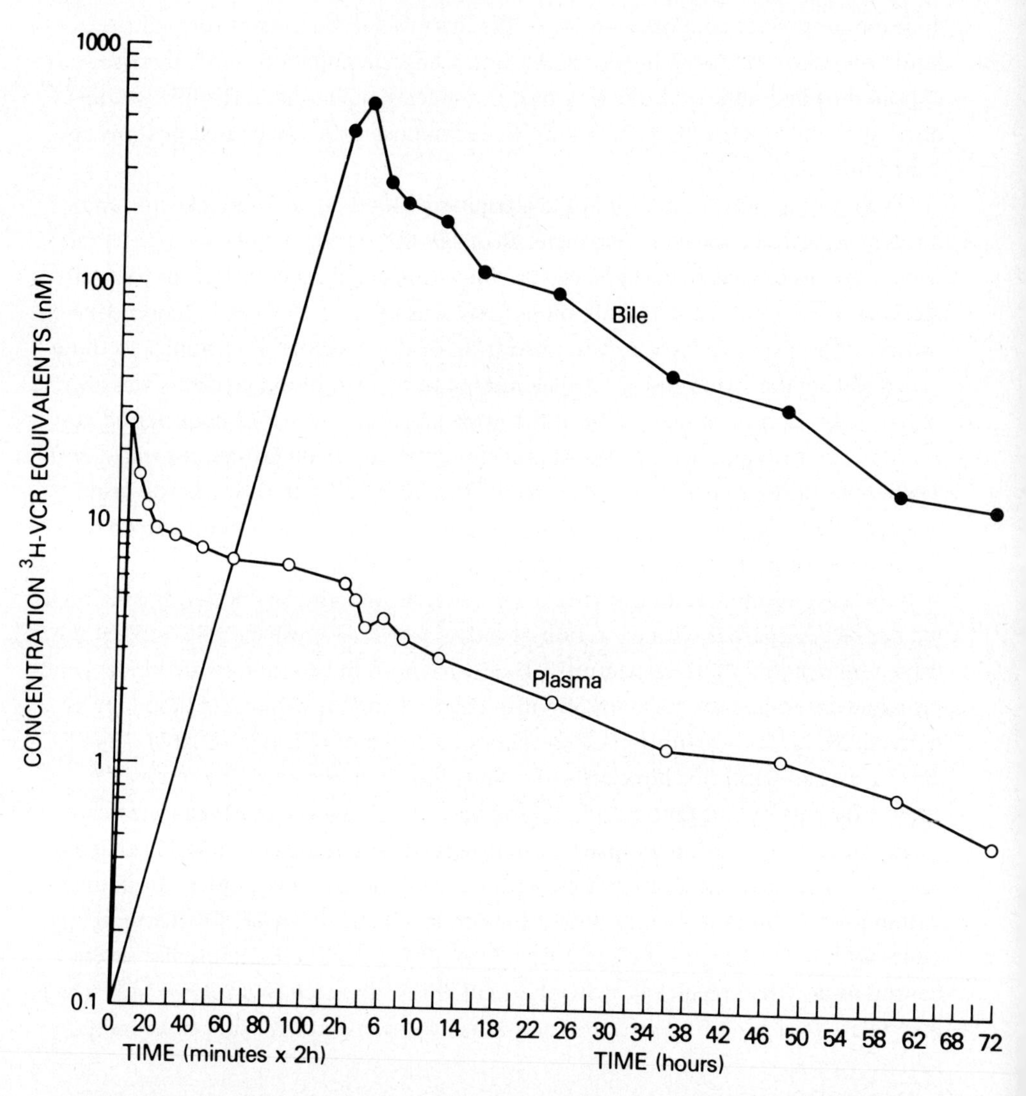

Fig. 3. Concentration of [^{3}H]-vincristine and its metabolic and/or decomposition products (nanomoles/liter) within the plasma (o— —o) and bile (o— —o) at various time points. (From Jackson et al. Clin. Pharmacol. Ther. 1978; in press.

about 5-20% of patients (1,20).Myelosuppression, neurotoxicity, and alopecia have also been noted in Phase I trials of vindesine (5-7).

Vinca alkaloid-induced neurotoxicity has been age and dose-related (44,49,50) and manifested by a peripheral, mixed sensory-motor neuropathy generally characterized by symmetrical neurologic signs and symptoms (43,45,46). The earliest and most consistent finding has been the loss of the deep tendon reflexes, followed by parethesias in the fingers and toes (42) which may progress, dependent on dose and schedule, to profound muscle weakness and sensory impairment (46,49). Paralytic ileus is the most frequent indication of autonomic neuropathy and may occur acutely or following chronic administration (45). Also, varying degrees of urinary retention and hypotension have been reported (45,46,51). Other neurologic changes associated with vincristine administration include cranial nerve palsies, confusion, depression, agitation, insomnia, hallucinations, psychosis, and hyponatremia as a result of inappropriate antidiuretic hormone secretion (42,43,45,46). Despite a wealth of neurologic manifestations and the principle pathologic finding of primary axonal degeneration (43,52), peripheral nerve conduction studies have generally been normal (42,45). The only known treatment has been discontinuation or reduction of the dose and/or frequency of administration of the vinca alkaloid. The known role of hepatic excretion in animals and man suggests that dose modification may be indicated in the presence of hepatic compromise.

Vincristine and vinblastine have generally been administered intravenously employing commonly used starting doses of 0.02 mg/kg and 0.1 mg/kg, respectively, with escalation according to tolerance. An oral preparation of vinblastine has been used erratic absorption and the necessity for large dosage made it impractical (1, 20).

EPIPODOPHYLLOTOXINS

Extracts of the roots and rhizomes of the May apple or mandrake plant, *Podophyllum peltatum*, have previously been used as a cathartic, emetic, antihelminthic, poison, and in the treatment of condylomata accuminata (8,53). Podophyllotoxin was identified as the main constituent possessing cytostatic activity as early as the 1940's. Initial clinical trials of two cytotoxic compounds derived from this substance, SP–I and SP–G, demonstrated a prohibitive degree of toxicity (54). Further research by Sandoz laboratories resulted in the production of two semisynthetic derivatives of podophyllotoxin, VM–26 and VP–16, whose structures are depicted in Fig. 4.

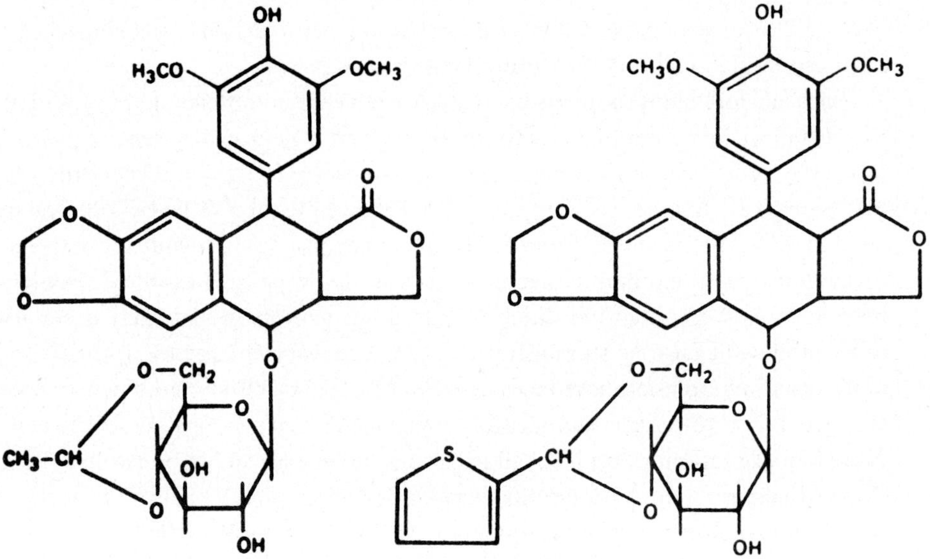

Fig. 4. Chemical structure of VP–16 (left) and VM–26 (right).

These agents have demonstrated antitumor activity against several experimental animal tumors including L1210 murine leukemia which has been relatively resistant to antitumor agents derived from plants (9,55,56).

Substantial antitumor responses in clinical trials of VP–16 and VM–26 have been noted in the Hodgkin's and non-Hodgkin's lymphomas, mycosis fungoides, acute nonlymphocytic leukemia, carcinoma of the bladder, small cell carcinoma of the lung, malignant gliomas of the brain, and malignant teratoma and hepatoma (57-62). In addition, the epipodophyllotoxins have produced encouraging responses in monocytic leukemia (63) and have exhibited lack of cross-resistance with the vinca alkaloids in the treatment of the lymphomas (8,64,65).

The mechanism of action of the epipodophyllotoxins appears to be distinct from the parent compound, podophyllotoxin, and from the vinca alkaloids. The latter compounds appear to exert their primary cytotoxic effect through disruption of microtubular function with subsequent arrest of cells in metaphase, whereas, polymerization of tubulin and microtubular structures remain intact following exposure to VP–16 and VM–26 (66,67). Arrest of cells in metaphase does not occur or is only a transient effect (22,56,66,68). On the contrary, in several cell lines *in vitro* these agents have produced a reduction of the mitotic index and result in a premitotic arrest with accumulation of cells in the G_2 phase of the cell cycle (22,66,68, 69). Moreover, this effect appears to be irreversible in contrast to the reversibility of podophyllotoxin and vinca alkaloid-induced mitotic arrest when cells are resuspended in fresh media (56,66). However, the molecular events leading to the premitotic block are not understood. Inhibition of nucleoside transport into HeLa cells in culture (67) and inhibition of nucleoside incorporation into the DNA and RNA of P–815 murine mastocytoma cells (22) have been demonstrated, but the relationship of these events to cytotoxicity remains unclear. The nonglucoside congener of VP–16, 4'demethyl epipodophyllotoxin, also inhibits nucleoside transport. However, unlike VP–16, this congener prevents microtubule assembly *in vitro* which suggests that the presence of the glucoside moiety in VP–16 may confer its inability to disrupt microtubular function (67). Single-stranded DNA breaks in a human tumor cell line (70) and chromosomal aberrations in various human hematopoietic cell lines (71) have also been seen following exposure to VP–16.

The human pharmacology of the epipodophyllotoxins has been examined by Allen and Creaven (72). Instantaneous mean peak blood levels of VM–26 and VP–16 given at maximally tolerated single intravenous doses of 67 mg/m^2 (73) and 290 mg/m^2 (74) were 14 μg/ml and 29 μg/ml, respectively (72). Plasma decay kinetics following intravenous injection of tritiated drug revealed a biphasic and triphasic pattern for VP–16 and VM–26, respectively. The terminal half-life was more prolonged for VM–26 (11-38.5 hours) than for VP–16 (13.5 hours) which may be related to the 10-fold greater binding of VM–26 to albumin and the 6-fold greater renal clearance of VP–16 (57,72). Over a 72 hour period, ~45% of the administered dose of both drugs was present in the urine of which 79% and 33% represented metabolites of VM–26 and VP–16, respectively. Fecal excretion during this period of observation accounted for less than 16% of the administered dose of both drugs. The fate of the retained fraction (~40% of the administered dose) remains undetermined but probably represents extensive tissue binding by these agents (72). Cerebrospinal fluid levels of radiolabeled VM–26 were less than 1% of the plasma levels 24 hours after injection, although this value was 27% in one patients who had had a prior craniotomy and cranial irradiation. VP–16 attained 1-10% of the plasma levels in the cerebrospinal fluid 2-26 hours after administration. Due to the high degree of lipid solubility and demonstration of increased survival of mice inoculated intracerebrally with L1210 leukemia (56), the poor penetration of the drugs into the cerebrospinal fluid was unexpected (72).

The major toxicities produced by the epipodophyllotoxins include gastrointestinal disturbances, myelosuppression, and alopecia (57). Following administration of VP–16, nausea and vomiting have been experienced by 25% of patients whether the drug was given intravenously (66,74) or orally (75). These disturbances after VM–26 have varied from 9 to 52% (57). Myelosuppression has been both schedule and dose-dependent and more frequently involves leukopenia than thrombocytopenia (57). Creaven et al. noted leukopenia ($<5{,}000/mm^3$) and thrombocytopenia ($<100{,}000/mm^3$) in 100% and 13% of patients, respectively, who received weekly intravenous VP–16 doses of 170 mg/m^2 (74). A daily schedule employing 50 mg/m^2 for five days produced leukopenia in only 16% of patients and thrombocytopenia in 7% (63). An approximate 3-fold lower maximally tolerated dose of VM–26 has been noted and may be related to the more rapid plasma and renal clearance of VP–16 (72). Other infrequent effects of these agents include stomatitis, phlebitis, fever, chills, bronchospasms and generalized erythema, anaphylaxis, and myocardial infarction (57). A unique toxicity of these agents appears to be related to the vehicle used for their intravenous administration. Immediate hypotension may be seen with rapid infusion rates and has generally responded briskly to either slowing the infusion rate or temporarily interrupting its administration (73,74,76).

Both agents are highly water-insoluble and can be given intravenously only after being solubilized in a detergent mixture. Although the intravenous route has been the most common mode of administration of the epipodophyllotoxins, VP–16 has been given orally in the form of capsules and drink ampules (57). The drink ampule form has produced a more predictable myelosuppressive response than the capsule form (75).

MAYTANSINE

In 1972, Kupchan et al. reported the isolation of maytansine, a new ansa macrolide (compounds which include streptovaricins and rifamycins) from the African shrub, *Maytenus oveatus* (77). Its structure is depicted in Fig. 5.

This agent has shown significant suppression of tumor growth in a number of animal tumors *in vitro* and *in vivo* employing doses in the nanomolar and μg/kg dose range, respectively (9,77-80). Similar to the vinca alkaloids, inhibition of tubulin polymerization, induction of mitotic arrest, and disruption of chromosomal organization appear to be the principle mechanisms of cytotoxicity (81,82). The vinca alkaloids and maytansine have been shown to share a common binding site on tubulin (83,84). In addition, maytansine has been demonstrated to occupy an additional binding site not shared by vincristine and exhibits tighter binding to tubulin than vincristine with association constants $1.5 \times 10^6 M^{-1}$ and $0.5 \times 10^6 M^{-1}$ respectively (84). These features may help to explain the greater potency of maytansine as an antitumor agent in animal tumor systems (80) and as an antimitotic

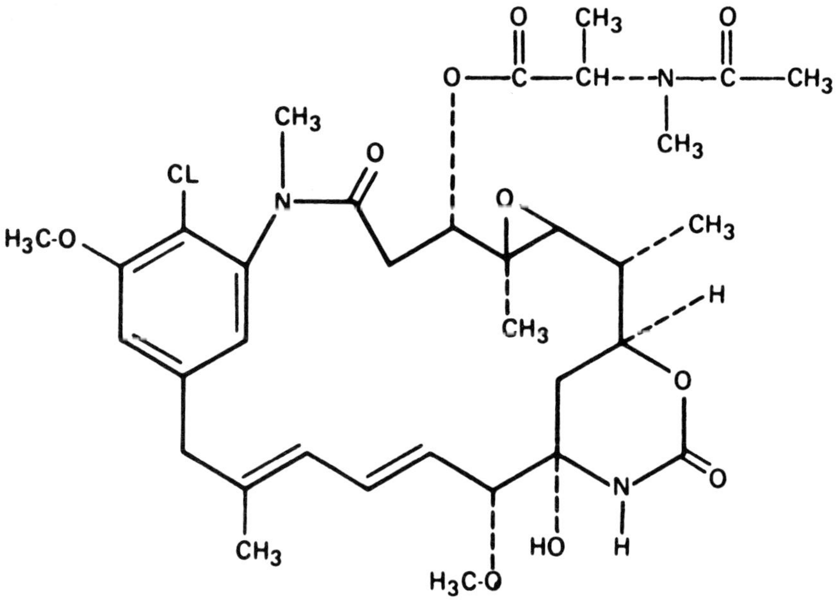

Fig. 5. Chemical structure of maytansine.

agent in sea urchin eggs (82) compared to vincristine. No increase in survival of mice bearing vincristine-resistant P388 murine leukemia has been produced by treatment with this drug which suggests that resistance to maytansine, like vincristine, may be due to impaired transport of the drug into the cell (24). Inhibition of DNA, RNA, and protein synthesis in animal tumors has also been demonstrated but its contribution to antitumor activity is unclear (80).

Several phase I clinical trials with maytansine have recently been completed (85-87). Gastrointestinal and neurologic side-effects have been the major limiting toxicities. Nausea, vomiting, and diarrhoea occurred at a dose level of 0.4 mg/m^2 given daily by intravenous infusion for 3-5 days (85,86) and 1.6 mg/m^2 with intravenous injection every three weeks (87). Stomatitis was seen infrequently. Patients who received a single injection of maytansine every three weeks experienced a syndrome of profound weakness, nausea, and vomiting following 1.6 - 2.0 mg/m^2 which generally lasted 3-5 days after administration (87). Neurologic complaints following the latter dose were otherwise minimal and included transient paresthesias in 14% of the patients. However, Blum et al. reported a dose-related neurotoxicity with central and peripheral findings in patients who received intravenous maytansine daily for three days and repeated every three weeks. Central nervous system toxicity manifested as lethargy, dysphoria, and insomnia occurred at doses of 0.5 mg/m^2 or greater and was reversible. The peripheral toxicity was similar to vinca alkaloid-induced neurotoxicity and increased in severity with increasing dosage. The majority of patients were affected at a dose level of 0.6 mg/m^2 (85). Patients without pre-existing liver disease had only minimal transaminase or bilirubin elevation following injection (85,87), but 3 patients with abnormal liver function tests prior to therapy became jaundiced due to worsening of hepatic function following doses of 0.6 - 0.9 mg/m^2 given daily for three days (86). One of the latter patients probably died as a direct result of exposure to the drug. Myelosuppression has been reported infrequently (87) but may be appreciable in patients who have abnormal liver function tests prior to therapy (86).

Antitumor responses following treatment with maytansine in phase I trials have been noted in patients with acute lymphoblastic leukemia, non-Hodgkin's lymphoma, melanoma, and carcinoma of the breast, head and neck, and ovary (85-87). Human pharmacologic data have not been reported thus far.

REFERENCES

1. Johnson, I.S., Armstrong, J.G., Gorman, M. and Burnett, J.P.Jr. (1963) Cancer Res., 23, 1390-1427.

2. Noble, R.L., Beer, C.T. and Cutts, J.H. (1959) Biochem. Pharmacol., I, 347-348.

3. Hodes, M.E., Rohn, R.J. and Bond, W.E. (1960) Cancer Res., 20, 1041-1049.

4. Karon, M., Freireich, E.J. and Frei, E. (1962) Pediatrics, 30, 791-796.

5. Blum, R.H. and Dawson, D.M. (1976) Proc. Am. Assoc. Cancer Res., 17, 108.

6. Bodey, G.P. and Freireich, E.J. (1976) Proc. Am. Assoc. Cancer Res., 17, 128.

7. Currie, V., Wong, P., Tan, R., Tan, C. and Krakoff, I. (1976) Proc. Am. Assoc. Cancer Res., 17, 174.

8. Carter, S.K. and Livingston, R.B. (1976) Cancer Treatment Rep., 60, 1141-1156.

9. Sieber, S.M., Mead, J.A.R. and Adamson, R.H. (1976) Cancer Treatment Rep. 60, 1127-1139.

10. Owellen, R.J., Owens, A.H.Jr., and Donigian, D.W. (1972) Biochem. Biophys. Res. Comm., 47, 685-691.

11. Owellen, R.J., Hartke, C.A., Dickerson, R.M.and Hains, F.O. (1976) Cancer Res., 36, 1499-1502.

12. Bruchovsky, N., Owen, A.A., Becker, A.J. and Till, J.E. (1965) Cancer Res., 25, 1232-1237.

13. Madoc-Jones, H. and Mauro, F. (1968) J. Cell. Physiol., 72, 185-196.

14. Tucker, R.W., Owellen, R.J. and Harris, S.B. (1977) Cancer Res., 37, 4346-4351.

15. Krishan, A. (1968) J. Natl. Cancer Inst., 41, 581-595.

16. Journey, L.J., Burdman, J. and George, P. (1968) Cancer Chemother. Rep., 52, 509-516.

17. Jellinghaus, W., Schultze, B. and Maurer, W. (1977) Cell Tissue Kinet., 10, 147-156.

18. Krishan, A. and Frei, E., III (1975) Cancer Res., 35, 497-501.

19. Schrek, R. (1974) Am. J. Clin. Path., 62, 1-7.

20. Creasey, W.A. (1975) in Antineoplastic and Immunosuppressive Agents II, Sartorelli, A.C. and Johns, D.G. eds., Springer-Verlag, New York, pp. 670-694.

21. Creasey, W.A., Bensch, K.G. and Malawista, S.E. (1971) Biochem. Pharmacol., 20, 1579-1588.

22. Grieder, A., Maurer, R. and Staehelin, H. (1977) Cancer Res., 37, 2998-3005.

23. Creasey, W.A. and Markiw, M.E. (1965) Biochim. Biophys. Acta, 103, 635-645.

24. Bleyer, W.A., Frisby, S.A. and Oliverio, V.T. (1975) Biochem. Pharmacol.,

24, 633-639.

25. Bender, R.A. and Nichols, A.P. (1978) Am. Assoc. Cancer Res., 19, 35.

26. Chu, M.Y. and Fisher, G.A. (1968) Biochem. Pharmacol. 17, 753-767.

27. Jackson, D.V.Jr. and Bender, R.A. (1978) Clin. Res., 26, 437A.

28. Wilkoff, L.J., Dulmadge, E.A. and Dixon, G.J. (1968) Proc. Soc. Exptl. Biol. Med., 127, 472-478.

29. Owellen, R.J., Root, M.A. and Hains, F.O. (1977) Cancer Res., 37, 2603-2607.

30. Bender, R.A., Castle, M.C., Margileth, D.A. and Oliverio, V.T. (1977) Clin. Pharmacol. Ther., 22, 430-438.

31. Castle, M.C., Margileth, D.A. and Oliverio, V.T. (1976) Cancer Res., 36, 3684-3689.

32. El Dareer, S.M., White, V.M., Chen, F.P., Mellet, L.B. and Hill, D.L. (1977) Cancer Treat. Rep., 61, 1269-1277.

33. Owellen, R.J. and Donigian, D.W. (1972) J. Med. Chem., 15, 894-898.

34. Jackson, D.V.Jr., Castle, M.C. and Bender, R.A. (1978) Clin. Pharmacol. Ther., in press.

35. Owellen, R.J., Hartke, C.A. and Hains, F.O. (1977) Cancer Res., 37, 2597-2602.

36. Donigian, D.W. and Owellen, R.J. (1973) Biochem. Pharmacol. 22, 2113-2119.

37. Echandia, E.L.R., Ramirez, B.U. and Fernandez, H.L. (1973) J. Neurocyt., 2, 149-156.

38. Wisniewski, H.M., Shelanski, M. and Terry, R. (1968) J. Cell Biol., 38, 224-229.

39. Daniels, M. (1975) Ann. N.Y. Acad. Sci., 253, 535-544.

40. Paulson, J.C. and McClure, W.O. (1975) Ann. N.Y. Acad. Sci., 253, 517-527.

41. Wooten, G.F., Kopin, I.J. and Axelrod, J. (1975) Ann. N.Y. Acad. Sci., 253, 528-534.

42. Sandler, S.G., Tobin, W. and Henderson, E.S. (1969) Neurology, 19, 367-374.

43. Bradley, W.G., Lassman, L.P., Pearce, G.W. and Walton, J.N. (1970) J. Neurol. Sci., 10, 107-131.

44. Carbone, P.P., Bono, V., Frei, E., III and Brindley, C.O. (1963) Blood, 21, 640-647.

45. Rosenthal, S.M. and Kaufman, S. (1974) Ann. Intern. Med., 80, 733-737.

46. Weiss, H.D., Walker, M.D. and Wiernik, P.H. (1974) N. Engl. J. Med., 291, 127-133.

47. Vaitkevicius, V.K., Talley, R.W., Tucker, J.L. and Brennan, M.J. (1962) Cancer, 15, 294-306.

48. Livingston, R.B. and Carter, S.K. (1970) Single Agents in Cancer Chemotherapy, Plenum Press, New York, p. 280.

49. DeVita, V.T., Serpick, A.A. and Carbone, P.P. (1970) Ann. Intern. Med., 73, 881-895.

50. Evans, A.F., Farber, S., Brunet, J. and Mariano, P.J. (1963) Cancer, 16, 1302-1306.

51. Hancock, B.W. and Naysmith, A. (1975) Brit. Med. J., 3, 207.

52. Gottschalk, P.G., Dyck, P.J. and Kiely, J.M. (1968) Neurology, 18, 875-882.

53. Kelly, M.G. and Hartwell, J.L. (1954) J. Natl. Cancer Inst., 14, 967-1010.

54. Vaitkevicius, V.K. and Reed, M.L. (1966) Cancer Chemother. Rep., 50, 565-571.

55. Dombernowsky, P. and Nissen, N.I. (1973) Arch. Path. Microbiol. Scand., 81, 715-724.

56. Staehelin, H. (1970) Europ. J. Cancer, 6, 303-311.

57. Rozencweig, M., Von Hoff, D.D., Henney, J.E. and Muggia, F.M. (1977) Cancer, 40, 334-342.

58. Cavalli, F., Sonntag, R.W. and Brunner, K.W. (1977) Lancet, 2, 362.

59. Crist, W.M., Ragab, A., Vietti, T.J., Ducos, R. and Chu, J.Y. (1976) Am. J. Dis. Child., 130, 639-642.

60. Mechl, Z., Rovny, F. and Sopkova, B. (1977) Neoplasma, 24, 411-414.

61. Newlands, E.S. and Bagshawe, K.D. (1977) Lancet, 2, 87.

62. Pouillart, P., Mathe, G., Thy, T.H., et al. (1976) Cancer, 38, 1909-1916.

63. E.O.R.T.C. (1973) Brit. Med. J., 3, 199-202.

64. Dombernowsky, P., Nissen, I. and Larsen, V. (1972) Cancer Chemother. Rep., 56, 71-82.

65. Nissen, N.I., Larsen, V., Pederson, H. and Thomsen, K. (1972) Cancer Chemother. Rep., 56, 769-777.

66. Krishan, A., Paika, K. and Frei, E., III (1975) J. Cell Biol., 66, 521-530.

67. Loike, J.D. and Horwitz, S.B. (1976) Biochem., 15, 5435-5442.

68. Drewinko, B. and Barlogie, B. (1976) Cancer Treat. Rep., 60, 1295-1306.

69. Misra, N.C. and Roberts, D. (1975) Cancer Res., 35, 99-105.

70. Loike, J.D. and Horwitz, S.B. (1976) Biochem., 15, 5443-5448.

71. Huang, C.C., Hou, Y. and Wang, J.J. (1973) Cancer Res., 33, 3123-3129.

72. Allen, L.M. and Creaven, P.J. (1975) Europ. J. Cancer, 11, 697-707.

73. Muggia, F., Selawry, O.S. and Hansen, H.H. (1971) Cancer Chemother. Rep., 55, 575-581.

74. Creaven, P.J., Newman, S.J., Selawry, O.S., Cohen, M.H. and Primack, A. (1974) Cancer Chemother. Rep., 58, 901-907.

75. Brunner, K.W., Sonntag, R.W., Ryssel, H.J. and Cavalli, F. (1976) Cancer Treat. Rep., 60, 1377-1379.

76. Sklansky, B.D., Mann-Kaplan, R.S., Reynold, A.F.Jr., Rosenblum, M.L. and Walker, M.D. (1974) Cancer, 33, 460-467.

77. Kupchan, S., Komoda, Y., Count, W.A., Thomas, G.J., Smith, R.M., Kavim, A., Gilmore, C.J., Haltiwanger, R.C. and Bryan, R.F. (1972) J. Am. Chem. Soc., 94, 1354-1356.

78. Sieber, S.M., Wolpert, M.K., Adamson, R.H., Cysyk, R.L., Bono, V.H. and Johns, D.G. (1976) in Comparative Leukemia Research 1975, Clemmensen, J.

and Yohn, D.S. eds., Karger, Basel, pp. 495-500.

79. Venditti, J.M. and Wolpert-DeFilippes, M.K. (1976) in Chemotherapy, Hellmann, K. and Connors, T.A. eds., Plenum Publishing Company, New York, pp. 129-147.

80. Wolpert-DeFilippes, M.K., Adamson, R.H., Cysyk, R.L. and Johns, D.G. (1975) Biochem. Pharmacol., 24, 751-754.

81. Wolpert-DeFilippes, M.K., Bono, V.H., Dion, R.L. and Johns, D.G. (1975) Biochem. Pharm. 24, 1735-1738.

82. Remillard, S., Rebhun, L.I., Howie, G.A. and Kupchan, S.M. (1975) Science, 189, 1002-1005.

83. Bhattacharyya, B. and Wolff, J. (1977) Fed. Europ. Biochem. Soc. Letters, 75, 159-162.

84. Mandelbaum-Shavit, F., Wolpert-DeFilippes, M.K. and Johns, D.G. (1976) Biochem. Biophys. Res. Comm., 72, 47-54.

85. Blum, R.H. and Kahlert, T. (1978) Cancer Treat. Rep., in press.

86. Cabanillas, F., Rodriguez, V., Hall, S.W., Burgess, M.A., Bodey, G.P. and Freireich, E.J. (1978) Cancer Treat. Rep., in press.

87. Chabner, B.A., Levine, A.S., Johnson, B.L. and Young, R.C. (1978) Cancer Treat. Rep., in press.

Clinical Pharmacology of Anti-Neoplastic Drugs
H. M. Pinedo, editor

THE CLINICAL PHARMACOLOGY OF CIS-DIAMMINEDICHLOROPLATINUM, A REVIEW

STANLEY T. CROOKE, M.D., Ph.D. Associate Director of Research and Development Bristol Laboratories, Syracuse, New York, U.S.A.
Assistant Professor of Pharmacology Baylor College of Medicine, Houston, Texas, U.S.A.
Clinical Assistant Professor Department of Medicine Upstate Medical Center, Syracuse, New York, U.S.A.
ARCHIE W. PRESTAYKO, Ph.D. Assistant Director of Research and Development, Bristol Laboratories
Assistant Professor of Pharmacology Baylor College of Medicine.

INTRODUCTION

Cis-diamminedichloroplatinum (II) (CDDP), is a recently developed antineoplastic agent representative of a group of heavy metal complexes in which increasing interest has developed as a result of the activities of CDDP. The structure of CDDP is shown in Fig. 1. It is a coordination complex of Pt (II) in which two amines and two chlorines occupy *cis* positions in a planar molecule (Rosenberg *et al.* (1).

CDDP has been demonstrated to be active in a variety of human malignancies. Employed in combination with vinblastin and bleomycin, CDDP has contributed to a complete remission rate of approximately 65%, and a marked prolongation of survival in patients with disseminated testicular carcinomas (Einhorn and Donohue (2)). Similar, but perhaps less positive, results in this disease have been reported for other regimens in which CDDP is employed (Cvitkovic *et al.* (3)). CDDP has been shown to be active as a single agent in ovarian cancer (Wiltshaw and Kroner (4)), and recently has shown activity in combination with adriamycin (Holland, J.F., personal communication). Other tumors for which CDDP has demonstrated activity include squamous cell carcinoma of the head and neck, disseminated bladder carcinoma, and certain pediatric solid tumors. It has failed to demonstrate activity against leukemias (Rozencweig *et al.* (5).

The principal toxicities of CDDP are hematologic, audiologic, gastrointestinal, and renal. To a very significant degree, the renal toxicities of CDDP, which were formerly dose-limiting, have been ameliorated by hydration with or without mannitol diuresis (Einhorn and Donohue (6)). At present the principal dose-limiting toxicities are nausea and vomiting and myelosuppression, and these are unaffected by hydration.

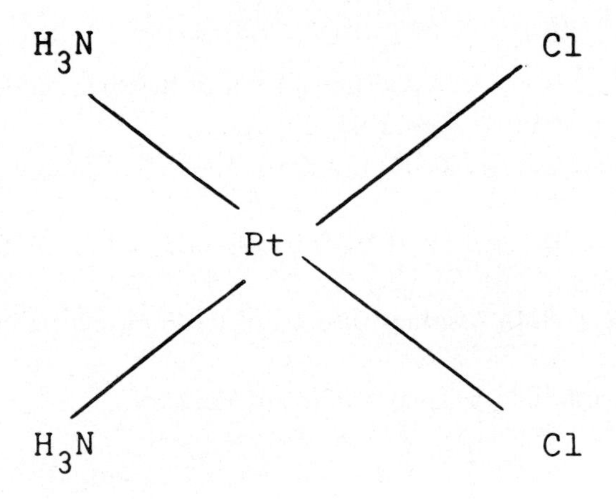

CIS-DIAMMINEDICHLOROPLATINUM II

Fig. 1. The structure of Cis-diamminedichloroplatinum II

METHODS OF ANALYSIS

Until recently the methods employed for clinical pharmacologic studies have determined the concentrations, in various fluids and tissues, of platinum. Most studies have employed flameless atomic absorption spectrometry. Employing this technique, the minimum assayable concentration of platinum is approximately 0.03-0.1 μg/ml plasma (Pera and Harder (7)).

Another method which has been employed is X-ray fluorescence. To improve the sensitivity of this method, protein-free CDDP was reacted with ethylene-diamine, and trapped on DEAE filters. This method allowed the concentration of relatively large sample volumes on 12 mm discs which were then analyzed by X-ray fluorescence. The maximum sensitivity of this method was reported to be approximately 0.24 μg/ml plasma, but X-ray spectroscopy is more rapid than atomic absorption (Bannister *et al.* (8)).

Recently, as a result of data reported in a clinical pharmacologic study employing radiolabeled CDDP, which showed that during the terminal elimination phase, 90% of the platinum was protein bound (DeConti *et al.* (9)), attention has focused on differentiation of protein-bound and free platinum. This has been effected by centrifugal ultrafiltration (Bannister *et al.* (8)).

Not reported as yet, however, are methods which can discriminate between intact CDDP and potential metabolites. However, two groups have independently developed high pressure liquid chromatographic techniques capable of separating CDDP from related compounds such as trans-DDP, and one group has coupled this technique with deproteinization, entrapment on DEAE filters and X-ray fluorescence.

A system currently being developed in our laboratory should provide the maximum sensitivity, and discriminate between intact drug and metabolites, and protein bound and protein-free CDDP. The method which we plan to employ is shown in Fig. 2. In essence, plasma and other fluids will be assayed by atomic absorption for total platinum concentration. The total platinum will then be fractionated into protein-bound and protein-free forms by centrifugal ultrafiltration. The protein-free drug will then be subjected to HPLC with known standards to determine the R_f of CDDP, and CDDP in each of the appropriate fractions will be trapped on DEAE filters by reacting the fractions with ethylene diamine. The CDDP trapped on the filters will then be assayed by atomic absorption. In many samples, it may be unnecessary to concentrate the HPLC effluent on DEAE filters since the atomic absorption technique is relatively sensitive.

PHARMACOKINETICS

Plasma Clearance

Employing [^{193m}Pt] labeled CDDP, DeConti and coworkers (9) showed that plasma clearance of platinum following intravenous administration of doses of 0.066 to 3.15 mg/kg to 10 patients with various malignancies, was biphasic. An initial half-life of 25.5 to 49.0 minutes, followed by a prolonged terminal phase which varied from 58.5 to 73.0 hours, was observed and was reported not to vary with varying doses. The peak plasma concentration increased with increasing doses to a peak of 10 μg/ml CDDP at a dose of 3.15 mg/kg.

Similar results were obtained by Wiltshaw and coworkers employing atomic ab-

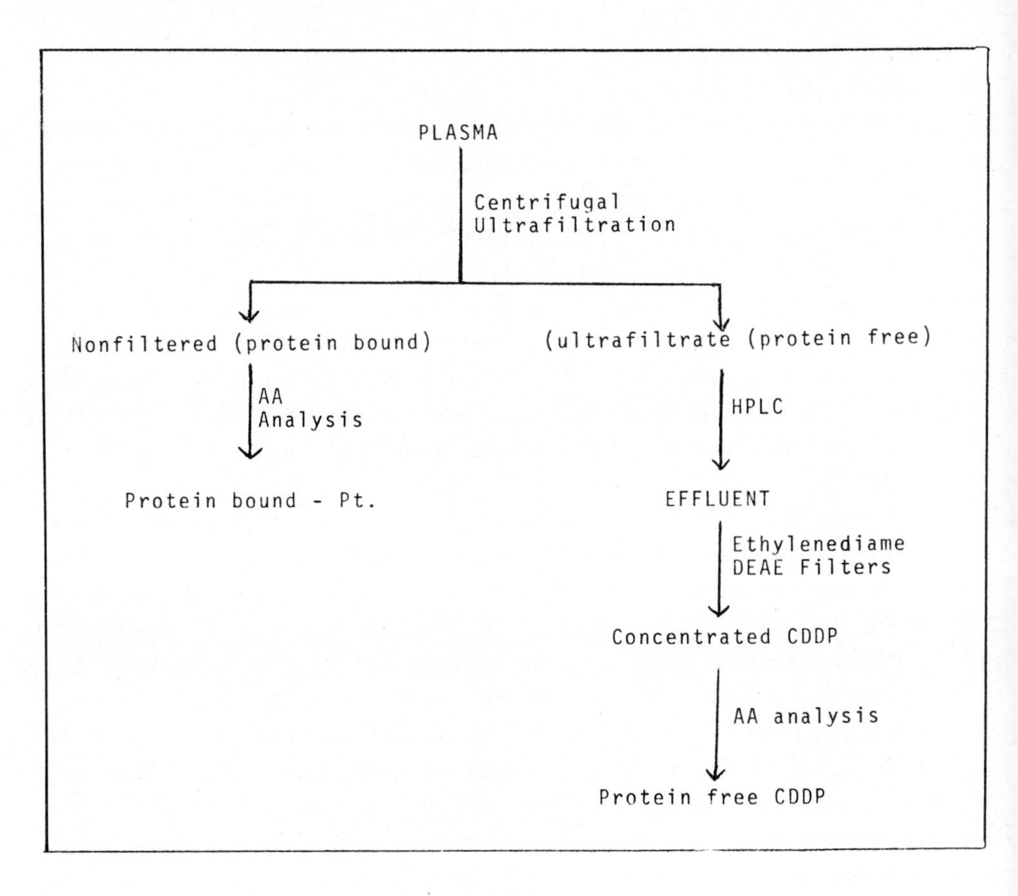

Fig. 2. Proposed Analytic scheme of CDDP

sorption analyses of serum (Wiltshaw, personal communication). In a group of 5 patients who received 20 or 30 mg/m^2 CDDP as an i.v. bolus, the serum concentration measured 5 minutes post injection varied from 0.5-1.7 μg/ml. In most patients the clearance was biphasic, but significant variability was encountered. Although initial and terminal half-lives were not reported, detectable platinum levels were present in all patients 20 hours post-administration. When the concentrations of platinum were examined from 0-5 minutes after administration of CDDP, the peak serum concentrations varied between 1-5 μg/ml, or 33-65% of the theoretical maxima.

The peak serum concentrations in patients who received 2.5 mg/kg CDDP varied from 5 μg/ml to 30 μg/ml. In one patient who was studied sufficiently, however, the terminal half-life appeared to approximate that observed in patients who were treated with lower doses of CDDP.

In none of the patients discussed in either of the two preceding studies, were serial creatinine clearance determinations or serum protein electrophoresis or liver function parameters reported. Thus, it is difficult to determine the degree to which variations were induced by variations in renal and hepatic function.

Recently, we have had the opportunity to study one patient in frank renal failure being treated with chronic hemodialysis. This patient had a creatinine clearance < 5 ml/min. The plasma decay curve obtained in this patient is shown in Fig. 3.

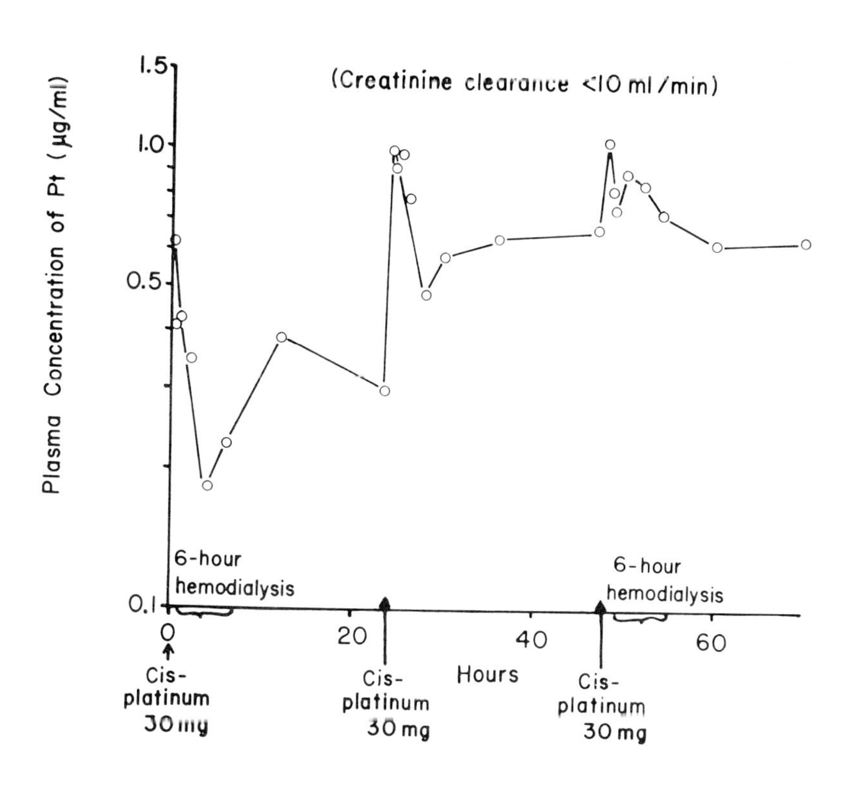

Fig. 3a. Plasma clearance of platinum in a patient with compromised renal function.

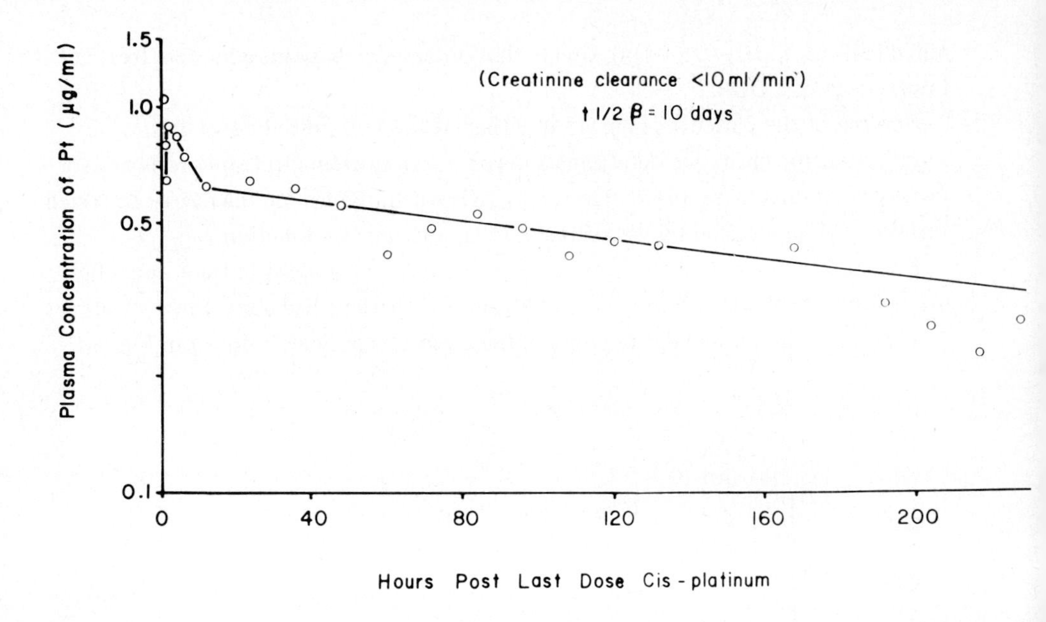

Fig. 3b.

The plasma concentration decayed in a biphasic fashion. The initial phase was rapid with a half-life of 35-45 minutes. However, the terminal phase was markedly prolonged with a half-life of 13 days. Thus, these data suggest that renal decompensation may markedly prolong the elimination of platinum from plasma (Prestayko *et al.* (10)).

Serum Protein Binding

Several studies have clearly shown that the platinum contained in CDDP binds to serum proteins. DeConti and coworkers (9) reported that 65 to 97% of the radioactive platinum in the plasma was protein-associated, and that the binding was time dependent. However, by the time the terminal elimination phase developed, the extent of protein binding was greater than 90%. They also demonstrated that protein binding was reversible, and unaffected by ionic strength, and suggested that protein

~~boun~~

bound drug might serve as a reservoir. In addition, they showed that the protein to which radiolabeled platinum bound was not albumin.

More recently, Bannister and coworkers (8), demonstrated that the binding of platinum from CDDP to serum proteins proceeded with a half-life of 156 minutes, and that 95-100% of the platinum added was protein bound within 7 hours. Other studies have demonstrated that the binding of platinum from CDDP to serum proteins is biphasic, with the slow phase half-life corresponding approximately to the initial half-life of CDDP in plasma (Hoogstraten, B., personal communication).

Absorption of CDDP

Very little information is available concerning the bioavailability of CDDP when administered by any route other than i.v. to human beings. Wiltshaw and coworkers have studied a few patients who received intrapleural or intraperitoneal CDDP. They found that the peak serum concentration was lower, and the time to peak serum concentration was longer when CDDP was administered by those routes than when administered intravenously. They also noted a prolongation of the elimination phase. However, the relative areas under the curves were not calculated so it is difficult to evaluate the bioavailability of CDDP when administered intraperitoneally or intrapleurally.

Excretion of CDDP

The only route of excretion which has been studied in man is renal excretion. In several studies, the urinary excretion of CDDP has been shown to account for only a fraction of the administered dose. DeConti and colleagues (9) reported that 15-27% of a dose was excreted in 24 hours, and only 27-45% was recovered within 5 days after a dose.

Similar results were obtained by Wiltshaw and colleagues. They noted significant variability in urinary excretion. In patients treated with 2.5 mg/kg CDDP, the percent of the total dose excreted in the urine was greater than in patients treated with 20 or 30 mg/m^2. Although this may have been related to vigorous hydration and mannitol diuresis, this concept is not supported by studies in dogs. The percent of a dose excreted in the urine in 24 hours varied from 5 to 30%.

CDDP was found to be dialyzable for only two hours after a dose in one patient in renal failure. This was probably due to binding to serum proteins.

Tissue Distribution of CDDP

Very little information concerning tissue distribution of CDDP in human beings is available. Wiltshaw and colleagues (Wiltshaw, E., personal communication), have shown that at all time points after a dose, the tissue which has the highest concentration of platinum in postmortem samples was the liver. The kidneys appeared to accumulate the next highest amount of platinum. In animals, the kidneys accumulated the greatest amount of platinum (Litterst *et al.* (11)).

CONCLUSIONS

It is apparent that very little is known about the clinical pharmacology of CDDP at present. However, the development of HPLC based techniques to discriminate intact CDDP from possible metabolites, and the use of ultrafiltration to discriminate between protein-bound and free CDDP, should in the near future allow a much better definition of the clinical pharmacology of CDDP.

Among the many questions to be answered are:

1) what are the metabolites of CDDP, and what are their activities
2) how is plasma clearance of CDDP affected by renal dysfunction, liver dysfunction or hypoproteinemia
3) what are the pharmacokinetic consequences of hydration and diuresis
4) what is the nature of the binding of CDDP to serum proteins, what is the significance of this binding, and to which proteins does CDDP bind
5) do pharmacokinetic alterations cause differences in the antitumor activity or toxicity of CDDP
6) with multiple courses, does CDDP accumulate in various tissues, and what are the consequences of tissue accumulation of CDDP.

ACKNOWLEDGEMENTS: We would like to thank Sue Ellen Briggs for typing the manuscript.

REFERENCES

1. Rosenberg, B., VanCamp, L., Krigas, T.: Inhibition of cell division in *Escherichia coli* by electrolysis products from a platinum electrode. *Nature (London) 205*: 698-699, 1965.

2. Einhorn, L.H. and Donohue, J.P.: Improved chemotherapy in disseminated testicular cancer. *J. Urol. 117*: 65-69, 1977.

3. Cvitkovic, E., Hayes, D. and Golbey, R.: Primary combination chemotherapy (VAB II) for metastatic or unresectable germ cell tumors. *Proc. Am. Assoc. Cancer Res. 17*: 296, 1976.

4. Wiltshaw, E. and Kroner, T.: Phase II study of cis-dichlorodiammineplatinum (II) in advanced adenocarcinoma of the ovary. *Cancer Treat. Rep. 60*: 55-60, 1976.

5. Rozencweig, M., VonHoff, D.D., Slavik, M. and Muggia, F.M.: Cis-diammine dichloroplatinum, a new anticancer drug. *Ann. Int. Med. 86*: 803-812, 1977.

6. Einhorn, L.H. and Donohue, J.P.: Cis-diamminedichloroplatinum, vinblastine, and bleomycin combination chemotherapy in disseminated testicular cancer. *Annals Int. Med. 87*: 293-298, 1977.

7. Pera, M.F. and Harder, H.C.: Analysis for platinum in biological material by flameless atomic absorption spectrometry. *Clin. Chem. 23*: 1245-1249, 1977.

8. Bannister, S.J., Sternson, L.A., Repta, A.J. and James, G.W.: Measurement of free-circulating cis-dichlorodiammineplatinum (II) in plasma. *Clin. Chem. 23*: 2258-2262, 1977.

9. DeConti, R.C., Tojtness, B.R., Lange, R.C. and Creasey, W.A.: Clinical and pharmacological studies with cis-diamminedichloroplatinum (II). *Cancer Res. 33*: 1310-1315, 1973.

10. Prestayko, A.W., Luft, F.C., Einhorn, L.H. and Crooke, S.T.: Cisplatinum pharmacokinetics in a patient with renal dysfunction. Submitted for publication, *Medical & Pediatric Oncology.*

11. Litterst, C.L., Gram, T.E., Dedrich, R.L., Leroy, A.F. and Guarino, A.M.: Distribution and disposition of platinum following intravenous administration of cis-diamminedichloroplatinum (II) to dogs. *Cancer Res. 36*: 2340-2344, 1976.

Summary of discussions on the papers presented in part II

FLUOROPYRIMIDINES
5-FU (Driessen, Timmermans, de Vos)

Two additional details in the GLC-technique were mentioned.
First, solid phase injection has been used to give sharper peaks; secondly the "flash technique" has been used to heat the injector.

It is thought that the inability to measure 5-FU metabolites separately with this assay method is a drawback. Metabolites of 5-FU are most important for the antineoplastic effect of the drug. The different patterns of the chromatograms (Fig. 4) could not be explained based on the presence of metabolites. The occasional extra peak (c) was also observed in control plasma at the same position. The extraction of plasma with ethyl acetate does not allow for selective extraction of the drug and its metabolites. Also, it is not known whether or not metabolites are co-elute with the 5-FU peak. These drawbacks indicate that samples should be measured by high performance liquid chromatography, a technique which is able to detect metabolites.

ADRIAMYCINS
Ara-C (van Prooyen)

Metabolism of Ara-C
The problem with an antimetabolite study of this nature is, simply that the rate of disappearance of the parent drug from the plasma must be considered. This rate of disappearance can be related to the anabolic uptake of the drug into the cells and to metabolism of the drug as well.
It does not seem wise to correlate this single aspect with the cytotoxicity of Ara-C, as many processes are involved. It should also be realized that the affinity of Ara-CTP can be quite different for the different DNA polymerases and that the relative amounts of the different polymerases may vary from cell to cell.
Kinase and deaminase levels have been measured in an attempt to use their ratio as a predictor of response to Ara-C. This parameter failed to predict the responders.

Deaminase is activated when cells are disrupted, i.e. by simply freezing and homogenising the cells. So, deaminase levels should be measured in intact cells. This may explain why measurable Ara-CTP levels have been found in cells with apparently very high deaminase levels.
This observation may also explain why no correlations with response have been found,

even when patients with leukemic cells with high kinase levels and low deaminase levels were specifically selected for Ara-C treatment.

Plasma half-life of Ara-C and resistance to the drug.
If failures (Table 2) were related to a shorter half-life, one might be able to overcome this problem by administration of the drug by infusion. Smyth studied 10 patients who had all become clinically resistant to Ara-C, each had increasing kinase/deaminase ratios during the development of resistance.

Adriamycin and daunorubicin and their hydroxyl metabolites (Eksborg)
Complexes of adriamycin are measured as the free drug. The complexes dissociate completely during the extraction procedure.

Clinical pharmacology of adriamycin (Wilkinson)
New analogues of adriamycin
AD32 (N-trifluoracetyl adriamycin-14-valerate) was, in the comparative studies, administered in the same vehicle as adriamycin. It was also more effective in Wistar Furth AML when given in this manner.
AD32 showed some binding to serum proteins but could readily be separated from the complex. For anthracyclines in general protein binding is not significant as it is for weakly acidic drugs such as methotrexate.

AD41 is N-trifluoracetyl adriamycin. AD41 and AD32 have very similar activities *in vitro.* There is, however, a solubility problem with AD41; as AD32 is more lipid soluble than AD41, a higher concentration of AD32 per unit of volume can be achieved. Both AD41 and AD32 are insoluble in water.

AD92 is the carbonyl reduced form of AD41. Given intraperitoneally it had no activity; it may have activity however, when administered intravenously.

Cardiotoxicity
A comparative study of adriamycin and AD32 has been performed in the rabbit with equal myelosuppressive doses (61). The adriamycin treated animals developed classically cardiotoxicity, whereas the AD32 animals were indistinguishable from control animals regarding body weight. At sacrifice some structural changes were noted, but no severe cardiac lesions were seen.

Weekly administration of lower doses of adriamycin is less cardiotoxic than regular three-weekly administration. This clinical observation has been confirmed in mouse studies in which cardiac uptake of the drug was considerably less in animals given low repetitive doses as compared to those given the same total dose as a single i.v.

push.
It is thought that the initial peak concentration causes the cardiotoxicity.

In mice it has been shown that treatment with α-tocopherol prior to administration of adriamycin protects the animals from cardiotoxicity.

Canellos reported that in a phase I clinical trial it seemed that the maximum tolerated dose of AD32 was about ten times higher than that of adriamycin. No cardiotoxicity was observed. There was some regression of tumors, even of an adenocarcinoma of the lung in a patient who had not been treated with any drug before. There might be a problem with lipid pulmonar embolism,which was, however, not encountered.

BLEOMYCIN (Crooke)

Assays

Results with the radioimmunoassays and the microbiological assay do not always correlate. This is not surprising as the RIA's detect active bleomycin as well as the metabolite amino bleomycin, which is about 35% as active as bleomycin A2.
If bleomycin B2 would be present as a metabolite, as *in vitro* data indicate, it can only be in very small amounts as no differences with time are observed in bleomycin concentrations. A new DNA assay is being developed for application in pharmacokinetic studies.

Tallysomycin B which is not a mixture of bleomycin derivatives will probably provide a convenient system for clinical metabolic studies. This drug and its metabolite can be studied by high performance liquid chromatography assay once tallysomycin is available for clinical use.

Toxicity

Up to now, no correlation has been found between creatinine clearance, bleomycin clearance and the development of pulmonary fibrosis or skin toxicity.
In studies in (worm-free) dogs pulmonary fibrosis could only be induced with higher rates of administration, contrary to previous data describing fibrosis in dogs at a low administration rate. It is, however, doubtful whether this was true bleomycin-induced pulmonary fibrosis as a similar fibrosis can be caused by worms infections which frequently occur in dogs. Any study on bleomycin pulmonary fibrosis in dogs should be performed in worm-free animals.

CYCLOPHOSPHAMIDE (Colvin)

Phosphoramide mustard is most likely the active alkylating metabolite. The proportion of phosphoramide mustard as a function of the administered dose of the parent drug until now has been studied in only 5 patients. The levels of phosphoramide mustard appeared to be higher in patients given 75 mg/kg cyclophosphamide than in those who received 60 mg/kg.

Activation by other drugs. In man it has been shown that the half-life of the parent compound can definitely be effected by administering a fairly large amount of phenobarbital. It has, however, never been shown that the clinical efficacy and the toxicity are different after administration of phenobarbital or any other drug along with cyclophosphamide.

The selectivity of cyclophosphamide may be due to the presence of aldehyde oxidase in normal tissues, where the drug can be transformed to inactive oxidation products. The effects of aldehyde oxidase in man have never been studied. The compound 4-methyl cyclophosphamide cannot be oxidized to the inactive intermediates and is more toxic and less effective as an antitumor agent than cyclophosphamide. These data have been presented as evidence for the selective deactivation of cyclophosphamide. It should be pointed out that bone marrow has virtually undetectable levels of aldehyde oxidase activity.

NITROSUREAS (Schein)

Chlorozotocin is one of the newer nitrosurea anticancer agents and is relatively bone marrow sparing.

Criteria for selecting the drug for clinical studies were

1) that blood levels were quite significant at a dose of 120 mg/m^2 and
2) that the alkylating activity delivered with the drug was substantial.

In phase I clinical trials therapeutic activity was shown at 80 mg/m^2 and at 35 mg/m^2 (Mayo Clinic). Ultimately, doses of 80 mg/m^2 or perhaps 100 mg/m^2 in combinations with other drugs may be used without the serious delayed myelosuppression that complicates the use of the other compounds of the nitrosurea group.

In cannot be predicted whether chlorozotocin will affect the bone marrow cells when given in combinations with other myelosuppressive agents (cf. bleomycin).

Chlorozotocin does cause an acute gastro-intestinal toxicity, although nausea and vomiting are somewhat less than with the other nitrosureas.This was also observed at the NCI and the Mayo Clinic.

In animals the principal lethal effect of chlorozotocin was found to be renal toxicity without evidence of bone marrow aplasia. Renal toxicity did not occur in the patient studies. Some elevation of transaminases was noted at week 4 after single drug administration, which did not appear to be associated with any clinical hepatotoxicity. There was no glucose intolerance.

Whether the difference in toxicity of chlorozotocin as compared to the other nitrosureas is due to differences in distribution patterns is difficult to investigate. The labelled compound appears to be rather inactive. As far as can be concluded from studies performed, there is no difference in penetration of the bone marrow. As a result of different solubility, however, CCNU enters the cerebrospinal fluid very rapidly, whereas chlorozotocin does not penetrate.

Since the lower dose of chlorozotocin is as effective as the higher dose, CCNU should now also be examined for effectiveness at lower doses. In general, we should now look towards evaluation of the toxicity of antineoplastic drugs in relation to dose requirement as appropriate drug assay become more available for pharmacokinetic studies. It is no longer necessarily true that the maximally tolerated dose should be given.

VINCA ALKALOIDS (Bender)

The molecular structures of vincristine and vinblastine differ only with respect to a formyl versus a methyl group. The intriguing question is whether there are differences in neurotoxicity as well as in myelosuppressive actions. It is attractive to presume that neurotoxicity involves the microtubular structures of the cells with the highest concentration of tubulin. There are conflicting results of differences in uptake of the drug into the cell.
Facilitated diffusion is certainly not the mechanism as there is actually some activation in the binding to tubulin.

CIS-PLATINUM (Crooke)

Toxicity

Nausea and vomiting are at present the dose-limiting toxicities. Renal toxicity is no longer dose-limiting with hydration (with or without mannitol diuresis).
Other regimens, e.g. drug infusion over an extended period of time, decrease the incidence of nausea and vomiting. As the half-life of the drug is much longer than the period of the infusion the concentration of the active drug will not be changed markedly. Bertino observed a plasma concentration of about 1 μg/ml with a dose of 8 mg/

m^2 given in a long term infusion of up to 24 h. He did not use diuretics besides hydration. About a quarter of the number of patients had no nausea at all. Nabolin seems to reduce nausea and vomiting to an acceptable level.

Cis-platinum can be detected in the urine for two months after administration of the drug. The probable excretion in saliva has not been measured appropriately. Neither is it known whether there is a measurable concentration of the drug in the CSF.

Pinedo observed that doses of furosemide as low as 10 mg are able to enhance diuresis in patients with an inappropriate water excretion due to vinblastine. This is important particularly in patients on a 5-day course of cis-platinum in whom forced diuresis is important to prevent toxicity.

LIST OF PARTICIPANTS

E. Balk	The Rotterdam Radio-Therapeutical Institute Rotterdam The Netherlands
C. Benckhuijsen	The Netherlands Cancer Institute Amsterdam The Netherlands
R. Bender	National Cancer Institute National Institutes of Health Bethesda U.S.A.
J. Bertino	Yale University School of Medicine New Haven U.S.A.
H. Beukers	University Hospital Lab. Medical Chemistry Leiden The Netherlands
*E. Boelsma	The Netherlands Cancer Society (KWF) Amsterdam The Netherlands
W. ten Bokkel Huinink	The Netherlands Cancer Institute Antoni van Leeuwenhoek Hospital Amsterdam The Netherlands
C. van Boxtel	University Hospital Lab. Pharmacology Leiden The Netherlands
J. Breed	University Hospital Dpt. of Internal Medicine Utrecht The Netherlands

Th. Brouwers	University Hospital Dpt. of Medical Microbiology Groningen The Netherlands
J. Buesa	c/o University Hospital Dpt. of Internal Medicine Utrecht The Netherlands
G. Canellos	Sidney Farber Cancer Institute Harvard School of Medicine Boston U.S.A.
F. Cleton	The Netherlands Cancer Institute Antoni van Leeuwenhoek Hospital Amsterdam The Netherlands
M. Colvin	Johns Hopkins Oncology Center Pharmacology Lab. Baltimore U.S.A.
S. Crooke	Bristol Laboratories Syracuse U.S.A.
J. Dankert	University Hospital Dpt. of Medical Microbiology Groningen The Netherlands
A. Drenthe	Sint Radboud Hospital Dpt. of Internal Medicine Nijmegen The Netherlands
*O. Driessen	University Hospital Pharmacology Lab. Leiden The Netherlands

S. Eksborg	Karolinska Apoteket Stockholm Sweden
L. van de Grint	University Hospital Dpt. of Internal Medicine Utrecht The Netherlands
K. Hande	National Institutes of Health National Cancer Institute Bethesda U.S.A.
K. Harrap	Institute of Cancer Research Royal Cancer Hospital Dpt. of Biochemical Pharmacology Surrey England
W. Haye	The Rotterdam Radio-Therapeutical Institute Rotterdam The Netherlands
*E. van Heemstra	The Netherlands Cancer Society (KWF) Amsterdam The Netherlands
A. Hoff	The Rotterdam Radio-Therapeutical Institute Rotterdam The Netherlands
S. van 't Hoff	The Netherlands Cancer Institute Amsterdam The Netherlands
B. Houwen	University Hospital Dpt. of Internal Medicine Groningen The Netherlands

K. Jonker	The Netherlands Cancer Institute Antoni van Leeuwenhoek Hospital Amsterdam The Netherlands
*E. van der Kleijn	Sint Radboud Hospital Dpt. of Pharmacy Nijmegen The Netherlands
J. de Koning	University Hospital Dpt. of Paediatrics Leiden The Netherlands
C. van Kralingen	Technological University Delft The Netherlands
J. Lankelma	Sint Radboud Hospital Dpt. of Clinical Pharmacy Nijmegen The Netherlands
P. Lelieveld	Radiobiological Institute Rijswijk The Netherlands
A. Leyva	University Hospital Dpt. of Internal Medicine Utrecht The Netherlands
R. Lippens	Sint Radboud Hospital Dpt. of Paediatrics Nijmegen The Netherlands
H. Maier-Lenz	Bristol Myers International Company Forschungsbüro Freiburg Freiburg Germany

J. Mulder	The Rotterdam Radio-Therapeutical Institute Rotterdam The Netherlands
C. Myers	National Cancer Institute National Institutes of Health Bethesda U.S.A.
A. Nederbragt	University Hospital Dpt. of Internal Medicine Utrecht The Netherlands
*H. Nieweg	University Hospital Dpt. of Haematology Groningen The Netherlands
A. van Oosterom	University Hospital Dpt. of Radiotherapy Leiden The Netherlands
J. Pasmooy	Sint Radboud Hospital Dpt. E.N.T. Nijmegen The Netherlands
*H. Pinedo	University Hospital Dpt. of Internal Medicine Utrecht The Netherlands
A. Postma	University Hospital Dpt. of Paediatrics Groningen The Netherlands

H. van Prooyen
Sint Radboud Hospital
Dpt. of Internal Medicine
Nijmegen
The Netherlands

L. van Putten
Radiobiological Institute
Rijswijk
The Netherlands

Ph. Schein
Georgetown University Hospital
Dpt. of Medical Oncology
Washington
U.S.A.

J. Schornagel
University Hospital
Dpt. of Internal Medicine
Utrecht
The Netherlands

*E. Schretlen
Sint Radboud Hospital
Dpt. of Paediatrics
Nijmegen
The Netherlands

J. Smyth
Institute of Cancer Research
Royal Marsden Hospital
Surrey
England

P. Sonneveld
Radiobiological Institute
Rijswijk
The Netherlands

C. Tromp
Sophia Children's Hospital
Rotterdam
The Netherlands

J. van Turnhout
University Hospital Dijkzigt
Dpt. of Haematology
Rotterdam
The Netherlands

P. Vendrik
University Hospital
Dpt. of Internal Medicine
Utrecht
The Netherlands

R. Versluis
University Hospital
Vrije Universiteit
Dpt. E.N.T.
Amsterdam
The Netherlands

D. de Vos
Sylvius Laboratories
Dpt. of Pharmacology
Leiden
The Netherlands

W. van der Vijgh
University Hospital
Vrije Universiteit
Dpt. of Internal Medicine
Amsterdam
The Netherlands

D. Wagener
Sint Radboud Hospital
Dpt. of Haematology
Nijmegen
The Netherlands

P. Wilkinson
Christie Hospital and Holt Radium Institute
Manchester
England

SUBJECT INDEX

M

N

O

P